CURRICULUM DEVELOPMENT FOR MEDICAL EDUCATION

CURRICULUM DEVELOPMENT FOR MEDICAL EDUCATION

A SIX-STEP APPROACH

Second Edition

Edited by

David E. Kern, M.D., M.P.H.

Patricia A. Thomas, M.D.

Mark T. Hughes, M.D., M.A.

The Johns Hopkins Faculty Development Program
The Johns Hopkins University School of Medicine
Baltimore, Maryland

THE JOHNS HOPKINS UNIVERSITY PRESS | BALTIMORE

The Johns Hopkins University Press
2715 North Charles Street
Baltimore, Maryland 21218-4363
www.press.jhu.edu

Library of Congress Cataloging-in-Publication Data

Curriculum development for medical education : a six-step approach /
edited by David E. Kern, Patricia A. Thomas, and Mark T. Hughes. — 2nd ed.
p. ; cm.
Includes bibliographical references and index.
ISBN-13: 978-0-8018-9366-7 (hardcover : alk. paper)
ISBN-10: 0-8018-9366-6 (hardcover : alk. paper)
ISBN-13: 978-0-8018-9367-4 (pbk. : alk. paper)
ISBN-10: 0-8018-9367-4 (pbk. : alk. paper)
1. Curriculum planning. 2. Medical education—United States—Curricula. 3. Medicine—
Study and teaching. I. Kern, David E. II. Thomas, Patricia A. (Patricia Ann), 1950–
III. Hughes, Mark T.
[DNLM: 1. Curriculum. 2. Education, Medical—methods. W 18 C975 2009]
R834.C87 1998
610.71'173—dc22   2009002889

A catalog record for this book is available from the British Library.

*Special discounts are available for bulk purchases of this book. For more information,
please contact Special Sales at 410-516-6936 or specialsales@press.jhu.edu.*

To the many faculty members
who strive to improve medical education
by developing, implementing, and evaluating
curricula in the health sciences.

Contents

Preface

Since the issuance of the first edition of this book in 1998, *Curriculum Development for Medical Education: A Six-Step Approach* has been widely used by educators in the health professions, not only in North America but also in other parts of the world. It has been translated into both Chinese and Japanese. Our assumption that medical educators would "benefit from learning a practical, generic, and timeless approach to curriculum development that can address today's as well as tomorrow's needs" has been supported by the book's readership and requests for related courses and workshops.

While it is true that the general principles of curriculum development remain timeless and are not changed in this second edition of the book, we have been surprised by the extent of the revisions. Throughout the second edition, we have updated the text and examples to reflect evolving accreditation standards and educational emphases. There are numerous new examples focusing on the core competencies of professionalism, practice-based learning and improvement, and systems-based practice. References have been extensively updated. The revised text and references reflect the growing use of technology and electronic resources to support health professions education. There is increasing emphasis on the application of what is learned beyond the environment of an isolated curricular experience in what has been termed the informal or hidden curriculum. While the book continues to focus on the practical aspects of curriculum development, implementation, and evaluation, this edition has an increased emphasis on opportunities for associated scholarship.

Revisions in a few chapters deserve specific mention. Chapter 3, previously "Needs Assessment of Targeted Learners," has been renamed "Targeted Needs Assessment" to emphasize that this step of curriculum development occurs at two levels: the level of the targeted learners and the level of the targeted institution or learning environment. We have also added a section on survey methodology, a common tool used for this step. In Chapter 4, "Goals and Objectives," we devote additional text to the classification and hierarchy of objectives. Chapter 5, "Educational Strategies," has new sections on promoting professionalism, practice-based learning and improvement, and systems-based practice. Chapter 7, "Evaluation and Feedback," has been revised to incorporate evolving concepts of evaluation, assessment, and validity evidence. Chapter 6, "Implementation," and Chapter 9, "Dissemination," now address the protection of human subjects and navigating institutional review boards, and Chapter 9 includes a section on intellectual property and copyright issues. Chapter 8, "Curriculum Maintenance and Enhancement," has an added section on accreditation standards. Appendix A includes one updated and two new full-length examples to reflect curricula at the medical student, house staff, and faculty levels. Finally, there are updated and much expanded sections on curricular, faculty development, and funding resources in Appendix B.

Since the first edition, Donna Howard has retired. Eric Bass has retired from editorship but remains a chapter author, focusing his attention on Chapters 2 and 9. We welcome Pamela Lipsett as the first author of our significantly revised chapter on evaluation and feedback. Barbara de Lateur, R. Samuel Mayer, Janice Ryden, Amit A. Shah, and Leah Wolfe contributed examples for Appendix A. Finally, Mark Hughes has joined David Kern and Patricia Thomas as the book's editors. The editors reviewed every chapter in detail, in addition to serving as chapter and/or appendix authors.

Contributors

Eric B. Bass, M.D., M.P.H., Professor, Departments of Medicine, Epidemiology, and Health Policy and Management, Division of General Internal Medicine, Codirector, Physician, and Society Course, Director, Johns Hopkins Evidence-based Practice Center, The Johns Hopkins University School of Medicine, Baltimore, Maryland

Barbara J. de Lateur, M.D., M.S., Distinguished Service Professor, Department of Physical Medicine and Rehabilitation, The Johns Hopkins University School of Medicine, Joint Professor, Health Policy and Management, The Bloomberg School of Public Health, Baltimore, Maryland

Mark T. Hughes, M.D., M.A., Assistant Professor, Department of Medicine, Division of General Internal Medicine, Core Faculty, Johns Hopkins Berman Institute of Bioethics, Director, Course on Research Ethics, The Johns Hopkins University School of Medicine, Facilitator, Program in Curriculum Development, The Johns Hopkins Faculty Development Program, Baltimore, Maryland

David E. Kern, M.D., M.P.H., Professor, Department of Medicine, The Johns Hopkins University School of Medicine, Director, Division of General Internal Medicine, Johns Hopkins Bayview Medical Center, Director, Program in Curriculum Development, The Johns Hopkins Faculty Development Program, Baltimore, Maryland

Pamela A. Lipsett, M.D., Professor, Departments of Surgery, Anesthesiology, and Critical Care Medicine, and School of Nursing, Director of Surgical Education, Program Director, General Surgery Residency Program, The Johns Hopkins University School of Medicine, Baltimore, Maryland

R. Samuel Mayer, M.D., Assistant Professor, Vice Chair, Education, Residency Program Director, Department of Physical Medicine and Rehabilitation, Johns Hopkins University School of Medicine, Baltimore, Maryland

Janice Ryden, M.D., Assistant Professor, Department of Medicine, Division of General Internal Medicine, The Johns Hopkins University School of Medicine, Baltimore, Maryland

Amit A. Shah, M.D., Assistant Professor, Department of Medicine, Division of General Internal Medicine, University of Texas Southwestern Medical School, Dallas, Texas

Patricia A. Thomas, M.D., Associate Professor, Department of Medicine, Division of General Internal Medicine, Associate Dean for Curriculum, The Johns Hopkins University School of Medicine, Facilitator, Program in Curriculum Development, The Johns Hopkins Faculty Development Program, Baltimore, Maryland

Leah Wolfe, M.D., Assistant Professor, Department of Medicine, Division of General Internal Medicine, The Johns Hopkins University School of Medicine, Baltimore, Maryland

CURRICULUM DEVELOPMENT FOR MEDICAL EDUCATION

Introduction

David E. Kern, M.D., M.P.H.

PURPOSE

The purpose of this book is to provide a practical, theoretically sound approach to developing, implementing, evaluating, and continually improving educational experiences in medicine.

TARGET AUDIENCE

This book is designed for use by curriculum developers and others who are responsible for the educational experiences of students, residents, fellows, faculty, and clinical practitioners. It should be particularly helpful to those who are planning to develop or are in the midst of developing a curriculum.

DEFINITION OF CURRICULUM

In this book, a curriculum is defined as *a planned educational experience.* This definition encompasses a breadth of educational experiences, from one or more sessions on a specific subject to a year-long course, from a clinical rotation or clerkship to an entire training program.

RATIONALE FOR THE BOOK

Faculty in the health professions often have responsibility for planning educational experiences, frequently without having received training or acquired experience in such endeavors, and usually in the presence of limited resources and significant institutional constraints. Accreditation bodies for each level of medical education in the United States, however, require written curricula with fully developed educational objectives, educational methods, and evaluation (1–3).

Ideally, medical education should change as our knowledge base changes and as the needs, or the perceived needs, of patients, medical practitioners, and society change. Some contemporary demands for change and curriculum development are listed in Table I.1. This book assumes that medical educators will benefit from learning a practical, generic, and timeless approach to curriculum development that can address today's as well as tomorrow's needs.

Table I.1.   Some Contemporary Demands for Medical Education

Content
- Train health care professionals as effective problem solvers who can efficiently access and apply an ever-evolving medical knowledge base.
- Motivate and help health care professionals to become self-directed, lifelong learners.
- Train health care professionals to access, assess, and apply the best scientific evidence to clinical practice (evidence-based medicine, or EBM).
- Train health care professionals to practice cost-effectively.
- Given the behavioral origins and emotional components of a large proportion of health problems, train physicians in effective communication, education, and behavioral change strategies.
- Train health care professionals in assessing and improving their own clinical practice (practice-based learning and improvement, or PBLI).
- Train health care professionals to understand, navigate, advocate for, and participate in improving health care systems (systems-based practice, or SBP).
- Train physicians as leaders, managers, and team members, in recognition of the increasing complexity of medical care delivery.
- Train health care professionals in population- and community-centered, as well as person-centered, approaches to providing health care.
- Improve training in professionalism.
- Improve training in chronic disease and disability.
- Improve training in nutrition and obesity.
- Improve training in preventive care.

Methods
- Train the number of primary care physicians and specialty physicians required to meet societal needs.
- Increase the quantity and quality of clinical training in ambulatory, subacute, and chronic care settings, while reducing the amount of training on inpatient services of acute hospitals, as necessary to meet training needs.
- Construct educational interventions based on the best evidence available (6, 7).
- Address the informal and hidden curricula of an institution that can promote or extinguish what is taught in formal curricula (8–10).
- Effectively integrate advancing technologies into medical curricula, such as simulation and interactive electronic interfaces.
- Develop faculty to meet contemporary demands.

Assessment
- Develop and use reliable and valid tools for assessing the cognitive, skill, and behavioral competencies of trainees. Certify competence in the six competency domains of medical knowledge, patient care, practice-based learning and improvement, systems-based practice, professionalism, and interpersonal/communication skills (11).
- Evaluate the efficacy of educational interventions.

BACKGROUND INFORMATION

The approach described in this book has evolved over the past 21 years, during which time the authors have taught curriculum development and evaluation skills to more than 220 faculty members and fellows in the Johns Hopkins University Faculty Development Program for Clinician-Educators (4, 5). Participants in the program's 10-month Longitudinal Program in Curriculum Development have developed and implemented more than 110 medical curricula in topics as diverse as preclerkship skills building, clinical reasoning and shared decision making, outpatient internal medicine, musculoskeletal disorders, office gynecology for the generalist, chronic illness and disability, geriatrics for nongeriatric faculty, surgical skills assessment, laparoscopic surgical skills, cross-cultural competence, and medical ethics. The authors have also developed and overseen the development of numerous curricula in their educational and administrative roles.

AN OVERVIEW OF THE BOOK

Chapter 1 presents an overview of a six-step approach to curriculum development. *Chapters 2 through 7* describe each step in detail. *Chapter 8* discusses how to maintain and improve curricula over time. *Chapter 9* discusses how to disseminate curricula and curricular products within and beyond institutions.

Throughout the book, *examples* are provided to illustrate major points. Most examples come from the real-life curricular experiences of the authors or their colleagues, although they may have been adapted for the sake of brevity or clarity. Some are taken from the literature. Those that are fictitious were designed to be realistic and to demonstrate an important concept or principle.

Chapters 2 through 9 end with *questions* that encourage the reader to review the principles discussed in each chapter and apply them to a desired, intended, or existing curriculum. In addition to lists of *specific references* that are cited in the text, these chapters include annotated lists of *general references* that can guide the reader who is interested in pursuing a particular topic in greater depth.

Appendix A provides examples of curricula that have progressed through all six steps and that range from newly developed curricula to curricula that have matured through repetitive cycles of implementation. *Appendix B* supplements the chapter references by providing the reader with a selected list of published and unpublished resources for curricular development, faculty development, and funding of curricular work.

REFERENCES

1. Liaison Committee on Medical Education. Available at www.lcme.org. Go to Accreditation Standards. Accessed March 1, 2009.
2. Accreditation Council for Graduate Medical Education. Available at www.acgme.org. Go to Program Directors & Coordinators, then Common Program Requirements. Accessed March 1, 2009.
3. Accreditation Council for Continuing Medical Education. Available at www.accme.org. Accessed March 1, 2009.

4. Windish DM, Gozu A, Bass EB, Thomas PA, Sisson SD, Howard DM, Kern DE. A ten-month program in curriculum development for medical educators: 16 years of experience. J Gen Intern Med. 2007;22:655–61.
5. Gozu A, Windish DM, Knight AM, Thomas PA, Kolodner K, Bass EB, Sisson SD, Kern DE. Long-term follow-up of a ten-month programme in curriculum development: a cohort study. Med Educ. 2008;42:684–92.
6. Harden RM, Grant J, Buckley G, Hart IR. Best evidence medical education. Adv Health Sci Educ Theory Pract. 2000;5:71–90.
7. The BEME Collaboration. Available at www.bemecollaboration.org/. Accessed March 1, 2009.
8. Hafferty FW, Ranks R. The hidden curriculum, ethics teaching, and the structure of medical education. Acad Med. 1994;69:861–71.
9. Hundert EM, Hafferty F, Christakis D. Characteristics of the informal curriculum and trainees' ethical choices. Acad Med. 1996;71:624–42.
10. Hafferty FW. Beyond curriculum reform: confronting medicine's hidden curriculum. Acad Med. 1998;73:403–7.
11. The ACGME (Accreditation Council on Graduate Medical Education) Outcome Project. Available at www.acgme.org/Outcome/. Accessed March 1, 2009.

Overview
A Six-Step Approach to Curriculum Development

David E. Kern, M.D., M.P.H.

RATIONALE AND ORIGINS

The six-step approach described in this monograph derives from the generic approaches to curriculum development set forth by Taba (1), Tyler (2), Yura and Torres (3), and others (4) and from the work of McGaghie et al. (5) and Golden (6), who advocated the linking of curricula to health care needs. Underlying assumptions are fourfold. First, educational programs have aims or goals, whether or not they are clearly articulated. Second, medical educators have a professional and ethical obligation to meet the needs of their learners, patients, and society. Third, medical educators should be held accountable for the outcomes of their interventions. And fourth, a logical, systematic approach to curriculum development will help achieve these ends. Accrediting bodies for undergraduate, graduate, and continuing medical education in the United States require formal curricula that include goals, objectives, and explicitly articulated educational and evaluation strategies (7–9). They are beginning to require outcome measurements (10).

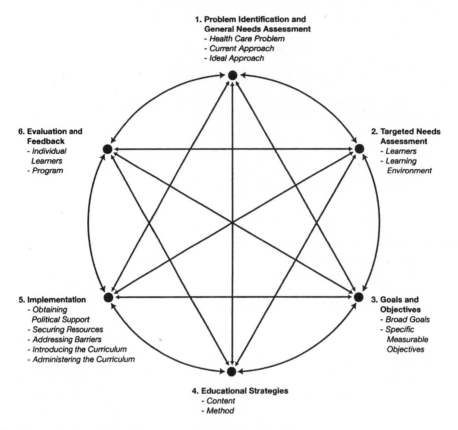

Figure 1.1. A Six-Step Approach to Curriculum Development

A SIX-STEP APPROACH (FIGURE 1.1)

Step 1: Problem Identification and General Needs Assessment

This step begins with the *identification and critical analysis of a health care need or other problem.* The need may relate to a specific health problem, such as the provision of care to patients infected with human immunodeficiency virus (HIV), or to a group of problems, such as the provision of routine gynecologic care by primary care physicians. It may relate to qualities of the physician, such as the need for health care providers to develop as self-directed, lifelong learners who can provide effective care as medical knowledge and practice evolve. Or it may relate to the health care needs of society in general, such as whether the quantity and type of physicians being produced are appropriate. A complete problem identification requires an analysis of the *current approach* of patients, practitioners, the medical education system, and society, in general, to addressing the identified need. This is followed by identification of an *ideal approach* that describes how patients, practitioners, the medical education system, and society should be addressing the need. The difference between the ideal approach and the current approach represents a *general needs assessment.*

Step 2: Targeted Needs Assessment

This step involves assessing the needs of one's targeted group of learners and their medical institution/learning environment, which may be different from the needs of learners and medical institutions in general.

> **EXAMPLE:** *Targeted Needs Assessment.* The *problem identification and general needs assessment* for a substance abuse curriculum for internal medicine residents revealed a high prevalence of substance abuse and consequent disorders in the United States, an increasing prevalence of methamphetamine abuse, underdiagnosis of substance abuse disorders, and underuse of evidence-based therapies by practicing physicians. The *targeted needs assessment* revealed a high prevalence of heroine abuse and low prevalence of methamphetamine abuse among patients using the targeted training center. The targeted learners were already being trained and felt competent in smoking cessation counseling. However, they received little training in the use of screening instruments for and the diagnosis and treatment of alcohol and other substance abuse disorders. Neither the residents nor their outpatient preceptors were trained or certified in the use of opioid agonist (buprenorphine) treatment, nor were they trained in the expert-recommended screening, brief intervention, referral, and treatment (SBIRT) approach to management.

Step 3: Goals and Objectives

Once the needs of targeted learners have been identified, goals and objectives for the curriculum can be written, starting with *broad or general goals* and then moving to *specific, measurable objectives.* Objectives may include cognitive (knowledge), affective (attitudinal), or psychomotor (skill and behavioral) objectives for the learner; process objectives related to the conduct of the curriculum; or even health, health care, or patient outcome objectives. The development of goals and objectives is critical because they help to determine curricular content and learning methods and help to focus the learner. They enable communication of what the curriculum is about to others and provide a basis for its evaluation. When resources are limited, prioritization of objectives can facilitate the rational allocation of those resources.

Step 4: Educational Strategies

Once objectives have been clarified, *curriculum content is chosen and educational methods are selected that will most likely achieve the educational objectives.*

> **EXAMPLE:** *Curriculum Content.* Based on the above example of a targeted needs assessment, two objectives of the substance abuse curriculum for residents were that residents and outpatient preceptors become 1) proficient in SBIRT and 2) proficient and certified in office-based opioid agonist use. Training in smoking cessation counseling, which would have been duplicative, was omitted.

> **EXAMPLES:** *Educational Methods.* Case-based, problem-solving exercises that actively involve learners are methods that are more likely to improve clinical reasoning skills than attendance at lectures.
>
> The development of physicians as effective team members is more likely to be promoted through their participation in and reflection on cooperative learning and work experiences than through reading and discussing a book on the subject.
>
> Interviewing, physical examination, and procedural skills will be best learned in an environment that supplements practice with self-observation, observation by others, feedback, and reflection.

Step 5: Implementation

Implementation of a curriculum has *several components*: obtaining political support; identifying and procuring resources; identifying and addressing barriers to implementation; introducing the curriculum (e.g., piloting the curriculum on a friendly audience before presenting it to all targeted learners, phasing in the curriculum one part at a time); administering the curriculum; and refining the curriculum over successive cycles. Implementation is critical to the success of a curriculum. It is *the step that converts a mental exercise to reality.*

Step 6: Evaluation and Feedback

This step has several components. It usually is desirable to assess the performance of both *individuals* (individual assessment) and the *curriculum* (called "program evaluation"). The purpose of evaluation may be *formative* (to provide ongoing feedback so that the learners or curriculum can improve) or *summative* (to provide a final "grade" or evaluation of the performance of the learner or curriculum).

Evaluation can be used not only to drive the ongoing learning of participants and the improvement of a curriculum but also to gain support and resources for a curriculum and, in research situations, to answer questions about the effectiveness of a specific curriculum or the relative merits of different educational approaches.

THE INTERACTIVE AND CONTINUOUS NATURE OF THE SIX-STEP APPROACH

In practice, curriculum development does not usually proceed in sequence, one step at a time. Rather, it is a dynamic, interactive process. Progress is often made on two or more steps simultaneously. Progress on one step influences progress on another (as illustrated by the bidirectional arrows in Figure 1.1). For example, limited resources (Step 5) may limit the number and nature of objectives (Step 3), as well as the extent of evaluation (Step 6) that is possible. Evaluation strategies (Step 6) may result in a refinement of objectives (Step 3). Evaluation (Step 6) may also provide information that serves as a needs assessment of targeted learners (Step 2). Time pressures, or the presence of an existing curriculum, may result in the development of goals, educational methods, and implementation strategies (Steps 3, 4, and 5) before a formal problem identification and needs assessment (Steps 1 and 2), so that Steps 1 and 2 are used to refine and improve an existing curriculum rather than develop a new one.

For a successful curriculum, curriculum development never really ends, as illustrated by the circle in Figure 1.1. Rather, the curriculum evolves, based on evaluation results, changes in resources, changes in targeted learners, and changes in the material requiring mastery.

REFERENCES

1. Taba H. *Curriculum Development: Theory and Practice*. New York: Harcourt, Brace, & World; 1962. Pp. 1–515.

2. Tyler RW. *Basic Principles of Curriculum and Instruction*. Chicago: University of Chicago Press; 1950. Pp. 1–83.
3. Yura H, Torres GJ, eds. *Faculty-Curriculum Development: Curriculum Design by Nursing Faculty*. New York: National League for Nursing; 1986. Publication No. 15–2164. Pp. 1–371.
4. Sheets KJ, Anderson WA, Alguire PC. Curriculum development and evaluation in medical education: annotated bibliography. *J Gen Intern Med.* 1992;7(5):538–43.
5. McGaghie WC, Miller GE, Sajid AW, Telder TV. *Competency Based Curriculum Development in Medical Education: An Introduction*. Geneva: World Health Organization; 1978. Pp. 1–99.
6. Golden AS. A model for curriculum development linking curriculum with health needs. In: Golden AS, Carlson DG, Hogan JL, eds. *The Art of Teaching Primary Care*. Springer Series on Medical Education, Vol. 3. New York: Springer Publishing Co.; 1982. Pp. 9–25.
7. Liaison Committee on Medical Education. Available at www.lcme.org. Go to Accreditation Standards. Accessed March 3, 2009.
8. Accreditation Council for Graduate Medical Education. Available at www.acgme.org. Go to Program Directors & Coordinators, then Common Program Requirements. Accessed March 3, 2009.
9. Accreditation Council for Continuing Medical Education. Available at www.accme.org. Accessed March 9, 2009.
10. ACGME outcomes project. Available at www.acgme.org/Outcome/. Accessed March 9, 2009.

Step 1
Problem Identification and General Needs Assessment

. . . building the foundation for meaningful objectives

Eric B. Bass, M.D., M.P.H.

Medical instruction does not exist to provide individuals with an
opportunity of learning how to make a living, but in order to make
possible the protection of the health of the public.
—Rudolf Virchow

DEFINITIONS

The first step in designing a curriculum is to identify and characterize the health care problem that will be addressed by the curriculum, how it is currently being addressed, and how it should be addressed. The difference between how the health care problem is currently being addressed, in general, and how it should be addressed is called a *general needs assessment*. Because the difference between the current and ideal approaches can be considered part of the problem that the curriculum will address, Step 1 is sometimes referred to, simply, as *problem identification*.

IMPORTANCE

The better a problem is defined, the easier it will be to design an appropriate curriculum to address the problem. All of the other steps in the curriculum development process depend on having a clear understanding of the problem (see Figure 1.1). Step 1 (problem identification and general needs assessment) and Step 2 (targeted needs assessment) are particularly helpful in focusing a curriculum's goals and objectives (Step 3), which in turn help to focus the curriculum's educational strategies and evaluation (Steps 4 and 6). Step 1 is especially important in justifying dissemination of a successful curriculum because it supports the generalizability of the curriculum. Last, Steps 1 and 2 provide a strong rationale that can help the curriculum developer obtain support for the curriculum (see Chapter 6: Step 5: Implementation).

IDENTIFICATION OF THE HEALTH CARE PROBLEM

The ultimate purpose of a curriculum in medical education is to address a problem that affects the health of the public or a given population (1–4). Frequently, the problem of interest is complex. Even the simplest health care problem, however, may be refractory to any educational or other intervention, if the problem has not been defined well. A comprehensive definition of the problem should consider the epidemiology of the problem, as well as the impact of the problem on patients, health care professionals, medical educators, and society (Table 2.1).

In defining the problem of interest, it is important to explicitly identify *whom* the problem affects. Does the problem affect people with a particular disease (e.g., frequent disease exacerbations requiring hospitalization in patients with asthma), or does the problem affect society at large (e.g., inadequate understanding of behaviors associated with acquiring the human immunodeficiency virus)? Does the problem directly or indirectly affect health professionals and their trainees (e.g., physicians inadequately prepared to provide ambulatory care or to teach in the ambulatory setting)? Does the

Table 2.1.   Identification and Characterization of the Health Care Problem

Whom does it affect?
    Patients
    Health care professionals
    Medical educators
    Society

What does it affect?
    Clinical outcomes
    Quality of life
    Quality of health care
    Use of health care and other resources
    Medical and nonmedical costs
    Patient and provider satisfaction
    Work and productivity
    Societal function

What is the *quantitative and qualitative importance* of the effects?

problem affect health care organizations or other corporate entities (e.g., failure to prac-tice cost-effective medicine)? The problem of interest may affect many different groups. The number of people affected has implications for curriculum development because a problem that affects many people may warrant more attention than a problem that affects relatively few people. Educators need to know who is affected by the problem, and their characteristics and behaviors, to choose the most appropriate target audience for a curriculum, formulate learning objectives, and develop curriculum content.

Once those who are affected by the problem have been identified, it is important to elaborate on *how* they are affected. What is the effect of the problem on clinical out-comes, quality of life, quality of health care, use of health care services, medical and nonmedical costs, patient and provider satisfaction, work and productivity, and the functioning of society? How common and how serious are these effects?

> **EXAMPLE:** *Partial Problem Identification for a Poverty in Health Care Curriculum.* "Thirty-seven million Americans live below the federal poverty threshold, representing 12.6% of the U.S. population. Even more—nearly 90 million Americans—live below 200% of the federal poverty threshold, an income at which many struggle to make ends meet. Given these reali-ties, most physicians will work with low-income patients, regardless of their specialty or practice location. Countless studies have shown that lower socioeconomic status (SES) is associated with unique challenges to health, higher disease burden and poorer health out-comes" (5).

GENERAL NEEDS ASSESSMENT (TABLE 2.2)

Current Approach

Having defined the nature of the health care problem, the next task is to assess current efforts to address the problem. The process of determining the current approach to a problem is sometimes referred to as a "job analysis" (1) because it is an assess-ment of the "job" that is currently being done to deal with a problem. To determine the current approach to a problem, the curriculum developer should ask what is being done by the following:

    a. Patients
    b. Health care professionals
    c. Medical educators
    d. Society

Knowledge of what *patients* are doing and not doing with regard to a problem may influence decisions about curriculum content. For example, are patients using nonef-fective treatments or engaging in activities that exacerbate a problem, behaviors that need to be reversed? Or, are patients predisposed to engage in activities that could alleviate the problem, behaviors that need to be encouraged?

Knowledge of how *health care professionals* are currently addressing the problem is especially relevant because they are frequently the target audience for medical curricu-la. In the general needs assessment, one of the challenges is in determining how health care professionals vary in their approach to a problem. Many studies have demon-strated substantial variations in clinical practice both within and between countries (6).

> **EXAMPLE:** *Limited Access to Antiretroviral Therapy in Many Countries.* More than 33 million people in the world are infected with human immunodeficiency virus (HIV),

95% of whom live in developing countries (7). Individuals with HIV infection need comprehensive health care, ideally involving appropriate antiretroviral therapy and measures to prevent opportunistic infections. However, in many countries, people living with HIV infection have limited access to effective medications. Given this information, an international curriculum on primary care of HIV-infected patients should address the availability of effective medications in targeted countries.

Most problems important enough to warrant a focused curriculum are encountered in many different places, so it is wise to explore what is currently being done by other *medical educators* to help patients and health care professionals address the problem. Much can be learned from the previous work of educators who have tried to tackle the problem of interest. For example, curricular materials may exist already for medical trainees and be of great value in developing a curriculum for one's own target audience. A dearth of relevant curricula will reinforce the need for innovative curricular work.

EXAMPLE: *Variability in Quality of Teaching of the Behavioral and Social Sciences.* Recognizing the impact of the behavioral and social sciences on health outcomes, as well as a burgeoning of new research in these sciences, the Institute of Medicine generated a report in 2004 that addressed the current approach to teaching the behavioral and social sciences in undergraduate medical education. The report concluded that there was wide variability in the time and content of courses in undergraduate medical education. The report proposed prioritized topics to address behavioral and social sciences effectively and presented the curricular approaches of several medical schools (8).

Curriculum developers should also consider what *society* is doing to address the problem. This will help to improve understanding of the societal context of current efforts to address the problem, taking into consideration potential barriers and facilitators influencing those efforts.

Table 2.2.   The General Needs Assessment

What is *currently* being done by the following?
    Patients
    Health care professionals
    Medical educators
    Society

What personal and environmental factors affect the problem?
    Predisposing
    Enabling
    Reinforcing

What *ideally* should be done by the following?
    Patients
    Health care professionals
    Medical educators
    Society

What are the key *differences* between the current and ideal approaches?

EXAMPLE: *Impact of Societal Approach on Curricular Planning.* In designing a curriculum to help health care professionals reduce the spread of HIV infection in a given society, it is necessary to know how the society handles the distribution of condoms and clean needles. If the distribution of either is prohibited, the curriculum will need to address the most appropriate options acceptable in that society.

To understand fully the current approach to addressing a health care problem, curriculum developers need to be familiar with the ecological perspective on human behavior. This perspective emphasizes multiple influences on behavior, including at the individual, interpersonal, institutional, community, and public policy levels (9). Interventions are more likely to be successful if they address multiple levels of influence on behavior. Most educational interventions will focus primarily on individual and/or interpersonal factors, but some may be part of larger interventions that also target other levels of influence.

When focusing on the individual and interpersonal levels of influence on behavior, curriculum developers should consider the fundamental principles of modern theories of human behavior change. While it is beyond the scope of this book to discuss specific theories in detail, three concepts are particularly important: 1) human behavior is mediated by what people know and think; 2) knowledge is necessary, but not sufficient, to cause a change in behavior; and 3) behavior is influenced by individual beliefs, motivations, and skills, as well as the environment (9).

In the light of these key concepts, curriculum developers need to consider *multiple types of factors* that may aggravate or alleviate the problem of interest. Factors that can influence the problem can be classified as predisposing factors, enabling factors, or reinforcing factors (10). *Predisposing factors* refer to knowledge, attitudes, and beliefs of people that influence their motivation to change (or not to change) behaviors related to a problem. *Enabling factors* generally refer to personal skills and societal or environmental forces that may help or hinder efforts to change a problem behavior. *Reinforcing factors* refer to the rewards and punishments that encourage continuation or discontinuation of a desired or undesired behavior.

EXAMPLE: *Predisposing, Enabling, and Reinforcing Factors.* In designing a curriculum for family practice residents on the prevention of smoking-related illness, curriculum developers identified predisposing, enabling, and reinforcing factors with multiple levels of influence on an individual's smoking behavior. Predisposing factors included an individual's self-defined readiness to quit, an individual's health concerns and beliefs regarding oneself and one's family, an individual's sense of personal efficacy or empowerment, and an individual's personal experiences related to smoking. Enabling factors included attitudes and behaviors of family, friends, and peers; prohibitions against smoking in restaurants, on airplanes, and at work places; economic factors; messages such as advertisements and government warnings; availability of cigarettes, cigars, and pipe tobacco; and costs of smoking. Reinforcing factors included the strength of physical and psychological addiction, personally defined benefits to smoking, personally defined motivators for stopping or not starting, and personally defined barriers to cessation. These factors were considered in designing a recommended approach for residents' participation in a school health program and for counseling individual pediatric, adolescent, and adult patients about smoking and smoking cessation.

By considering all aspects of how a health care problem is addressed, one can determine the most appropriate role for an educational intervention in addressing the problem, keeping in mind the fact that an educational intervention by itself usually cannot solve all aspects of a complex health care problem.

Ideal Approach

After examination of the current approach to the problem, the next task is to determine the ideal approach to the problem. Determination of the ideal approach will require careful consideration of the multiple levels of influence on behavior, as well as the same fundamental concepts of human behavior change described in the preceding section. The process of determining the ideal approach to a problem is sometimes referred to as a "task analysis," which can be viewed as an assessment of the specific "tasks" that need to be performed to appropriately deal with the problem (1, 11). To determine the ideal approach to a problem, the curriculum developer should ask what each of the following groups should do to deal most effectively with the problem:

a. Patients
b. Health care professionals
c. Medical educators
d. Society at large

To what extent should *patients* be involved in handling the problem themselves? In many cases, the ideal approach will require education of patients affected by or at risk of having the problem.

> **EXAMPLE:** *Role of Patients.* An educational program that is designed to prevent atherosclerotic cardiovascular disease in high-risk young adults should address their understanding of and adherence to effective preventive behaviors related to diet, exercise, and smoking.

Which *health care professionals* should deal with the problem and what should they be doing? Answering these questions can help the curriculum developer to appropriately target learners and define the content of a curriculum. If more than one type of health care professional typically encounters the problem, the curriculum developer must decide what is most appropriate for each type of provider and whether the curriculum will be modified to meet the needs of each type of provider or target just one type of provider.

> **EXAMPLE:** *Role of Health Care Professionals.* The design of a curriculum on management of common gynecologic problems should account for differences in the competencies expected of gynecologists, family practitioners, and internists. The curriculum might focus on the needs of residents in family medicine and internal medicine, while acknowledging potential differences regarding which patients, with what specific problems, should be referred to a gynecologist.

What role should *medical educators* have in addressing the problem? Determining the ideal approach for *medical educators* involves identifying the appropriate target audiences, the appropriate content, the best educational strategies, and the best evaluation methods to ensure effectiveness. Reviewing previously published curricula that address the health care problem often uncovers elements of best practices in educational methods and evaluation methods that can be used in new curricular efforts.

> **EXAMPLE:** *Identifying Best Practices.* Since publication of the Institute of Medicine's Report, *Unequal Treatment* (12), there has been increasing attention to addressing health care disparities in undergraduate medical education. A review of the literature found two approaches to the problem. In one school, an interactive workshop at the start of a family medicine clerkship used didactics, as well as skill-building exercises on effective cross-cultural doctor-

patient interactions, and demonstrated an increase in student cultural awareness on a validated cultural awareness scale (13). Another school used a curriculum in which students received basic science education at the school of medicine and completed all required clinical rotations in an underserved urban community. Analysis of 1071 graduates found that 53% were practicing in underserved areas, with participation in this program as an independent predictor of future practice in medically underserved areas (14).

Keep in mind, however, that educators may not be able to solve the problem by themselves. When the objectives are to change the behavior of patients or health care professionals, educators should define their role relative to other interventions that may be needed to stimulate and sustain behavioral change.

What role should *society* have in addressing the problem? While curriculum developers usually are not in the position to effect *societal* change, some of their targeted learners may be, now or in the future. A curriculum, therefore, may choose to address not only current societal factors that contribute to a problem but also those societal changes that might alleviate the problem.

EXAMPLE: *Social Action Influenced by a Curriculum.* Some residents who took part in a curriculum on violence became involved in local and national efforts to reduce the incidence of domestic and gun-related violence.

The ideal approach should serve as an important, but not rigid, guide to developing a curriculum. One needs to be flexible in accommodating others' views and the many practical realities related to curriculum development. For this reason, it is useful to be transparent about the basis for one's "ideal" approach: individual opinion, consensus, the logical application of established theory, or scientific evidence. Obviously, one should be more flexible in espousing an "ideal" approach based on individual opinion than an "ideal" approach based on strong scientific evidence.

Differences between Current and Ideal Approaches

Having determined the current and ideal approaches to a problem, the curriculum developer should identify the differences between the two approaches. The differences identified by this *general needs assessment* should be the main target of any plans for addressing the health care problem. As mentioned above, the differences between the current and ideal approaches can be considered part of the problem that the curriculum will address, which is why Step 1 is sometimes referred to, simply, as *problem identification*.

OBTAINING INFORMATION ABOUT NEEDS

Each curriculum has unique needs for information about the problem of interest. In some cases, substantial information already exists and simply needs to be identified. In other cases, much information is available, but it needs to be systematically reviewed and synthesized. Frequently, the information available is insufficient to guide a new curriculum, in which case new information must be collected. Depending on the availability of relevant information, different methods can be used to identify and characterize a health care problem and to determine the current and ideal approaches to that problem (1–3). The most commonly used methods are listed in Table 2.3.

Table 2.3.   Methods for Obtaining the Necessary Information

Review of Available Information
    Evidence-based reviews of educational and clinical topics
    Published original studies
    Clinical practice guidelines
    Published recommendations on expected competencies
    Reports by professional organizations or government agencies
    Documents submitted to educational clearinghouses
    Curriculum documents from other institutions
    Patient education materials prepared by foundations or professional organizations
    Patient support organizations
    Public health statistics
    Clinical registry data
    Administrative claims data

Use of Consultants/Experts
    Informal consultation
    Formal consultation
    Meetings of experts

Collection of New Information
    Surveys of patients, practitioners, or experts
    Focus group(s)
    Nominal group technique
    Group judgment methods (Delphi method)
    Daily diaries by patients and practitioners
    Observation of tasks performed by practitioners
    Time and motion studies
    Critical incident reviews
    Study of ideal performance cases or role-model practitioners

By carefully obtaining information about the need for a curriculum, educators will demonstrate that they are using a scholarly approach to curriculum development. This is an important component of educational scholarship, as defined by a consensus conference on educational scholarship that was sponsored by the Association of American Medical Colleges (15). A scholarly approach is valuable because it will help to convince learners and other educators that the curriculum is based on up-to-date knowledge of the published literature and existing best practices.

Finding and Synthesizing Available Information

The curriculum developer should start with a *well-focused review of information that is already available.* A *review of the medical literature*, including journal articles and textbooks, is generally the most efficient method for gathering information about a health care problem, what is currently being done to deal with it, and what should be done to deal with it. A medical librarian can be extremely helpful in accessing the medical and relevant nonmedical (e.g., educational) literature, as well as in accessing the increasing number of computerized databases that contain relevant, but unpublished, information. However, the curriculum developer should formulate specific questions to guide the review and the search for relevant information. Without focused questions, the review will be inefficient and less useful.

The curriculum developer should look for published *reviews* as well as any *original studies* about the topic. If a systematic review has been performed recently, it may be possible to rely on that review with just a quick look for new studies performed since the review was completed. The Best Evidence in Medical Education (BEME) Collaboration is a good source of high-quality evidence-based reviews of topics in medical education (16). Depending on the topic, other evidence-based medicine resources may also contain valuable information, especially the Cochrane Collaboration, which produces evidence-based reviews on a wide variety of clinical topics (17). If a systematic review has not been done previously, it will be necessary to search systematically for relevant original studies. In such cases, the curriculum developer has an opportunity to make a scholarly contribution to the field by performing a *systematic review* of the topic. A systematic review of a medical education topic should include a carefully documented and comprehensive search for relevant studies, with explicitly defined criteria for inclusion in the review, as well as a verifiable methodology for extracting and synthesizing information from eligible studies (18). By examining historical and social trends, the review may yield insights regarding future needs, in addition to current needs.

For many clinical topics, it is wise to look for pertinent *clinical practice guidelines* because the guidelines may clearly delineate the ideal approach to a problem. In some countries, practice guidelines can be accessed easily through a governmental health agency, such as the Agency for Healthcare Research and Quality in the United States or the National Institute for Health and Clinical Excellence in the United Kingdom, each of which sponsors a clearinghouse for practice guidelines (19, 20). With so many practice guidelines available, it is likely that curriculum developers will find one or more guidelines for a clinical problem of interest. Sometimes guidelines conflict in their recommendations. When that happens, the curriculum developer should critically appraise the methods used to develop the guidelines to determine which recommendations should be included in the ideal approach (21, 22).

When designing a curriculum, educators need to be aware of any recommendations or statements by accreditation agencies or professional organizations about the *competencies* expected of practitioners. For example, any curriculum for internal medicine residents in the United States should take into consideration the core competencies set by the Accreditation Council for Graduate Medical Education (ACGME), requirements of the Internal Medicine Residency Review Committee, and the evaluation objectives of the American Board of Internal Medicine (ABIM) (23, 24). Similarly, any curriculum for medical students in the United States or Canada should take into consideration the accreditation standards of the Liaison Committee on Medical Education (LCME) (25). Within any clinical discipline, a corresponding professional society may issue a consensus statement about core competencies that should guide training in that discipline. A good example is the Society of Hospital Medicine, the national professional organization of hospitalists, which commissioned a task force to prepare a framework for curriculum development based on the core competencies in hospital medicine (26). Often, the ideal approach to a problem will be based on this sort of authoritative statement about expected competencies.

EXAMPLE: *Use of Accreditation Body, Professional Organization, and Systematic Review.* Medical students and residents need training in the methods of quality improvement because the ACGME and the Institute of Medicine now consider this an important competency area (27, 28). To guide the development of new curricula for medical trainees on the use of quality improvement methods in clinical practice, a group of educators performed a systematic review of the effectiveness of published quality improvement curricula for clinicians (29). The group found that most quality improvement curricula demonstrated improvement in knowledge or confidence to perform quality improvement, but additional studies were needed to determine whether such programs have meaningful clinical benefits.

Educational clearinghouses can be particularly helpful to the curriculum developer because they may provide specific examples of what is being done by other medical educators to address a problem. The most useful educational clearinghouses tend to be those that have sufficient support and infrastructure to have some level of peer review, as well as some process for keeping them up to date. One particularly noteworthy clearinghouse for medical education is the growing MedEdPORTAL run by the Association of American Medical Colleges (30). This database includes a wide variety of educational documents and materials that have been prepared by educators from many institutions. Clearinghouses are also maintained by some specialty and topic-oriented professional organizations (see Appendix B).

Other sources of available information also should be considered, especially when the published literature is sparse (see Appendix B, Curricular Resources). For example, the Association of American Medical Colleges (AAMC) maintains a Curriculum Management and Information Tool (CurrMIT), where most U.S. and Canadian medical schools enter information such as curricular objectives, educational content, educational methods, resources, and assessment methods for their curricula (31, 32). One can access CurrMIT to find out what is happening in other medical schools with respect to a topic of interest. Other sources of information include *reports by professional societies or governmental agencies*, which can highlight deficiencies in the current approach to a problem or make recommendations for a new approach to a problem. In some cases, it may be worthwhile to contact *colleagues at other institutions* who are performing related work and who may be willing to share information that they have developed or collected. For some health care problems, *patient education materials* have been prepared by foundations or professional organizations, and these materials can provide information about the problem from the patient's perspective, as well as material to use in one's curriculum.

Public health statistics, *clinical registry data*, and *administrative claims data* can be used for obtaining information about the incidence or prevalence of a problem. Most medical libraries have reports on the vital statistics of the population, which are published by the federal government. Clinical registry data may be difficult to access directly, but reports from clinical registries can be identified by searching the medical literature on a particular clinical topic. In the United States, the federal government and many states maintain administrative claims databases that provide data on the use of inpatient and outpatient medical services. Such data can help to define the magnitude of a clinical problem. Because of the enormous size of most claims databases, special expertise is needed to perform analyses of such data (33). Despite their potential value in defining a problem, these types of databases rarely have the depth of information that is needed to guide curriculum planning.

Even though the curriculum developer may be expert in the area to be addressed by the curriculum, it frequently is necessary to ask other experts how they interpret the information about a problem, particularly when the literature gives conflicting information or when there is uncertainty about the future direction of work in that area. In such cases, *expert opinions* can be obtained by consultation, or by organizing a meeting of experts to discuss the issues. For most curricula, this can be done on a relatively informal basis with local experts. Occasionally, the problem is so controversial or important that the curriculum developer may wish to spend the additional time and effort necessary to obtain formal input from outside experts.

Collecting New Information

When the available information about a problem is so inadequate that curriculum developers cannot draw reasonable conclusions, it is desirable to *collect new information* about the problem. *In-person interviews* with a small sample of patients, students, practitioners, medical educators, or experts can yield information relatively quickly but may or may not be representative. Such interviews may be conducted individually or in the format of a *focus group* of 8–12 people, where the purpose is to obtain in-depth views regarding the topic of concern (34–36). Obtaining consensus of the group is not the goal; rather, it is to elicit a range of perspectives. Another small group method occasionally used in needs assessment is the *nominal group technique,* which employs a structured, sometimes iterative approach to identifying issues, solutions, and priorities (37). The outcome of this technique is an extensive list of brainstormed and rank-ordered ideas. When the objective is not only to generate ideas or answers to a question but also to move a group toward agreement, an iterative process, called the *Delphi method*, can be used with participants who either meet repeatedly or respond to a series of questions over time. Participant responses are fed back to the group on each successive cycle to promote consensus (38). When quantitative and representative data are desired, it is customary to perform a systematic *questionnaire or interview survey* (39–41) by mail, telephone, Internet, or in person. (See Chapter 3 for more information on survey methodology.)

Sometimes, more intensive methods of data collection are necessary. When little is known about the current approach to a clinical problem, educators may ask practitioners or patients to complete *daily diaries or records of activities.* Alternatively, they may use *observation* by work sampling (1, 2), which involves direct observation of a sample of patients, practitioners, or medical educators in their work settings. Other options are *time and motion studies* (which involve observation and detailed analysis of how patients and/or practitioners spend their time) (1), *critical incident reviews* (in which cases having desired and undesired outcomes are reviewed to determine how the process of care relates to the outcomes) (1, 2, 42, 43), and *review of ideal performance cases*. The latter methods require considerable time and resources but may be valuable when detailed information is needed about a particular aspect of clinical practice.

Regardless of what methods are used to obtain information about a problem, it is necessary to synthesize that information in an efficient manner. A logical, well-organized report, with tables that summarize the collected information, is one of the most common methods for accomplishing the synthesis. A well-organized report has the advantages of efficiently communicating this information to others and being available for quick reference in the future. Collected reference materials and resources can be filed for future access. A less common but useful method for synthesizing information related to a specific aspect of a problem is the use of a fishbone diagram (44).

> **EXAMPLE:** *Synthesis of Information Using Fishbone Diagram.* A number of methods were used to determine the current and ideal approaches to training physicians to address the ethical aspects of clinical decision making in ambulatory settings. A literature review was conducted. The review identified important issues that had been raised by recent developments in genomics and genetic testing but did not reveal enough data on how different approaches to genetic testing affect clinical outcomes and quality of life. Experts were consulted and provided opinions about how ethical dilemmas in genetic testing should be handled, but there was still a lack of objective information on how patients are affected. Finally, curriculum developers collaborated with other investigators on a survey to collect new information about how patients and practitioners in their local settings view genetic testing. The types of information important to clinical decision making that were obtained from these methods were summarized in a fishbone diagram (Figure 2.1).

TIME AND EFFORT

Those involved in the development of a curriculum must decide how much they are willing to spend, in terms of time, effort, and other resources, for problem identification and general needs assessment. A commitment of too little time and effort runs the risk of having a curriculum that is poorly focused and unlikely to address adequately the problem of concern, or of "reinventing the wheel" when an effective curriculum already exists. A commitment of too much time and effort runs the risk of leaving insufficient resources for the other steps in the curriculum development process. Careful consideration of the nature of the problem is necessary to achieve an appropriate balance.

Some problems are complex enough to require a great deal of time to adequately understand them. On the other hand, less complex problems that have been less well studied may require more time and effort than more complex problems that have been well studied because original data may need to be collected.

One of the goals of this step is for the curriculum developer to become expert enough in the area to make decisions about curricular objectives and content. The curriculum developer's prior knowledge of the problem area, therefore, will also determine the amount of time and effort he/she needs to spend on this step.

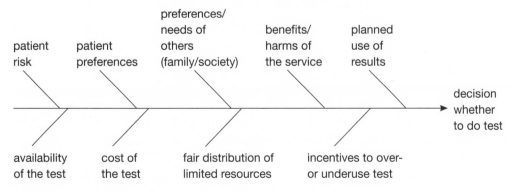

Figure 2.1.   Fishbone Diagram

The time and effort spent on defining the problem of interest in a scholarly manner may yield new information or new perspectives that warrant publication in the medical literature (see Chapter 9: Dissemination). However, the methods employed in the problem identification and general needs assessment must be rigorously applied and described if the results are to be published in a peer-reviewed journal. The curriculum developer must decide whether the academic value of a scholarly publication is worth the time and effort that would be diverted from the development of the curriculum itself. A sound, if less methodologically rigorous, problem identification and needs assessment that is used for planning the curriculum could also be used for the introduction and discussion of a scholarly publication about evaluation results or novel educational strategies.

Time pressures, or the inheritance of an existing curriculum, may result in a situation in which the curriculum is developed before an adequate problem identification and general needs assessment. In such situations, a return to this step may be helpful in explaining or improving an existing curriculum.

CONCLUSION

To effectively and efficiently address a health care problem, a curriculum developer must define the problem carefully and determine the current and ideal approaches to the problem. A curriculum by itself may not solve all aspects of the problem, particularly if the problem is a complex one. Nevertheless, this step is essential in focusing a curriculum so that it can make a meaningful contribution to solving the problem.

The conclusions drawn from the general needs assessment may or may not apply to the particular group of learners or institution(s) targeted by a curriculum developer. For this reason, it is necessary to assess the specific needs of one's targeted learners and institution(s) (see Chapter 3) before proceeding with further development of a curriculum.

QUESTIONS

For the curriculum you are coordinating, planning, or would like to be planning, please answer or think about the following questions:

1. Identify a health care problem that is (will be) addressed by this curriculum.

2. *Whom* does the problem affect?

3. *What* effects does the problem have on these people?

4. How important is the problem, *quantitatively and qualitatively*?

5. Based on your current knowledge, use the top row of the table below to list some of the things that patients, health care professionals, educators, and society at large are doing *currently* to address the problem.

	Patients	Health Care Professionals	Medical Educators	Society
Current Approach				
Ideal Approach				

6. Based on your current knowledge, use the bottom row of the table above to list key things that patients, health care professionals, educators, and society should *ideally* be doing to address the problem.

7. Perform a *general needs assessment* by identifying the differences between the current and ideal approaches.

8. Identify key areas in which your knowledge has been deficient for this exercise. Given your available resources, what *methods* would you use to correct these deficiencies? (See Table 2.3.)

GENERAL REFERENCES

Altschuld JW, Witkin BR. *From Needs Assessment to Action: Transforming Needs into Solution Strategies.* Thousand Oaks, Calif.: SAGE Publications; 2000.
Reviews earlier work (Witkin and Altschuld, see below), addresses value of multiple/mixed method approach to needs assessment, including both qualitative and quantitative methods, then focuses on the prioritization of needs and the transformation of needs assessments into action. Provides real-world examples. 282 pages.

Golden AS. A model for curriculum development linking curriculum with health needs. In: Golden AS, Carlson DG, Hogan JL, eds. *The Art of Teaching Primary Care*. Springer Series on Medical Education, Vol. 3. New York: Springer Publishing Co.; 1982.
Addresses the role of task and job analysis in the development of competency-based curricula. Pp. 9–25.

Green LW, Kreuter MW. *Health Promotion Planning: An Educational and Environmental Approach*. Mountain View, Calif.: Mayfield Publishing Co.; 1991.
Provides a sound conceptual basis for developing plans to change health behaviors. 506 pages.

Witkin BR, Altschuld JW. *Planning and Conducting Needs Assessments: A Practical Guide*. Thousand Oaks, Calif.: Sage Publications; 1995.
Readable yet comprehensive book with information and examples organized in two major sections: 1) planning/managing the needs assessment, and 2) methods used for conducting a needs assessment. The methods section is particularly useful as it covers the following: records and social indicators (including mapping); surveys; interviews; the critical incident technique; nominal group technique; focus groups; mailed Delphi survey and modified (or group) Delphi process; strategic planning; and causal analysis including fishboning, cause and consequence analysis, and fault tree analysis. The organizational and community examples are easily translatable to medical care settings. 302 pages.

SPECIFIC REFERENCES

1. Golden AS. A model for curriculum development linking curriculum with health needs. In: Golden AS, Carlson DG, Hogan JL, eds. *The Art of Teaching Primary Care*. Springer Series on Medical Education, Vol. 3. New York: Springer Publishing Co.; 1982. Pp. 9–25.
2. McGaghie WC, Miller GE, Sajid AW, Telder TV. *Competency Based Curriculum Development in Medical Education: An Introduction*. Geneva: World Health Organization; 1978. Pp. 21–41.
3. Harden RM. Ten questions to ask when planning a course or curriculum. *Med Educ.* 1986;20:356–65.
4. Ludmerer KM. *Time to Heal: American Medical Education from the Turn of the Century to the Era of Managed Care*. Oxford: Oxford University Press; 1999.
5. Doran KM, Kirley K, Barnosky AR, Williams JC, Cheng JE. Developing a novel Poverty in Healthcare curriculum for medical students at the University of Michigan Medical School. *Acad Med.* 2008;83:5–13.
6. Wennberg J. Practice variations and health care reform: connecting the dots. *Health Affairs* (Millwood). 2004; Suppl Web Exclusives: VAR140–44.
7. Worldwide HIV and AIDS Statistics Commentary. Available at www.avert.org/worlstatinfo.htm. Accessed March 3, 2009.
8. Cuff PA, Vanselow NA, eds. Board on Neuroscience and Behavioral Health, Institute of Medicine of the National Academies. *Improving Medical Education: Enhancing the Behavioral and Social Science Content of Medical School Curricula*. Washington, D.C.: National Academies Press; 2004.
9. Glanz K, Rimer BK. *Theory at a Glance: A Guide for Health Promotion Practice*, 2nd ed. Washington, D.C.: Department of Health and Human Services; 2005. Pp. 10–26.
10. Green LW, Kreuter MW. *Health Promotion Planning. An Educational and Environmental Approach*. Mountain View, Calif.: Mayfield Publishing Co.; 1991. Pp. 22–31.
11. Arsham GM, Colenbrander A, Spivey BE. A prototype for curriculum development in medical education. *J Med Educ.* 1973;48:78–84.
12. Smedley BD, Stith AY, Nelson AR, eds. Committee on Understanding and Eliminating Racial and Ethnic Disparities in Health Care, Board on Health Sciences Policy, Institute of Medicine. *Unequal Treatment: Confronting Racial and Ethnic Disparities in Health Care*. Washington, D.C.: National Academies Press; 2003.
13. Carter MM, Lewis EL, Sbrocco T, Tanenbaum R, Oswald JC, Sykora W, Williams P, Hill LD. Cultural competency training for third-year clerkship students: effects of an interactive workshop on student attitudes. *J Natl Med Assoc.* 2006;98:1772–78.
14. Ko M, Heslin KC, Edelstein RA, Grumbach K. The role of medical education in reducing health care disparities: the first ten years of the UCLA/Drew Medical Education Program. *J Gen Intern Med.* 2007;22:625–31.
15. Simpson D, Fincher RM, Hafler JP, Irby DM, Richards BF, Rosenfeld GC, Viggiano TR. Advancing educators and education: defining the components and evidence of educational scholarship. *Med Educ.* 2007;41:1002–9.
16. Best Evidence in Medical Education Collaboration. www.bemecollaboration.org. Accessed March 3, 2009.
17. The Cochrane Collaboration. www.cochrane.org. Accessed March 3, 2009.
18. Reed D, Price EG, Windish DM, Wright SM, Gozu A, Hsu EB, Beach MC, Kern D, Bass EB. Challenges in systematic reviews of educational intervention studies. *Ann Intern Med.* 2005;142:1080–89.
19. National Guideline Clearinghouse, sponsored by the Agency for Healthcare Research and Quality. Available at www.guideline.gov. Accessed March 3, 2009.
20. National Institute for Health and Clinical Excellence. Available at www.nice.org.uk. Accessed March 3, 2009.

21. Hayward RSA, Wilson MC, Tunis SR, Bass EB, Guyatt GH. Users' guides to the medical literature. VIII. How to use clinical practice guidelines. Part A. Are the results valid? Evidence-based Medicine Working Group. *JAMA.* 1995;274:570–74.
22. Wilson MC, Hayward RSA, Tunis SR, Bass EB, Guyatt GH. Users' guides to the medical literature: VIII. How to use clinical practice guidelines. Part B. What are the recommendations, and will they help you in caring for your patients? Evidence-based Medicine Working Group. *JAMA.* 1995;274:1630–32.
23. Accreditation Council for Graduate Medical Education. Available at www.acgme.org. Go to Outcome Project and the relevant Residency Review Committee. Accessed March 3, 2009.
24. American Board of Internal Medicine, Internal Medicine Certification Examination Blueprint. Available at www.abim.org/pdf/blueprint/im_cert.pdf. Or can be reached through ABIM home at www.abim.org, go to Take the Exam, then Specific Information about Each Exam, then Internal Medicine, then Internal Medicine Certification exam blueprint (pdf). Accessed March 3, 2009.
25. Liaison Committee on Medical Education. Go to Accreditation Standards. Available at www .lcme.org. Accessed March 3, 2009.
26. McKean SCW, Budnitz TL, Dressler DD, Amin AN, Pistoria MJ. How to use the Core Competencies in Hospital Medicine: a framework for curriculum development. *J Hospital Medicine.* 2006;1:57–67.
27. Accreditation Council for Graduate Medical Education Outcomes Project. Available at www .acgme.org/Outcome/. Accessed March 3, 2009.
28. Greiner AC, Knebel E, eds. Institute of Medicine; Committee on Health Professions Education Summit. *Health Professions Education: A Bridge to Quality.* Washington, D.C.: National Academy Press; 2003. Pp. 45–96.
29. Boonyasai RT, Windish DM, Chakraborti C, Feldman LS, Rubin HR, Bass EB. Effectiveness of teaching quality improvement to clinicians. A systematic review. *JAMA.* 2007;298:1023–37.
30. MedEdPORTAL. Available at www.aamc.org/mededportal. Accessed March 3, 2009.
31. Curriculum Management and Information Tool. Available at www.aamc.org/meded/curric/start.htm. Accesssed March 3, 2009.
32. Salas AA, Anderson MB, LaCourse L, Allen R, Candler CS, Careon T, Lafferty D. CurrMIT: a tool for managing medical school curricula. *Acad Med.* 2003;78:275–79.
33. Romanov PS, Luft HS. Getting the most out of messy data: problems and approaches for dealing with large administrative data sets. In: Geady ML, Schwartz H, eds. *Medical Treatment Effectiveness Research Data Methods.* Rockville, Md.: U.S. Department of Health and Human Services; 1992. AHCPR Publication No. 92-0056.
34. Krueger RA, Casey MA. *Focus Groups: A Practical Guide for Applied Research,* 3rd ed. Thousand Oaks, Calif.: Sage Publications; 2000.
35. Stewart DW, Shamdasani PN, Rook DW. *Focus Groups: Theory and Practice,* 2nd ed. Thousand Oaks, Calif.: SAGE Publications; 2007.
36. Morgan DL, Krueger RA, King JA. *The Focus Group Kit.* Thousand Oaks, Calif.: SAGE Publications; 1998.
37. Witkin BR, Altschuld JW. *Conducting Needs Assessments: A Practical Guide.* Thousand Oaks, Calif.: Sage Publications; 1995. Pp. 167–71.
38. Witkin BR, Altschuld JW. *Conducting Needs Assessment: A Practical Guide.* Thousand Oaks, Calif.: Sage Publications; 1995. Pp. 187–88, 193–203.
39. Fink A. *How to Conduct Surveys: A Step-by-Step Guide,* 3rd ed. Thousand Oaks, Calif.: SAGE Publications; 2006.
40. Fink A. *The Survey Kit,* 2nd ed. Thousand Oaks, Calif.: SAGE Publications; 2003.
41. Dillman DA. *Mail and Internet Surveys: The Tailored Design Method,* 2nd ed. Hoboken, N.J.: John Wiley & Sons; 2000.

42. Witkin BR, Altschuld JW. *Planning and Conducting Needs Assessments: A Practical Guide.* Thousand Oaks, Calif.: Sage Publications; 1995. Pp. 150–51.
43. Flanagan JC. The critical incident technique. *Psychological Bulletin.* 1954;51:327–58.
44. Witkin BR, Altschuld JW. *Planning and Conducting Needs Assessments: A Practical Guide.* Thousand Oaks, Calif.: Sage Publications; 1995. Pp. 243–49.

Step 2
Targeted Needs Assessment

. . . refining the foundation

Mark T. Hughes, M.D., M.A.

DEFINITION

A targeted needs assessment is a process by which curriculum developers apply the knowledge learned from the general needs assessment to their particular learners and learning environment. In Step 2, curriculum developers identify specific needs by assessing *the differences between ideal and actual characteristics of the targeted learner group and the differences between ideal and actual characteristics of their environment.*

IMPORTANCE

The targeted needs assessment serves many functions. Rather than just throwing resources at a problem, it allows the problem to be framed properly and for stakeholders to be involved in the process of finding solutions. Done appropriately, the targeted needs assessment prevents duplication of what is already being done, teaching what is already known, or teaching above the level of the targeted learners. In addition, "a needs assessment can align resources with strategy, build relationships among those who have a stake in the situation, motivate learners, clarify problems or opportunities, set goals for future action, and provide data for decision making" (1).

The targeted needs assessment should occur at two levels: 1) the targeted learners (their current and past experiences; their strengths and weaknesses in knowledge, attitudes, skills, and performance); and 2) the targeted learning environment (the existing curriculum; other characteristics of the learner's environment that influence whether/how learning occurs and is reinforced; the needs of key stakeholders).

The needs of a curriculum's targeted learners, whether they are patients, practitioners, practitioners in training, or students, are likely to be somewhat different from the needs of learners identified in the general needs assessment (see Chapter 2). A curriculum's targeted learners may already be proficient in one area of general need but have particular learning needs in another area. Some objectives may already be taught in other parts of the overall teaching program but need to be further developed in the new curriculum. Stakeholders, such as clerkship or program directors, may want specific learner objectives or competencies to interact with and reinforce topics addressed in other curricula. Sometimes aspects of the environment, such as the informal or hidden curriculum (2–4), will inhibit translating what has been learned in a specific curriculum into actual clinical practice. Unless curriculum developers assess the needs of their targeted learners and their learners' environment, their curriculum may be inefficient, because it devotes unnecessary resources to areas already addressed and mastered, or suboptimally effective, because it has devoted insufficient resources or attention to other areas of need.

EXAMPLE: *Learners and Existing Curriculum.* Curriculum developers planning an ethics curriculum for PGY–2 and PGY–3 residents during an ambulatory medicine rotation reviewed previous curricula to which the residents had been exposed in the residency, spoke individually to several residents, and surveyed all targeted residents about their previous training, perceived competencies, and perceived needs. They discovered that the residents had been exposed to considerable training related to autonomy, beneficence, substituted judgment, advance directives, and end-of-life decisions, but not at all to clinical decision making in the context of competing interests such as patient versus family versus societal needs, or to reimbursement structures for ambulatory health care. All of the residents' training had centered on inpatient cases. The curriculum developers, therefore, decided to focus their curriculum on clinical decision making, with an emphasis on the ambulatory setting.

EXAMPLE: *Environment, Other Stakeholders.* Curriculum developers designing a curriculum on the pelvic exam for internal medicine residents found that the clinic rooms were inadequately stocked with the supplies needed to perform a pelvic exam and Pap smear. Consequently, the residents were more likely to refer their patients to gynecology for routine women's preventive health measures. After meeting with the clinic director and the nursing staff, the curriculum developers were able to assure that the clinic rooms were properly stocked and staffed, so that residents could offer their female patients the option of getting the pelvic exam in the medicine clinic. The curriculum developers could then concentrate their curricular efforts on the proper techniques for performing a pelvic exam.

EXAMPLE: *Environment, Informal Curriculum.* Curriculum developers designing a curriculum in palliative care surveyed learners about their attitudes toward prescribing opioid analgesics. They found that while the trainees conceptually understood the selection and dosing of opioid analgesics, there was resistance in prescribing them, especially in high doses or to those patients with a history of substance abuse disorders. The resistance was prevalent among nursing and attending staff as well. One of the objectives of the curriculum therefore became addressing attitudinal barriers in prescribing opiates.

IDENTIFICATION OF TARGETED LEARNERS

Before curriculum developers can proceed with the needs assessment of targeted learners, they must identify their targeted learners. Ideally, this choice of targeted learners would flow from the problem identification and general needs assessment (see Chapter 2). The targeted learners would be the group most likely, with further learning, to contribute to the solution of the problem. Frequently, however, curriculum developers have already been assigned their targeted learners, such as medical students or resident physicians in training. In this case, it is worth considering whether an educational intervention directed at one's targeted learners could contribute to solving the health care problem of concern.

CONTENT

Content about Targeted Learners

The first step in the needs assessment of targeted learners, once they have been identified, is to decide on the information that is most needed. Such information might include previous and already planned training and experiences; expectations regarding the scope of knowledge and skills needed (which will differ, for instance, between a medical student and a senior resident); existing proficiencies (cognitive, affective, psychomotor); perceived deficiencies and needs (from evaluators' and/or learners' perspectives); measured deficiencies in knowledge or skills; reasons for past poor performance; learners' capacities and motivations to improve performance; attitudes about the curricular topic; learning styles; preferred learning methods; and targeted learners' experiences regarding different learning strategies (Table 3.1). For learners in a work environment, it may also be important to learn the scope of their work responsibilities, the competencies necessary to fulfill those responsibilities, and the training and nontraining requirements required for the learner to become competent (5).

Content about the Targeted Learning Environment

Concomitant with acquiring information about the learners, curriculum developers must also understand the environment in which their curriculum is to be delivered. For instance, does a curriculum addressing the problem already exist, and if so, what has been its track record (in terms of both learner satisfaction and achievement of learning objectives)? Curriculum developers may discover that the existing curriculum is adequate to meet learners' knowledge and skill needs, but that programmatic or system changes are needed to facilitate subsequent application of the knowledge and skills in clinical settings. They may find that the trainees' clinical training experiences do not match their learning needs.

Table 3.1.   Content Potentially Relevant to a Targeted Needs Assessment

---

Content about Targeted Learners

Previous training and experiences relevant to the curriculum
Already planned training and experiences relevant to the curriculum
Existing characteristics/proficiencies/practices
    Cognitive: knowledge, problem-solving abilities
    Affective: attitudes, values, beliefs, role expectations
    Psychomotor: skills/capabilities (e.g., history, physical examination, procedures,
        counseling); current behaviors/performance/practices
Perceived deficiencies and learning needs
Preferences and experiences regarding different learning strategies
    Synchronous (educator sets time, such as with noon lecture)
    Asynchronous (learner decides on learning time, such as with computer learning)
    Duration (amount of time learner thinks is needed to learn or that they can devote to
        learning)
    Methods (e.g., lectures, readings, Web-based computer interactive modules, case-based
        discussions, group learning, role plays/simulations, supervised experience)

Content about Targeted Learning Environment

Related existing curricula
Needs of stakeholders other than the learners (course directors, clerkship directors, residency
    program directors, accrediting bodies, others)
Barriers, enabling, and reinforcing factors that affect learning by the targeted learners
    The informal and hidden curriculum
    Incentives
    Resources
        Patients and clinical experiences
        Faculty
        Information resources
        Computers
        Audiovisual equipment
        Role models, teachers, mentors
        Other

EXAMPLE: *Inadequate Case Mix and Supervision of Clinical Experience.* Curriculum developers designing a curriculum on the musculoskeletal exam in an internal medicine residency program found that residents working in their continuity clinic had little exposure to clinicians with expertise in musculoskeletal medicine. Because of inadequate case mix, they were not learning about the management of common musculoskeletal problems or gaining proficiency in injection techniques in their rheumatology or elective orthopedic clinic experiences. In addition to updating already existing workshop, lecture, and syllabus materials, the curriculum developers instituted a separate, concentrated primary care musculoskeletal clinic supervised by internal medicine preceptors with a special interest in musculoskeletal medicine, to which other primary care practitioners referred patients for diagnosis and injection. The clinic enabled residents to gain supervised experience in diagnosing and managing common musculoskeletal disorders, such as back, shoulder, elbow, hip, knee, and foot pain; to perform procedures; and to see role models in action (6).

Other information about the environment might include the needs of key stakeholders other than the learners (faculty, educational leaders, accrediting bodies). For instance, curriculum developers may find that faculty are not prepared to teach what needs to be learned, and faculty development thus becomes an important factor in the targeted needs assessment. It is also important to understand the barriers, enabling factors, and reinforcing factors (see Chapter 2) in the environment that affect learning by the targeted learners. For example, is a resident too busy with clinical responsibilities to devote time to educational pursuits? Are there only limited designated time slots (e.g., noon conference) for delivering the curriculum? Does the informal or hidden curriculum promote or inhibit the application of learning? Are there incentives for learning or improving performance? Are there sufficient resources for learning and applying what is learned in practice? (See Table 3.1.)

> **EXAMPLE:** *Inadequate Active Learning, Need for Faculty Development.* Curriculum developers for a preclinical undergraduate curriculum wanted to increase active learning and reduce lecture time. A framework for basic science course time was developed that included delivery of e-lectures, to be viewed before formal class time, and development of cases for small group work. Successful implementation required identification of information technology resources, learning management software, appropriate conference room space, and training of faculty in facilitating case-based small group work.

The problem identification and general needs assessment can be used to identify the information that is most relevant for the targeted needs assessment. Curriculum developers may already have some of the information about their targeted learners and their environment; other information may have to be acquired.

METHODS

General Considerations

Data already in existence, such as the results of questionnaires (e.g., Association of American Medical Colleges' matriculation and graduation questionnaires), standardized examinations (e.g., in-service training and specialty board examinations), procedure and experience logs, other curricula to which the targeted learners are exposed, and audit results, may provide information relevant to curriculum developers and obviate the need for independent data collection. Curriculum management software is another source of already collected data that can help curriculum developers determine what is happening in their institution with respect to a topic of interest. Such software is used to track information regarding a school's curricula, information that is increasingly being required by accreditation bodies. Many U.S. and Canadian schools use the Association of American Medical Colleges' Curriculum Management and Information Tool (CurrMIT), which can be accessed by medical school faculty (7, 8).

When the desired information about the targeted learners is not already available or known by the curriculum developers, they must decide how to acquire it. As with problem identification and general needs assessment (see Chapter 2), curriculum developers must decide *how much time, effort, and resources should be devoted to this step.* A commitment of too little time and effort risks development of an inefficient or ineffective curriculum. A commitment of too much time and effort can diminish the resources available for other critical steps, such as the development of effective educational strategies, successful implementation of the curriculum, and evaluation. Because resources are almost always limited, the curriculum developers will need to *prioritize* their information needs.

Once the information that is required has been decided on, the curriculum developers should decide what the *best method is to obtain this information, given available resources*. In making this decision, they should ask the following questions:

1. What standards of representativeness and accuracy will be required?
2. Will *subjective or objective, quantitative or qualitative data* be preferable?

If there is strong disagreement within the group responsible for developing the curriculum about the knowledge, attitude, skill, or performance deficits of the targeted learners, a more rigorous, representative, objective, and quantitative assessment of learner needs may be required. If a curriculum developer is new to an institution and needs to get a "big picture" sense of the learners and learning environment, collection and analysis of in-depth qualitative data gathered from a sample of selected learners and faculty may be most useful.

If the curriculum developers have limited or no experience using a needs assessment method, it is wise to seek *advice or mentorship from those with expertise* in the method. Before applying a method formally to the group of targeted learners, it is important to *pilot* the data collection instrument on a convenient, receptive audience.

> **EXAMPLE:** *Piloting an Instrument.* A questionnaire was developed to assess the perceived learning needs and preferences of a targeted group of resident physicians. It was piloted on a few friendly residents and faculty, one with expertise in survey methodology. Feedback from the pilot revealed that the questionnaire was too long and that some of the questions were worded in a confusing manner. Feedback provided specific suggestions on improved wording and format, on what questions could be cut, and on one new question that the curriculum developers decided to add. If the original questionnaire had been sent out without revision, much of the data would have been unusable.

If publication or dissemination of the findings of one's targeted needs assessment is anticipated, the work is likely to be considered educational research. Issues related to the protection of human subjects may need to be considered, and one's institutional review board should be consulted before collecting data (see Chapters 6 and 9).

Specific Methods

Specific methods commonly used in the needs assessment of targeted learners include informal discussion or formal interviews with individual learners, their supervisors or observers, and other stakeholders; small group or focus group discussions with proposed participants in the curriculum; formal interviews and questionnaires; direct observation of targeted learners; pretests of knowledge, attitudes, or skills; audits of current performance; and strategic planning sessions for the curriculum (9). Strategic planning sessions can promote success in implementation of the curriculum by engaging stakeholders (see Chapter 6). Strategic planning (10–13) is a team-building process that involves key individuals in the brainstorming and discussion of existing strengths and weaknesses; the prioritization of needs, goals, and objectives; the assignment of responsibilities; and the establishment of timetables.

The advantages and disadvantages of each method of targeted needs assessment are displayed in Table 3.2.

Table 3.2.   Advantages/Disadvantages of Different Needs Assessment Methods

Method	Advantages	Disadvantages
Informal discussion (in-person, over phone, or by e-mail)	Convenient Inexpensive Rich in detail and qualitative information Method for identifying stakeholders	Lack of methodological rigor Variations in questions Interviewer biases
Formal interviews	Standardized approach to interviewee Methodological rigor possible Questions and answers can be clarified With good response rate, can obtain data representative of entire group of targeted learners Quantitative and/or qualitative information Means of gaining support from stakeholders	Methodological rigor requires trained interviewers and measures of reliability Costly in terms of time and effort, especially if methodological rigor is required Interviewer bias and influence on respondent
Focus group discussions	Efficient method of "interviewing" several at one time (especially those with common trait) Learn about group behavior that may affect job performance (especially helpful to understand team-based learning) Group interaction may enrich or deepen information obtained Qualitative information	Requires skilled facilitator to control group interaction and minimize facilitator influence on responses Need note taker or other means of recording information (e.g., audiotape) Views of quiet participants may not be expressed No quantitative information Information may not be representative of all targeted learners Time and financial costs involved in data collection and analysis
Questionnaires	Standardized questions Methodological rigor relatively easy With good response rate, can obtain representative data Quantitative and/or qualitative information Can assess affective traits (attitudes, beliefs, feelings) Respondents can be geographically dispersed (Internet questionnaires increase the ease of reaching geographically dispersed respondents)	Requires skill in writing clear, unambiguous questions Answers cannot be clarified without resurveying Requires time and effort to ensure methodological rigor in survey development, data collection, and data analysis Dependent on adequate response rate (and resources devoted to achieving this) Requires time, effort, and skill to construct valid measures of affective traits

Table 3.2.   *(continued)*

Method	Advantages	Disadvantages
Direct observation	Best method for assessing skills and performance Can be informal or methodologically rigorous Informal observations can sometimes be accomplished as part of one's teaching or supervisory role	Can be time-consuming, especially if methodological rigor is desired Guidelines must be developed for standardized observations Observer generally must be knowledgeable of behavior being observed Observer bias Impact of observer on observed Assesses ability, not real-life performance (unless observations are unobtrusive)
Tests	Efficient, objective means of assessing cognitive or psychomotor abilities Tests of key knowledge items relatively easy to construct	Requires time, effort, and skill to construct valid tests of skills and higher order cognitive abilities Test anxiety may affect performance Assesses ability, not real-life performance
Audits of current performance	Useful for medical record keeping and the provision of recorded care (e.g., tests ordered, provision of discrete preventive care measures, prescribed treatments) Unobtrusive Assesses real-life performance Can be methodologically rigorous with standards, instructions, and assurance of inter- and intra-rater reliability	Requires development of standards Requires resources to pay and train auditors, time and effort to perform audit oneself May require permission from learner and/or institution to audit records Difficult to avoid or account for recording omissions Addresses only indirect, incomplete measures of care
Strategic planning sessions for the curriculum	Can involve targeted learners as well as key faculty Can involve brainstorming of learner needs, as well as current program strengths and weaknesses Can involve prioritization as well as generation of needs Creates sense of involvement and responsibility in participants Part of a larger process that also identifies goals, objectives, and responsibilities	Requires skilled facilitator to ensure participation and lack of inhibition by all participants Requires considerable time and effort to plan and conduct successful strategic planning sessions and to develop the associated report

Surveys

Surveys are collections and/or reviews of data that are usually systematically performed. Three types of survey frequently used in curriculum development are interviews (questions asked and recorded by an interviewer), focus groups, and questionnaires (usually self-administered). Curriculum developers can decide which method best suits their needs. In designing a survey, curriculum developers must decide on the sample population to be surveyed, whether the sample is randomly or purposively selected, and the design of the survey (cross-sectional vs. longitudinal). Regardless of the type of survey administered, each question should have clearly delineated objectives and justification for its inclusion in the survey. The length of a survey and/or the sensitivity of its questions will influence the response rate by the sample population. Because response rates are critical for acquisition of representative data, curriculum developers should generally include only questions that can be acted on (14). The sample population being surveyed should be notified about the survey, its purpose, what their responses will be used for, whether responses will be considered confidential, and the time needed to conduct the survey.

Interviews can be conducted in person, by phone, or by computer technology (e.g., instant messaging). Interviews can be structured, unstructured, or semi-structured. Structured interviews allow for consistency of questions across respondents so that they can be compared/contrasted, whereas unstructured or semi-structured interviews allow spontaneity and on-the-spot follow-up of interesting responses. Several caveats should be kept in mind when developing, preparing for, and conducting an interview (Table 3.3) (15).

Table 3.3.   Tips for Developing, Preparing for, and Conducting an Interview

1. Decide how information will be recorded (hand-written, typed into a computer, audiotaped) and the time needed to document responses.

2. If multiple interviewers are used, develop an interview guide.

3. Structure interview questions to facilitate conversation, with more general, open-ended questions up front, important questions toward the beginning, and sensitive questions at the end.

4. Cluster questions with a common theme in a logical order.

5. Clarify responses when necessary (use prompts such as the following: "Describe for me...." "Tell me more...." "Can you say more about that...?" "Can you give me an example?").

6. Maintain a neutral attitude and avoid biasing interviewee responses (e.g., by discussing the responses of another interviewee).

7. At the end of the interview, express gratitude and ask the interviewee whether he has any additional questions or comments.

8. Time permitting, summarize key points and ask interviewee whether he can be contacted for follow-up questions.

Source: Gupta et al., pp. 44–49 (15).

Focus groups bring together people with a common attribute to share their collective experience with the help of a skilled facilitator. Focus groups should be of a manageable size (7 ± 2 is a good rule) and should engender an atmosphere of openness and respectful sharing. The facilitator should be familiar with the topic area and use language understandable to focus group participants (their typical jargon if a specialized group or layperson language if a mixed group). The facilitator should encourage participation, acknowledge responses nonjudgmentally, manage those who are more or less willing to engage in the discussion, foster brainstorming in response to participant answers, and keep track of time. After the focus group is completed, a report should be generated highlighting the key findings from the session (16).

Questionnaires, as opposed to interviews and focus groups, are completed by the individual alone or with minimal assistance from another. They can be paper-based or online (e.g., www.surveymonkey.com). A questionnaire must contain instructions on how to answer questions. It is also generally advisable to have a cover letter with the questionnaire explaining the rationale of the questionnaire and what is expected of the respondent. *Pilot-testing* to assure clarity and understandability in both the format and the content of the questions is especially important, as no interviewer is present to explain the meaning of ambiguously worded questions.

When representative data are desired, response rate is critical. Overall questionnaire response rates will depend on the amount of burden (time, opportunity costs, etc.) placed on respondents in completing the questionnaire. Questionnaire designers have to decide on incentives for completion of the questionnaire and the location where the questionnaire will be administered (e.g., at the end of a mandatory training session when learners are still a "captive audience" or at home so that respondents can complete the questionnaire at their own pace). Methods for following up with questionnaire nonrespondents also have to be considered, as this may entail additional time and resources (17). Curriculum developers must also be cognizant of the potential for nonresponse to particular questions on the questionnaire (18).

Questions should relate to the questionnaire's objectives, and the respondent should be aware of the rationale for each question. How questions are worded in a survey greatly affects the value of the information gleaned from them. Table 3.4 (19, 20) provides tips to keep in mind when writing questions.

Once information is collected, the data need to be systematically analyzed (see Chapter 7 for more detail on data analysis). Regardless of whether curriculum developers are analyzing quantitative (21) or qualitative data (22, 23), the curriculum developers must always keep in mind that the targeted needs assessment is intended to focus the problem in the context of their learners and their learning environment and to help shape the subsequent steps in curriculum development.

RELATION TO OTHER STEPS

The information one chooses to collect as part of the targeted needs assessment may be influenced by what one expects will be a *goal or objective* of the curriculum or by the *educational* and *implementation strategies* being considered for the curriculum. Subsequent steps, such as *Goals and Objectives, Educational Strategies, Implementation, and Evaluation*, are likely to be affected by what is learned in the targeted needs assessment. The process of conducting a needs assessment can serve as

Table 3.4.   Tips for Writing and Administering Questionnaire Questions

1. Ask for only one piece of information. The more precise and unambiguous the question is, the better.

2. Avoid biased, leading, or negatively phrased questions.

3. Avoid abbreviations, colloquialisms, or phrases not easily understood by respondents.

4. For paper-based questionnaires, make sure questions follow a logical order, key items are highlighted with textual elements (boldface, italics, underline), the overall format is not visually complex or distracting, and the sequence of questions/pages is easy to follow.

5. Decide whether an open-ended or closed-ended question will elicit the most fitting response. Open-ended answers (e.g., fill in the blank) will require more data analysis, so they should be used in a limited fashion when surveying a large sample. Closed-ended questions are used when the surveyor wants an answer from a prespecified set of response choices.

6. Make categorical responses (e.g., race) mutually exclusive and exhaust all categories (if necessary, using "other") in the offered list of options.

7. When more than one response is possible, offer the option of "check all that apply."

8. In using ordinal questions (responses can be ordered on a scale by level of agreement, frequency, intensity, or comparison), make the scale meaningful to the topic area and easy to complete and understand based on the question thread and instructions. For potentially embarrassing or sensitive questions, it is generally best to put the negative end of the scale first.

9. For attitudinal questions, decide whether it is important to learn how respondents feel, how strongly they feel, or both.

10. If demographic questions are asked, know how this information will influence the data analysis, what the range of answers will be in the target population, how specific the information needs to be, and whether it will be compared to existing data sets (in which case common terms should be used). Sometimes asking respondents to answer in their own words or numbers (e.g., date of birth, zip code, income) allows the surveyor to avoid questions with a burdensome number of response categories.

Source: Adapted from Fink, pp. 1–91 (19), Gupta et al., p. 61 (20).

advance publicity for a curriculum, engage stakeholders, and ease a curriculum's *implementation.* Information gathered as part of the targeted needs assessment can serve as *"pre-" or "before" data for evaluation* of the impact of a curriculum. For all of these reasons, it is wise to think through other steps, at least in a preliminary manner, before investing time and resources in the targeted needs assessment.

> **EXAMPLE:** *Interaction with Implementation.* A targeted needs assessment of internal medicine residents revealed performance barriers in terms of space, equipment, and support staff, as well as skill deficits, that prevented residents from including cervical cancer screening in the care of their ambulatory continuity patients. The curriculum developers were able to convince the clinic administrator to purchase the necessary equipment and to redefine nursing staff roles with respect to availability for pelvic examinations. Space needs were incorporated into planning for the new ambulatory building.

EXAMPLE: *Interaction with Evaluation.* On the first day of a pediatrics clerkship, medical students were administered a knowledge and problem-solving test. They performed better than expected in some areas, such as managing otitis media in the toddler, and less than expected in other areas, such as interpretation of growth charts. This information was used to tailor subsequent learning sessions. Test data were used as part of a pre-post evaluation of the learners' cognitive achievements in the clerkship.

It is also worth realizing that one can learn a lot about a curriculum's targeted learners in the course of conducting the curriculum. This information can then be used as a targeted needs assessment for the next cycle of the curriculum.

EXAMPLE: *Evaluation that Serves as Targeted Needs Assessment.* During an ambulatory medicine rotation, it was noted that residents were, for the most part, unskilled in incorporating preventive care into office visits and in motivating patients to follow treatment plans. Focused training in these areas was developed for the next cycle of the ambulatory medicine rotation.

SCHOLARSHIP

A well-done targeted needs assessment allows curriculum developers to provide specific information about learners and the learning environment that facilitates adoption of the curriculum by other institutions or training programs. This is a critical step in the dissemination of the curriculum beyond one's own institution. (See Chapter 9.)

CONCLUSION

By clarifying the characteristics of one's targeted learners and their environment, the curriculum developer can help assure that the curriculum being planned not only addresses important general needs but also is relevant and applicable to the specific needs of its learners and their learning institution. Steps 1 and 2 provide a sound basis for the next step, choosing the goals and objectives for the curriculum.

QUESTIONS

For the curriculum you are coordinating, planning, or would like to be planning, please answer or think about the following questions:

1. *Identify your targeted learners.* From the point of view of your problem identification and general needs assessment, will training this group as opposed to other groups of learners make the greatest contribution to solving the health care problem? If not, who would be a better group of targeted learners? Are these learners an option for you? Notwithstanding these considerations, is it nevertheless important to train your original group of targeted learners? Why?

2. To the extent of your current knowledge, *describe your targeted learners and their environment.* What are your targeted learners' previous training experiences, existing proficiencies, past and current performance, attitudes about the topic area and/or

curriculum, learning style and needs, and familiarity with and preferences for different learning methods? In the targeted learning environment, what other curricula exist or are being planned, what are the enabling and reinforcing factors and barriers to development and implementation of your curriculum, and what are the resources for learning? Who are the stakeholders (course directors, faculty, school administrators, clerkship and residency program directors, and accrediting bodies) and what are their needs with respect to your curriculum?

3. *What information* about your learners and their environment *is unknown* to you? *Prioritize* your information needs.

4. *Identify one or more methods* (e.g., informal and formal interviews, focus groups, questionnaires) by which you could obtain the most important information. For each method, *identify the resources* (time, personnel, supplies, space) required to develop the necessary data collection instruments and to collect and analyze the needed data. To what degree do you feel that each method is feasible?

5. Identify individuals on whom you could *pilot* your needs assessment instrument(s).

GENERAL REFERENCES

Needs Assessment

Altschuld JW, Witkin BR. *From Needs Assessment to Action: Transforming Needs into Solution Strategies.* Thousand Oaks, Calif.: Sage Publications; 2000.
Reviews earlier work (Witkin and Altschuld, see below), addresses value of multiple/mixed method approach to needs assessment, including both qualitative and quantitative methods, and then focuses on the prioritization of needs and the transformation of needs assessments into action. Provides real-world examples. 282 pages.

Green LW, Kreuter MW, Deeds SG, Partridge KB. *Health Education Planning: A Diagnostic Approach.* Palo Alto, Calif.: Mayfield Publishing; 1980.
Basic text in health education program planning that includes the importance and role of the needs assessment in determining a social/quality-of-life diagnosis and in identifying health problems (epidemiologic diagnosis) for a targeted population. 306 pages.

Gupta K, Sleezer CM, Russ-Eft DF. *A Practical Guide to Needs Assessment (Essential Knowledge Resource).* Hoboken, N.J.: John Wiley & Sons (published by Pfeiffer); 2007.
Practical how-to handbook on conducting a needs assessment, with case examples and toolkit in hard copy and CD-ROM. 336 pages.

Morrison GR, Ross SM, Kemp JE. *Designing Effective Instruction,* 5th ed. Hoboken, N.J.: John Wiley & Sons; 2007.
A general book on instructional design, including needs assessment, instructional objectives, instructional strategies, and evaluation. Chapters 2–4 (pp. 28–101) deal with needs assessment. 441 pages.

Rossett A. *Training Needs Assessment.* Englewood Cliffs, N.J.: Educational Technology Publications; 1987.
Practical book focusing on determining the training needs of employees in organizations, with the concepts, examples, and needs assessment methods easily transferable to all levels of health care workers and professionals. Written from an instructional design perspective. 294 pages.

Witkin BR, Altschuld JW. *Planning and Conducting Needs Assessments: A Practice Guide.* Thousand Oaks, Calif.: Sage Publications; 1995.

Readable yet comprehensive book with information and examples organized into two major sections: 1) planning/managing the needs assessment; and 2) methods used for conducting a needs assessment. The methods section is particularly useful as it covers records and social indicators (including mapping); surveys; interviews; the critical incident technique; nominal group technique; focus groups; mailed Delphi survey and modified (or group) Delphi process; strategic planning; and causal analysis including fishboning, cause and consequence analysis, and fault tree analysis. The organizational and community examples are easily translatable to medical care settings. 302 pages.

Survey Design

Books

Biemer PP, Lyberg LE. *Introduction to Survey Quality (Wiley Series in Survey Methodology).* Hoboken, N.J.: John Wiley & Sons; 2003.

A comprehensive review of survey methodology focusing on sources of error in collecting information and how to address these errors. Once the sources of error have been identified, the authors give tips on how surveyors can evaluate the effects of error on total survey quality. 424 pages.

Couper MP, Baker RP, Bethlehem J, Clark CZF, Martin J, Nicholls WL, O'Reilly JM, eds. *Computer Assisted Survey Information Collection.* Hoboken, N.J.: John Wiley & Sons; 1998.

Multiauthored 29 chapter text from a conference on this subject. 653 pages.

Dillman DA. *Mail and Internet Surveys: The Tailored Design Method,* 2nd ed. Hoboken, N.J.: John Wiley & Sons; 2000.

Topics include writing questions, constructing questionnaires, survey implementation and delivery, mixed mode surveys, and Internet surveys. Presents a stepwise approach to survey implementation that incorporates strategies to improve rigor and response rates. Clearly written with many examples. 464 pages.

Fink A. *How to Conduct Surveys: A Step-by-Step Guide,* 3rd ed. Thousand Oaks, Calif.: Sage Publications; 2006.

Short, basic text that covers question writing, questionnaire format, sampling, survey administration design, data analysis, creating code books, and presenting results. 107 pages.

Fink A. *The Survey Kit,* 2nd ed. Thousand Oaks, Calif.: Sage Publications; 2003.

Practical 10 volume set: 1. Fink A. *The Survey Handbook.* 2. Fink A. *How to Ask Survey Questions.* 3. Bourque LB, Fielder EP. *How to Conduct Self-Administered and Mail Surveys.* 4. Bourque LB, Fielder EP. *How to Conduct Telephone Surveys.* 5. Oishi SM. *How to Conduct In-Person Interviews for Surveys.* 6. Fink A. *How to Design Survey Studies.* 7. Fink A. *How to Sample in Surveys.* 8. Litwin MS. *How to Assess and Interpret Survey Psychometrics.* 9. Fink A. *How to Manage, Analyze, and Interpret Survey Data.* 10. Fink A. *How to Report on Surveys.*

Fowler FJ. *Survey Research Methods (Applied Social Research Methods),* 3rd ed. Thousand Oaks, Calif.: Sage Publications; 2001.

Short text on survey research methods including chapters on sampling, nonresponse, data collection, designing questions, evaluating survey questions and instruments, interviewing, data analysis, and ethical issues. Focuses on reducing sources of error. 178 pages.

Groves RM, Dillman DA, Eltinge JL, Little RJA. *Survey Nonresponse* (Wiley Series in Survey Methodology). Hoboken, N.J.: John Wiley & Sons; 2001.

Multi-authored text that compiles theoretical and empirical research on survey nonresponse by experts in the field. 500 pages.

Groves RM, Fowler FJ, Couper MP, Lepkowski JM, Singer E, Tourangeau R. *Survey Methodology* (Wiley Series in Survey Methodology). Hoboken, N.J.: John Wiley & Sons; 2004.

Written by experts in the field, this detailed book describes the principles of survey design discovered in methodological research and offers guidance for making successful decisions in the design and execution of high-quality surveys. Detailed text that can serve as a reference and text for researchers and advanced students. 424 pages.

Krueger RA, Casey MA. *Focus Groups: A Practical Guide for Applied Research,* 3rd ed. Thousand Oaks, Calif.: Sage Publications; 2000.
Practical how-to book that covers uses of focus groups, planning, developing questions, determining focus group composition, moderating skills, data analysis, and reporting results. 215 pages.

Lepkowski JM, Tucker C, Brick JM, De Leeuw ED, Japec L, Lavrakas PJ, Link MW, Sangster RL. *Advances in Telephone Survey Methodology.* Hoboken, N.J.: John Wiley & Sons; 2008.
Multi-authored text, emanating from 2006 International Conference on Telephone Survey Methodology, providing state-of-the-art view of field, 683 pages.

Morgan DL, Krueger RA, King JA. *The Focus Group Kit.* Thousand Oaks, Calif.: Sage Publications; 1998.
Practical six-volume set: 1. Morgan DL. *The Focus Group Guidebook.* 2. Morgan DL. *Planning Focus Groups.* 3. Krueger RA. *Developing Questions for Focus Groups.* 4. Krueger RA. *Moderating Focus Groups.* 5. Krueger RA., Kin JA. *Involving Community Members in Focus Groups.* 6. Krueger RA. *Analyzing & Reporting Focus Group Results.*

Stewart DW, Shamdasani PN, Rook DW. *Focus Groups: Theory and Practice,* 2nd ed. Thousand Oaks, Calif.: Sage Publications; 2007.
Short text that provides a systematic treatment of the design, conduct, and interpretation of focus group discussions in the context of social science research and theory. 188 pages.

Internet Resources

American Association of Public Opinion Research
The American Association for Public Opinion Research (AAPOR) is a U.S. professional organization of public opinion and survey research professionals, with members from academia, media, government, the nonprofit sector, and private industry. It provides educational opportunities in survey research, provides resources for researchers on a range of survey and polling issues, and publishes the journal *Public Opinion Quarterly.* Available at www.aapor.org. Accessed March 11, 2009.

Survey Research Methods Section, American Statistical Association
Provides downloadable "What is a survey" booklet on survey methodology and links to other resources. Available at www.amstat.org/sections/SRMS/index.html. Accessed March 11, 2009.

SPECIFIC REFERENCES

1. Gupta K, Sleezer CM, Russ-Eft DF. *A Practical Guide to Needs Assessment (Essential Knowledge Resource).* Hoboken, N.J.: John Wiley & Sons (published by Pfeiffer); 2007. P. 20.
2. Hafferty FW, Ranks R. The hidden curriculum, ethics teaching, and the structure of medical education. *Acad Med.* 1994;69:861–71.
3. Hundert EM, Hafferty F, Christakis D. Characteristics of the informal curriculum and trainees' ethical choices. *Acad Med.* 1996;71:624–42.
4. Hafferty FW. Beyond curriculum reform: confronting medicine's hidden curriculum. *Acad Med.* 1998;73:403–7.
5. Gupta K, Sleezer CM, Russ-Eft DF. *A Practical Guide to Needs Assessment (Essential Knowledge Resource).* Hoboken, N.J.: John Wiley & Sons (published by Pfeiffer); 2007. Pp. 105–55.

6. Houston TK, Connors RL, Cutler N, Nidiry MA. A primary care musculoskeletal clinic for residents: success and sustainability. *J Gen Intern Med.* 2004 May;19(5 Pt 2):524–29.

7. CurrMIT (Curriculum Management and Information Tool). Available at www.aamc.org/meded/curric/. Accessed March 11, 2009.

8. Salas AA, Anderson MB, LaCourse L, Allen R, Candler CS, Careon T, Lafferty D. CurrMIT: a tool for managing medical school curricula. *Acad Med.* 2003;78:275–79.

9. Witkin BR, Altschuld JW. *Planning and Conducting Needs Assessments: A Practical Guide.* Thousand Oaks, Calif.: Sage Publications; 1995. Pp. 101–274.

10. Witkin BR, Altschuld JW. *Planning and Conducting Needs Assessments: A Practical Guide.* Thousand Oaks, Calif.: Sage Publications; 1995. Pp. 210–17.

11. Allison M, Kaye J. *Strategic Planning for Nonprofit Organizations: A Practical Guide and Workbook,* 2nd ed. San Francisco: John Wiley & Sons; 2005.

12. Barry BW. *Strategic Planning Workbook for Nonprofit Organizations.* St. Paul, Minn.: Amherst H. Wilder Foundation; 1997. Pp. 1–131.

13. Goodstein LD, Nolan TM, Pfeiffer JW. *Applied Strategic Planning: An Introduction.* San Diego: Pfeiffer & Co.; 1992. Pp. 1–61.

14. Fink A. *How to Conduct Surveys: A Step-by-Step Guide,* 3rd ed. Thousand Oaks, Calif.: Sage Publications; 2006. Pp. 11–29.

15. Gupta K, Sleezer CM, Russ-Eft DF. *A Practical Guide to Needs Assessment (Essential Knowledge Resource).* Hoboken, N.J.: John Wiley & Sons (published by Pfeiffer); 2007. Pp. 44–49.

16. Gupta K, Sleezer CM, Russ-Eft DF. *A Practical Guide to Needs Assessment (Essential Knowledge Resource).* Hoboken, N.J.: John Wiley & Sons (published by Pfeiffer); 2007. Pp. 46–51.

17. Fink A. *The Survey Kit,* 2nd ed. *Volume 9: How to Manage, Analyze, and Interpret Survey Data.* Thousand Oaks, Calif.: Sage Publications; 2003. Pp. 1–24.

18. Groves RM, Dillman DA, Eltinge JL, Little RJA. *Survey Nonresponse* (Wiley Series in Survey Methodology). Hoboken, N.J.: John Wiley & Sons; 2001.

19. Fink A. *The Survey Kit,* 2nd ed. *Volume 2: How to Ask Survey Questions.* Thousand Oaks, Calif.: Sage Publications; 2003. Pp. 1–91.

20. Gupta K, Sleezer CM, Russ-Eft DF. *A Practical Guide to Needs Assessment (Essential Knowledge Resource).* Hoboken, N.J.: John Wiley & Sons (published by Pfeiffer); 2007. Pp. 61–62.

21. Fink A. *The Survey Kit,* 2nd ed. *Volume 9: How to Manage, Analyze, and Interpret Survey Data.* Thousand Oaks, Calif.: Sage Publications; 2003. Pp. 25–121.

22. Miles MB, Huberman AM. *Qualitative Data Analysis: An Expanded Sourcebook,* 2nd ed. Thousand Oaks, Calif.: Sage Publications; 1994.

23. Morse JM, ed. *Critical Issues in Qualitative Research Methods.* Thousand Oaks, Calif.: Sage Publications; 1994.

Additional references on specific methods are cited under "Obtaining the Necessary Information" in Chapter 2, Step 1: Problem Identification and General Needs Assessment.

CHAPTER FOUR

Step 3
Goals and Objectives

. . . focusing the curriculum

Patricia A. Thomas, M.D.

DEFINITIONS

Once the needs of the learners have been clarified, it is desirable to target the curriculum to address these needs by setting goals and objectives. *A goal or objective is defined as an end toward which an effort is directed. In this book, the term "goal" will be used when broad educational objectives are being discussed. The term "objective" will be used when specific measurable objectives are being discussed.*

EXAMPLE: *Goal versus Specific Measurable Objective.* A *goal* (or broad educational objective) of a gynecology curriculum for internal medicine residents is that internal medicine residents develop the knowledge, attitudes, and skills necessary to diagnose, manage, and appropriately refer women who present to primary care settings with gynecologic needs or complaints. A *specific measurable objective* of the curriculum might be that, by the end of the gynecology curriculum, each resident will have demonstrated, at least once, the appropriate technique, as defined on a check sheet, for obtaining a Pap smear and cervical cultures.

IMPORTANCE

Goals and objectives are important because they do the following:

- help direct the choice of curricular content and the assignment of relative priorities to various components of the curriculum;
- suggest what learning methods will be most effective;
- enable evaluation of learners and the curriculum, thus permitting demonstration of the effectiveness of a curriculum;
- suggest what evaluation methods are appropriate;
- clearly communicate to others, such as learners, faculty, program directors, department chairs, and individuals from other institutions, what the curriculum addresses and hopes to achieve.

Broad educational goals communicate the overall purposes of a curriculum and serve as criteria against which the selection of various curricular components can be judged. The development and prioritization of *specific measurable objectives* permit further refinement of the curricular content and guide the selection of appropriate educational and evaluation methods.

WRITING OBJECTIVES

Writing educational objectives is an underappreciated skill. Despite the importance of objectives, learners, teachers, and curriculum planners frequently have difficulty in formulating or explaining the objectives of a curriculum. Poorly written objectives can result in a poorly focused and inefficient curriculum, prone to "drift" over time from its original goals.

A key to writing useful educational objectives is to make them *specific and measurable. Five basic elements* should be included in such objectives (1):

Who will do how much (how well) of what by when?

1)   2)   3)   4)   5)

EXAMPLE: *Specific Measurable Objective.* The example provided at the beginning of the chapter contains these elements: Who (each resident) will do (demonstrate, obtain) how much/how well (once/the appropriate technique per checklist) of what (obtaining a Pap smear and cervical cultures) by when (by the end of the curriculum)? That objective could be measured by observation using a checklist.

In other words, the specific measurable objective should include a verb (2) and a noun (4) that describe a *performance,* as well as a *criterion* (3) and *conditions* of the performance (3 and 5). In writing specific measurable objectives (as opposed to goals), one should *use verbs that are open to few interpretations* (e.g., to list or demonstrate) rather than words that are open to many interpretations (e.g., to know or be able). Table 4.1 lists more and less precise words to use in writing objectives. Finally, it is important to *have people who are not involved in the curriculum review the objectives*, to ensure that others can accurately describe what the objectives are intended to convey. Table 4.2 provides some examples of poorly written and better written objectives.

Table 4.1.   Verbs Open to More and Fewer Interpretations

Verbs Open to More Interpretations	Verbs Open to Fewer Interpretations	
Verbs that frequently apply to cognitive objectives:		
	Taxonomy of cognitive objectives (2, 3)	Verb
know	*Remember* (recall of facts)	identify list recite define recognize retrieve
understand	*Understand*	define contrast interpret classify describe sort explain illustrate
be able know how appreciate	*Apply*	implement execute use (a model, method) complete
	Analyze	differentiate distinguish organize deconstruct discriminate
	Evaluate	detect judge critique test
know how	*Create*	design hypothesize construct produce
Verbs that frequently apply to affective objectives:		
appreciate grasp the significance of	rate as valuable, rank as important	
believe	identify, rate, or rank as a belief or opinion	
enjoy	rate or rank as enjoyable	
internalize	use one of above terms	

Table 4.1.   *(continued)*

Verbs that frequently apply to psychomotor objectives:

Skill/Competence:

be able	demonstrate
know how	show

Behavior/Performance

Internalize	use or incorporate into performance (as measured by)

Other Verbs:

learn	(use one of the above terms)
teach	(use one of the above terms; do not confuse the teacher and the learner in writing learner objectives)

TYPES OF OBJECTIVE

In constructing a curriculum, one should be aware of the different types and levels of objective. *Types of objective* include objectives related to the learning of *learners*, to the educational *process* itself, and to health care and other *outcomes* of the curriculum. These types of objective can be written at the level of the *individual learner* or at the level of the *program* or of all learners in *aggregate*. Table 4.3 provides examples of the different types of objective for a curriculum on smoking cessation.

Learner Objectives

Learner objectives include objectives that relate to learning in the cognitive, affective, and psychomotor domains. Learner objectives that pertain to the *cognitive* domain of learning are often referred to as "knowledge" objectives. The latter terminology, however, may lead to an overemphasis on factual knowledge. Objectives related to the cognitive domain of learning should take into consideration a spectrum of mental skills relevant to the goals of a curriculum, from simple factual knowledge to higher levels of cognitive functioning, such as problem solving and clinical decision making.

> **EXAMPLE:** *Cognitive Objective.* By the end of the neurology curriculum, the learner will describe in writing a cost-effective approach to the initial evaluation and management of a patient presenting with dementia (an approach that includes at least six of the eight elements listed on the handout).

Bloom's taxonomy was the first attempt to describe this potential hierarchy of mental skills (2). The elegance of Bloom's taxonomy of cognitive learning objectives lay in the realization that cognitive learning occurred through a series of steps, which were referred to as six levels in the cognitive domain: knowledge (i.e., recall of facts), comprehension, application, analysis, synthesis, and evaluation (2). These categories were revised by Anderson et al. to incorporate modern concepts in cognitive psychology and understanding of learning (3). This version presents cognitive processes as follows:

Table 4.2.   Examples of Less-Well-Written and Better-Written Objectives

Less-Well-Written Objectives	Better-Written Objectives
▪ Residents will learn the techniques of joint injections. [*The types of injection to be learned are not specified. The types of resident are not specified. It is unclear whether cognitive understanding of the technique is sufficient, or whether skills must be acquired. It is unclear by when the learning must have occurred, and how proficiency could be assessed. The objective on the right addresses each of these concerns.*]	▪ By the end of the residency, each family practice resident will have demonstrated at least once (according to the attached proto- col) the proper techniques for the following: - subacromial, bicipital, and intra-articular shoulder injection; - intra-articular knee aspiration and/or injection; - injections for lateral and medial epicondylitis; - injections for deQuervain's tenosynovitis; - aspiration and/or injection of at least one new bursa, joint, or tendinous area, using appropriate references and supervision.
▪ By the end of the internal medicine clerkship, each third-year medical student will be able to diagnose and manage common ambulatory medical disorders. [*This objective specifies "who" and "by when" but is vague about what it is the medical students are to achieve. The two objectives on the right add specificity to the latter.*]	▪ By the end of the internal medicine ambula- tory medicine clerkship, each third-year medical student will have achieved cogni- tive proficiency in the diagnosis and man- agement of hypertension, diabetes, angina, chronic obstructive pulmonary disease, hyperlipidemia, alcohol and drug abuse, smoking, and asymptomatic HIV infection, as measured by acceptable scores on inter- im tests and the final examination. ▪ By the end of the internal medicine clerkship, each third-year medical student will have seen and discussed with the preceptor, or discussed in a case conference with colleagues, at least one patient with each of the above disorders.
▪ Physician practices, whose staff com- plete the three-session communication skills workshops, will have more satisfied patients. [*This objective does not specify the comparison group or what is meant by "satisfied." The objective on the right specifies more precisely which practices will have more satisfied patients, what the comparison group will be, and how satis- faction will be measured. It specifies one aspect of performance as well as satis- faction. One could look at the satisfaction questionnaire and telephone manage- ment monitoring instrument for a more precise description of the outcomes being measured.*]	▪ Physician practices, which have ≥50% of their staff complete the three-session communication skills workshops, will have lower complaint rates, higher patient satisfaction scores on the yearly questionnaire, and better telephone management, as measured by random simulated calls, than practices that have lower completion rates.

Table 4.3.   Types of Objective: Examples from a Smoking Cessation Curriculum for Residents

	Individual Learner	Aggregate or Program
Learner		
Cognitive (knowledge)	By the end of the curriculum, each resident will be able to list the five-step approach to effective smoking cessation counseling.	By the end of the curriculum, ≥80% of residents will be able to list the five-step approach to effective smoking cessation counseling, and ≥90% will be able to list the four critical (asterisked) steps.
Affective (attitudinal)	By the end of the curriculum, each primary care resident will rank smoking cessation counseling as an important and effective intervention by primary care physicians (≥3 on a 4-point scale).	By the end of the curriculum there will have been a statistically significant increase in how primary care residents rate the importance and effectiveness of smoking cessation counseling by primary care physicians.
Psychomotor (skill or competence)	During the curriculum, each primary care resident will demonstrate in role-play a smoking cessation counseling technique that incorporates the attached five steps.	During the curriculum, ≥80% of residents will have demonstrated in role-play a smoking cessation counseling technique that incorporates the attached five steps.
Psychomotor (behavioral or performance)	By 6 months after completion of the curriculum, each primary care resident will have negotiated a plan for smoking cessation with ≥60% of his/ her smoking patients or have increased the percentage of such patients by ≥20% from baseline.	By 6 months after completion of the curriculum, there will have been a statistically significant increase in the percentage of GIM residents who have negotiated a plan for smoking cessation with their patients.
Process	Each primary resident will have attended both sessions of the smoking cessation workshop.	≥80% of primary care residents will have attended both sessions of the smoking cessation workshop.
Patient outcome	By 12 months after completion of the curriculum, the smoking cessation rate (for ≥6 months) for the patients of each primary care resident will increase twofold or more from baseline or be ≥10%.	By 12 months after completion of the curriculum, there will have been a statistically significant increase in the percentage of primary care residents' patients who have quit smoking (for ≥6 months).

1. *Remember*: To recall or recognize relevant knowledge.
2. *Understand:* To construct meaning from information; to interpret, explain, compare, or summarize communications.
3. *Apply:* To execute or implement a procedure in a given situation.
4. *Analyze:* To break material into its constituents and determine how parts relate to each other; to organize, differentiate, or assign an attribution.
5. *Evaluate*: To make judgments based on criteria and standards.
6. *Create:* To put elements together; reorganize; generate hypotheses; plan a project.

Marzano and Kendall further refined the taxonomy based on their review of the literature (4). They identify four levels: retrieval of knowledge, comprehension, analysis, and use of knowledge. They also emphasize the importance of learner motivation, beliefs and emotions (self-system), and goal setting and self-monitoring (metacognition) in learning.

To some extent, these taxonomies are hierarchical. Curriculum planners usually specify the highest level objective expected of the learner. The level of objectives is implied by the choice of verbs (see Table 4.1). Planners should also recognize that there are *enabling objectives* necessary to attain a certain level. In the example above, learners will need to know the differential diagnosis of dementia and the operating characteristics of diagnostic tests before they can implement a cost-effective approach. Understanding the need for these enabling objectives will help curricular developers to plan educational strategies.

Learner objectives that pertain to the *affective* domain are frequently referred to as "attitudinal" objectives. They may refer to specific attitudes, values, beliefs, biases, emotions, or role expectations that can affect a learner's learning or performance. Affective objectives are usually more difficult to express and to measure than cognitive objectives (5). Indeed, some instructional design experts maintain that because attitudes cannot be accurately assessed by learner performance, attitudinal objectives should not be written (6). Affective objectives, however, are implicit in most educational programs for medical students, physicians, and other providers. Nearly every curriculum, for instance, holds as an affective objective that learners will value the importance of learning the curriculum, which is critical to attainment of other learner objectives. This objective relates to Marzano and Kendall's "self-system" (see above), which includes motivation, emotional response, perceived importance, and efficacy, and which they argue is an important underpinning of learning. Because attitudes and practices that are reinforced by actual experiences within and outside medical institutions (termed the "informal" and "hidden" curricula) may run counter to what is formally taught (7, 8), it behooves curriculum developers to recognize and address such attitudes and practices. Therefore, to the extent that a curriculum involves learning in the affective domain, curriculum planners should develop objectives in this domain. Such objectives can help direct educational strategies, even when there are insufficient resources to objectively assess their achievement.

EXAMPLE: *Affective Objective.* By the end of the HIV curriculum, all residents will have identified their attitudes and beliefs regarding HIV patients who abuse substances, and discussed with their colleagues and attending physicians how these might influence their management of such patients.

Learner objectives that relate to the *psychomotor* domain of learning are often referred to as "skill" or "behavioral" objectives. These objectives refer to specific psychomotor tasks or actions that may involve hand or body movements, vision, hearing, speech, or the sense of touch. History taking, patient education, interpersonal communication, physical examination, record keeping, and procedural skills fall into this domain. In writing objectives for relevant psychomotor skills, it is helpful to indicate whether learners are expected only to achieve the ability to perform a skill (a "skill" or "competence" objective) or to incorporate the skill into their continuing behavior (a "behavioral" or "performance" objective). Whether a psychomotor skill is written as a skill or behavioral objective has important implications for the choice of evaluation strategies and may influence the choice of educational strategies (see Chapter 5).

> **EXAMPLE:** *Skill or Competence Objective.* By the end of the curriculum, all medical students will have demonstrated proficiency in assessing alcohol use using all four of the CAGE questions with one simulated and one real patient. (This skill or competence objective can be assessed by direct or videotaped observation by an instructor.)

> **EXAMPLE:** *Behavioral or Performance Objective.* All students who have completed the curriculum will routinely (>80% of time) use the CAGE questions to assess their patients' alcohol use. (This performance or behavioral objective might be indirectly assessed by reviewing a random sample of student write-ups of the new patients they work up during their core medical clerkship.)

Another way to envision the learner objectives related to clinical competence is in the hierarchy implied by Miller's assessment pyramid (9). The pyramid implies that clinical competence begins with building a knowledge base (knows) and proceeds to learning a related skill (knows how), demonstrating the skill (shows how), and finally performing in actual clinical practice (does). While the learning objective may be stated as the highest objective of the pyramid, it is important again to recognize that there are enabling objectives necessary to achieve this objective that may require the attention of the curriculum developer. Attainment of a skill objective usually implies attainment of prerequisite knowledge. Attainment of a performance objective implies attainment of prerequisite knowledge, attitudes, and skills. Because some objectives encompass more than one domain, efficiency may be achieved by clearly articulating the highest order objective, without separately articulating the underlying cognitive, affective, and skill objectives. From the evaluation perspective, achievement of a performance objective implies achievement of the prerequisite underlying objectives. However, educational strategies must still address the knowledge, attitudes, and skills that the learner requires to perform well.

> **EXAMPLE:** *Multidomain Objective.* At the completion of a continuing medical education course, "Update in Cardiology," participants will uniformly implement the ACC/AHA clinical practice guidelines for care of adults with ST-elevation myocardial infarction. (This objective implies knowledge of guidelines, valuing the importance of the guideline in improving patient outcomes, and skill in patient care.)

In North American medical education especially, there has been increasing interest in describing learning objectives across the continuum of medical education in terms of *competency-based outcomes*, driven in large part by the ACGME Outcome Project and the adoption of the language of the six core competencies in 1999 (10). As of 2002, all ACGME-accredited graduate medical education programs must relate their objectives to these six competencies, which are felt to best describe the expertise of modern clinical practice. The six competencies, which are detailed on the ACGME Web site, are patient care, medical knowledge, interpersonal and communication skills, practice-based learning and improvement, professionalism, and systems-based care.

EXAMPLE: *Practice-based Learning and Improvement.* A residency program has as one of its learning goals that residents will develop lifelong learning skills and seek out continuous improvement. The program adopts the use of personal learning plans, which encourage residents to systematically collect information on their performances throughout the training program and to develop strategies for improvement (11).

EXAMPLE: *Systems-based Care.* A monthly case-based conference was designed to improve residents' understanding of medical reimbursement and billing, to improve attitudes toward management of hospital resources, and to increase collaboration between health care team members to deliver more efficient and effective care (12).

Knowledge of the various domains of learner objectives is valuable because it helps one to understand the complexity of learning related to any educational goal and to choose objectives and educational strategies wisely.

Process Objectives

Process objectives relate to the implementation of the curriculum. They may indicate the degree of participation that is expected from the learners (see Table 4.3). They may indicate the expected response or satisfaction of learners or faculty to a curriculum. In the *logic model* approach, which creates a visual representation of causal links between program objectives and outcomes, the process objectives may be referred to as "outputs." Outputs in this model are conceptualized as the direct results of a program or curriculum, such as the number of participants receiving the curriculum (13).

EXAMPLE: *Individual Process Objective.* Each resident during the PGY–2 year will participate in a critical incident root cause analysis as part of a multidisciplinary team. (This objective falls under the ACGME competency of systems-based care.)

EXAMPLE: *Program Process Objectives.* By the end of this academic year, 90% of PGY–2 residents will have participated in a critical incident root cause analysis and in a hospital patient safety initiative.

EXAMPLE: *Logic Model.* In a faculty development program for medical educators, the number of faculty participants and number of hours spent on program activities are "outputs" of the program; participants' belief that the program was "transformational" and increased identity as medical educators are participant "outcomes" of the program (14).

Outcome Objectives

In this book we use the term *outcome objectives* to refer to *health, health care, and patient outcomes* (i.e., the impact of the curriculum beyond those delineated in its learner and process objectives). Outcomes might include health outcomes of patients or career choices of physicians. More proximal outcomes might include changes in the behaviors of patients, such as smoking cessation (15). Outcome objectives relate to the health care problem that the curriculum addresses. Unfortunately, the term "outcome objectives" is not consistently used, and learner cognitive, affective, and psychomotor objectives are sometimes referred to as outcomes, e.g., as knowledge, attitudinal, or skill outcomes. A case in point is the "logic model" example above, which refers to an affective "outcome." To avoid confusion, it is best to describe the objective using precise language that includes the specific type of outcome that will be measured.

> **EXAMPLE:** *Career Outcome Objective.* Eighty percent or more of the graduates of our primary care residency programs will be pursuing careers in primary care 5 years after graduation.

> **EXAMPLE:** *Behavioral and Health Outcome Objectives.* Physicians who have completed the two-session continuing education course on basic interviewing skills will demonstrate, during audiotaped doctor-patient encounters 1 to 2 months later, a significantly greater use of taught skills in their practice setting than control group physicians *(learner psychomotor behavioral objective).* Their emotionally disturbed patients, as determined by General Health Questionnaire (GHQ) scores of 5 or more, will show significantly greater improvement in GHQ scores at 2 weeks, 3 months, and 6 months following the audiotaped encounters than patients of control group physicians *(health outcome objective)* (16).

It is often unrealistic to expect medical curricula to have easily measurable effects on quality of care and patient outcomes. (Medical students, for example, may not have responsibility for patients until years after completion of a curriculum.) However, most medical curricula should be designed to have positive effects on quality of care and patient outcomes. Even if outcomes will be difficult or impossible to measure, the inclusion of some health outcome objectives in a curriculum plan will emphasize the ultimate aims of the curriculum and may influence the choice of curricular content and educational methods.

> **EXAMPLE:** *Rationale for Including Health Outcome Objectives.* Including health outcome objectives for patients who present with a common problem may lead to emphasis in a curriculum on the content and clinical decision making skills that are expected to affect those patient outcomes.

At this point, it may be useful to review Table 4.3 for examples of each type and level of objective.

ADDITIONAL CONSIDERATIONS

While educational objectives are an important part of any curriculum, it is important to remember that *most educational experiences encompass much more than a list of preconceived objectives* (17, 18). For example, on clinical rotations much learning derives from unanticipated experiences with individual patients. In many situations, the most useful learning derives from learning needs identified and pursued by individual learners and their mentors. An exhaustive list of objectives in such settings can be overwhelming for learners and teachers alike, stifle creativity, and limit learning related to individual needs and experiences. On the other hand, if no goals or objectives are articulated, learning experiences will be unfocused and important cognitive, affective, or psychomotor objectives may not be achieved.

Goals provide desired overall direction for a curriculum. An important and difficult task in curriculum development is to develop a *manageable number of specific measurable objectives* that:

- interpret the goals;
- focus and prioritize curricular components that are critical to the realization of the goals; and
- encourage (or at least do not limit) creativity, flexibility, and nonspecified learning relevant to the curriculum's goals.

EXAMPLE: *Use of Goals and Objectives to Encourage Learning from Experience.* A broad goal for a residency in general internal medicine might be for learners to become proficient in the cost-effective diagnosis and management of common clinical problems. Once these clinical problems have been identified, patient case mix can be assessed to determine whether or not the settings used for training provide the learners with adequate clinical experience.

Broad goals for clinical rotations in the same residency might be that residents develop as self-directed learners, develop sound clinical reasoning skills, and use evidence-based and patient-centered approaches in the care they provide. Specific measurable process objectives could promote the achievement of these goals without being unnecessarily restrictive. One such objective might be that each resident, during the course of a one-month clinical rotation, present a 15-minute report on a patient management question encountered that month that incorporates principles of clinical epidemiology, evidence-based medicine, clinical decision making, cost-effectiveness, and an assessment of patient or family preferences. A second objective might be that, each week during the rotation, each resident identifies a question relevant to the care of one of their patients and briefly reports during morning rounds the sources used, the search time required, and the answer to their question.

Usually, several cycles of writing objectives are required to achieve a manageable number of specific measurable objectives that truly match the needs of one's targeted learners.

EXAMPLE: *Refining and Prioritizing Objectives.* Faculty developing a curriculum on diabetes for the residency in the above example might begin with the following objectives:

1. By the end of the curriculum, each resident will be able to list each complication of diabetes mellitus.
2. By the end of the curriculum, each resident will be able to list atherosclerotic cardiovascular disease, retinopathy/blindness, nephropathy, neuropathy, and foot problems/amputation as complications of diabetes and be able to list specific medical interventions that prevent each of these complications or their sequelae.
3. By the end of the curriculum, each resident will be able to list all of the medical and sensory findings seen in each of the neuropathies that can occur as a complication of diabetes mellitus. (Similar objectives might have been written for other complications of diabetes.)
4. Residents will know how to use insulin.

After reflection and input from others, objective 1 might be eliminated because remembering every complication of diabetes regardless of prevalence or management implications is felt to be of little value. Objective 3 might be eliminated as being too many in number and containing detail unnecessary for management by the generalist. Objective 4 might be rejected as being too general and could be rewritten in specific measurable terms. Objective 2 might be retained because it is felt that it is sufficiently detailed and relevant to the goal of training residents to be proficient in the cost-effective diagnosis and management of clinical problems commonly encountered in medical practice. In the above process, the curriculum team would have reduced the number of objectives while ensuring that the remaining objectives are sufficiently specific and relevant to direct and focus teaching and evaluation.

CONCLUSION

Writing goals and objectives is a critically important skill in curriculum development. Well-written goals and objectives define and focus a curriculum. They provide direction to curriculum developers in selecting educational strategies and evaluation methods.

QUESTIONS

For the curriculum you are coordinating, planning, or would like to be planning, please answer or think about the following questions:

1. Write one to three broad educational goals.

2. Write one specific measurable educational objective of each type, using the template provided.

Level of Objective

	Individual Learner	Aggregate or Program
Learner (cognitive, affective, or psychomotor)		
Process		
Health, health care, or patient outcome		

Check each objective to make sure that it includes all five elements of a specific measurable objective (<u>Who</u> <u>will do</u> <u>how much</u> <u>of what</u> <u>by when</u>?). Check to see that the words you used are precise and unambiguous (Table 4.1). Have someone else read your objectives and see if they can explain them to you accurately.

3. Do your specific measurable objectives support and further define your broad educational goals? If not, you need to reflect further on your goals and objectives and change one or the other.

4. Reflect on how your objectives, as worded, will focus the content, educational methods, and evaluation strategies of your curriculum. Is this what you want? If not, you may want to rewrite, add, or delete some objectives.

GENERAL REFERENCES

Accreditation Council for Graduate Medical Education. *ACGME Outcome Project*. Available at www.acgme.org/Outcome/. Accessed March 7, 2009.
This site contains a wealth of information regarding definitions, tools for implementation and assessment, and annotated bibliographies for each of the six core competencies.

Anderson LW, Krathwhol DR, eds. *A Taxonomy for Learning, Teaching and Assessing: A Revision of Bloom's Taxonomy of Educational Objectives.* New York: Longman; 2001.
A revision of Bloom's taxonomy of cognitive objectives that presents a two-dimensional framework for cognitive learning objectives. Written by cognitive psychologists and educators, with many useful examples to illustrate the function of the taxonomy. 302 pages.

Bloom BS. *Taxonomy of Educational Objectives: A Classification of Educational Objectives. Handbook 1: Cognitive Domain.* New York: Longman; 1984.
Classic text that presents a detailed classification of cognitive educational objectives. A condensed version of the taxonomy is included in an appendix for quick reference. 207 pages.

Green L, Kreuter M, Deeds S, Partridge K. *Health Education Planning: A Diagnostic Approach*. Palo Alto, Calif.: Mayfield Publishing; 1980.
Basic text of health education program planning that includes the role of objectives in program planning. 306 pages.

Gronlund NE. *Writing Instructional Objectives for Teaching and Assessment,* 7th ed. Upper Saddle River, N.J.: Pearson/Merrill/Prentice Hall; 2004.
Comprehensive and well-written reference that encompasses the cognitive, affective, and psychomotor domains of educational objectives. It provides a useful updating of Bloom's and Krathwohl's texts with many examples and tables. 136 pages.

Krathwohl DR, Bloom BS, Masia BB. *Taxonomy of Educational Objectives: Affective Domain*. New York: Longman; 1964.
Classic text that presents a detailed classification of affective educational objectives. A condensed version of the taxonomy is included in an appendix for quick reference. 196 pages.

Mager RF. *Preparing Instructional Objectives: A Critical Tool in the Development of Effective Instruction,* 3rd ed. Atlanta: CEP Press; 1997.
Readable, practical guidebook for writing objectives. Includes examples. Popular reference for professional educators, as well as health professionals who develop learning programs for their students. 185 pages.

Marzano RJ, Kendall JS. *The New Taxonomy of Educational Objectives*, 2nd ed. Thousand Oaks, Calif.: Corwin Press; 2007.
Yet another revision of Bloom's taxonomy. Based on three domains of knowledge: information, mental procedures, and psychomotor procedures. Well-written and thoughtful, this work argues for well-researched models of knowledge and learning. 167 pages.

SPECIFIC REFERENCES

1. Green L, Kreuter M, Deeds S, Partridge K. *Health Education Planning: A Diagnostic Approach*. Palo Alto, Calif.: Mayfield Publishing; 1980. Pp. 48, 50, 64–65.
2. Bloom BS. *Taxonomy of Educational Objectives: Cognitive Domain*. New York: Longman; 1984.
3. Anderson LW, Krathwohl DR, eds. *A Taxonomy for Learning, Teaching, and Assessing: A*

Revision of Bloom's Taxonomy of Educational Objectives. New York: Addison Wesley Longman; 2001.

4. Marzano RJ, Kendall JS. *The New Taxonomy of Educational Objectives,* 2nd ed. Thousand Oaks, Calif.: Corwin Press; 2007.

5. Henerson ME, Morris LL, Fitz-Gibbon CT. How to measure attitudes (Book 6). In: Herman JL, ed. *Program Evaluation Kit.* Newbury Park, Calif.: Sage Publications; 1987. Pp. 9–13.

6. Mager RF. *Preparing Instructional Objectives: A Critical Tool in the Development of Effective Instruction,* 3rd. ed. Atlanta: CEP Press; 1997. Pp. 151–54.

7. Hafferty FW. Beyond curriculum reform: confronting medicine's hidden curriculum. *Acad Med.* 1998;73:403–7.

8. Hundert EM, Hafferty FW, Christakis D. Characteristics of the informal curriculum and trainees' ethical choices. *Acad Med.* 1996;71:624–33.

9. Miller G. The assessment of clinical skills/competence/performance. *Acad Med.* 1990;65(Suppl):S63–67.

10. Accreditation Council for Graduate Medical Education. *ACGME Outcome Project.* Available at www.acgme.org/Outcome/. Accessed March 7, 2009.

11. Challis M. AMEE Medical Education Guide No. 19: Personal learning plans. *Med Teach.* 2000;22:225–36.

12. Kravet SJ, Wright SM, Carrese JA. Teaching resource and information management using an innovative case-based conference. *J Gen Intern Med.* 2001;16:399–403.

13. W.K. Kellogg Foundation. *Using Logic Models to Bring Together Planning, Evaluation and Action: Logic Model Development Guide.* Battle Creek, Mich.: W.K. Kellogg Foundation; 2004.

14. Armstrong EG, Barsion SJ. Using an outcomes-logic-model approach to evaluate a faculty development program for medical educators. *Acad Med.* 2006;81:483–88.

15. Cornuz J, Humair JP, Seematter L, et al. Efficacy of resident training in smoking cessation: a randomized control trial of a program based on application of behavioral theory and practice with standardized patients. *Ann Intern Med.* 2002;136:429–37.

16. Roter DL, Hall JA, Kern DE, Barker LR, Cole KA, Roca RP. Improving physicians' interviewing skills and reducing patients' emotional distress: a randomized clinical trial. *Arch Intern Med.* 1995;155:1877–84.

17. Ende J, Atkins E. Conceptualizing curriculum for graduate medical education. *Acad Med.* 1992;67:528–34.

18. Ende J, Davidoff F. What is curriculum? *Ann Intern Med.* 1992;116:1055–57.

Step 4
Educational Strategies

. . . accomplishing educational objectives

Patricia A. Thomas, M.D.

Education is not the filling of a pail, but the lighting of a fire.
—William Butler Yeats

True teaching is not an accumulation of knowledge; it is an awakening
of consciousness which goes through successive stages.
—from a temple wall inside an Egyptian pyramid

Education is what survives when what has been learned
has been forgotten.
—B. F. Skinner

DEFINITIONS

Once the goals and specific measurable objectives for a curriculum have been determined, the next step is to *develop the educational strategies* by which the curricular objectives will be achieved. Educational strategies involve both content and methods. *Content* refers to the specific material to be included in the curriculum. *Methods* are the ways in which the content is presented.

IMPORTANCE

Educational strategies provide the means by which a curriculum's objectives are achieved. They are the heart of the curriculum, the educational intervention itself. There is a natural tendency to think of the curriculum in terms of this step alone. As we shall see, the groundwork of Steps 1 through 3 guides the selection of educational strategies.

LEARNING THEORY

As the curriculum developers think through the educational strategies that will be employed, they should be aware of some of the principles and issues related to learning, and to learning by adults in particular. (See Brookfield et al. in General References.) *Teaching* is what educators do, but *learning* is what happens within the learner. The job of curriculum developers, therefore, is largely to *facilitate* learning in curriculum participants. Adult learners tend to be goal-oriented and motivated to learn what is necessary to accomplish a desired task or solve a relevant problem. They are more likely than children to take responsibility for, direct, and evaluate their own learning (*self-directed learning*), especially if they have the requisite skills and resources. They bring a wealth of different *experiences and cultures* to the learning situation that shape their interpretation of reality and their approach to learning, and that should be recognized and used to facilitate learning. *Reflection* on previous experiences, or new experiences built into a curriculum, is a key component of *experiential learning*. *Transformative learning* occurs when the learners change in meaningful ways. It usually involves experiences that promote the questioning of assumptions, beliefs, and values, as well as the consideration of multiple points of view. Such change tends to be resisted. It is promoted by skillful facilitation and a safe and supportive *learning environment*. The quotations at the beginning of the chapter remind us that a goal of combining educational objectives with congruent and resourceful educational strategies should be to stimulate learning that is meaningful, profound, and enduring.

DETERMINATION OF CONTENT

The content of the curriculum flows from its learning objectives. Listing the nouns used in these objectives (see Chapter 4) should outline the content of the curriculum. The amount of material presented to the learners should not be too little to lack substance, too much to overwhelm, or more detailed than is necessary to achieve the desired objectives and outcomes. For some curricula, it is helpful to group or sequence objectives and their associated content in a manner that is logical and promotes under-standing. It is usually helpful to construct a *syllabus* for the curriculum that includes 1) an explicit statement of learning objectives and methods to help focus learners; 2) a schedule of the curriculum events and other practical information, such as locations and directions; 3) written curricular materials (e.g., readings, cases, questions); and 4) suggestions/resources for additional learning. The use of learning management soft-ware has allowed course directors to easily provide and update these resources using Web-based software. When using software to deliver online content, however, it is important to attend to the issues of interface design and "cognitive load" (1). Developers should partner with an expert in multimedia instructional design to plan for efficient use of electronic resources.

CHOICE OF EDUCATIONAL METHODS

General Guidelines (Table 5.1)

It is helpful to keep the following general principles in mind when considering edu-cational methods for a curriculum:

- *Maintain Congruence between Objectives and Methods:* Choose educational meth-ods that are most likely to achieve a curriculum's goals and objectives. One way to approach the selection of educational methods is to group the specific measurable objectives of the curriculum as cognitive, affective, or psychomotor objectives (see Chapter 4) and select educational methods most likely to be effective for the type of objective (see Table 5.2).

  EXAMPLE: *Cognitive Objective.* If an objective is to improve learners' higher cognitive skills, such as clinical decision making, then facilitated case discussions that require learners to apply concepts are likely to be more effective than having a faculty member analyze the case for the learners.

  EXAMPLE: *Affective Objective.* If an objective is attitudinal change, then selected real-life experiences, combined with group discussion and reflection on the experiences, are more likely to achieve this goal than lectures or didactic pronouncements.

  EXAMPLE: *Psychomotor Objective.* If an objective of a curriculum is to improve residents' ability to perform a procedure correctly (i.e., a skill or competence objective), such as obtain-ing a Pap smear, supervised practice with feedback and discussion of technique is likely to be more effective than lectures about technique. If an additional objective is that, following the above instruction, residents will obtain adequate Pap smears when indicated in their outpatient practice (i.e., a behavioral or performance objective), congruent educational strat-egies would be to have appropriate equipment and support for pelvic and Pap exams read-ily available in the practice and to provide feedback on the adequacy of the Pap smears obtained (2).

Table 5.1.   Guidelines for Choosing Educational Methods

- Maintain congruence between objectives and educational methods
- Use multiple educational methods
- Choose educational methods that are feasible in terms of resources

Table 5.2.   Matching Educational Methods to Objectives

Educational Method	Type of Objective				
	Cognitive: Knowledge	Cognitive: Problem Solving	Affective: Attitudinal	Psychomotor: Skills or Competence	Psychomotor: Behavioral or Performance
Readings	+++	+	+	+	
Lectures	+++	+	+	+	
Programmed learning	+++	++		+	
Discussion	++	++	+++	+	+
Reflection on experience			+++	+++	+++
Feedback on performance	+	++	++	+++	+++
Small group learning	++	++	++	+	+
Problem-based learning	++	+++	+		+
Team-based learning	+++	+++	++	+	+
Learning projects	+++	+++	+	+	+
Role models		+	++	+	++
Demonstration	+	+	+	++	++
Role-plays	+	+	++	+++	+
Artificial models and simulation	+	++	++	+++	+
Standardized patients	+	++	++	+++	+
Real-life experiences	+	++	++	+++	+++
Audio or video review of learner	+			+++	+
Behavioral/ environmental interventions*			+	+	+++

Note: blank = not recommended; + = appropriate in some cases, usually as an adjunct to other methods; ++ = good match; +++ = excellent match (consensus ratings by author and editors).
*Removal of barriers to performance; provision of resources that promote performance; reinforcements that promote performance.

• *Use Multiple Educational Methods:* Individuals have different preferences for learning, sometimes referred to as *learning styles* (3). A study of engineering students led to one model of differential learning styles, which has been subsequently validated with other higher education students (4). The model uses four dimensions of learning preferences: 1) sensing (concrete) or intuitive (abstract), 2) visual (seeing) or verbal (hearing), 3) active or reflective, and 4) sequential (left brain) or global (right brain). A 44 item *Index of Learning Styles* (ILS) questionnaire, which provides individuals and groups with information on their preferred learning styles, is available on the Web (5). Choosing an educational method that meets the learner's preference for learning is essential to developing a learner-centered curriculum (see below) and avoids a mismatch between the educational method and the learner, which would impair successful learning. Ideally, the curriculum would use those methods that work best for individual learners. However, few curricula can be that malleable; often a large number of learners need to be accommodated in a short period of time. The use of different educational methods helps to overcome the problem of different learning styles.

   The use of different educational methods also helps to maintain *learner interest* and provides opportunities for *reinforcement of learning*. Such reinforcement can deepen learning, promote retention, and enhance the application of what has been learned. It is particularly relevant for curricula extending over longer time periods.

   Finally, for *curricula attempting to achieve higher order or complex objectives that span several domains* (see Chapter 4), the use of multiple educational methods is necessary to achieve congruence between objectives and methods.

   EXAMPLE: *Higher Order Objective Requiring Multiple Educational Methods.* A gynecology curriculum for internal medicine residents has as one objective that PGY–3 residents will appropriately perform 80% of indicated screening Pap smears themselves on their continuity clinic patients (behavioral or performance objective that requires prerequisite knowledge, attitude, and skill training). The curriculum includes knowledge-based *lectures* discussing cervical cancer risk, the importance of Pap smears, and compliance with screening by primary care physicians. Residents receive supervised training in the technique of Pap smears with live models in a PGY–1 workshop and with real patients during a PGY–2 ambulatory gynecology rotation (*experiential learning*). Their attitudes regarding the role of primary care physicians in screening for cervical cancer are discussed at the beginning and end of the curriculum (*discussion*). Yearly *audit* results are given to individual residents on their performance of Pap smears on their continuity practice patients.

• *Choose Educational Methods That Are Feasible in Terms of Resources:* Resource constraints may limit the implementation of the ideal approach in this step, as well as in other steps. Curriculum developers will need to consider faculty time, space, availability of clinical material and experiences, and costs, as well as the availability of learner time. Faculty development may be an additional consideration, especially if an innovative instructional method is chosen, such as role-play or the use of multimedia. Use of technology may involve initial cost but save faculty resources over the time course of the curriculum. When resource limitations threaten the achievement of curricular outcomes, objectives and/or educational strategies (content and methods) will need to be further prioritized and selectively limited. The question then becomes, what is the most that can be accomplished, given the resource limitation?

When one selects education methods for a curriculum, it is helpful to consider the advantages and disadvantages of each method under consideration. Advantages and disadvantages of commonly used educational methods are summarized for the reader in Table 5.3. Specific methods are discussed below, in relation to their function.

Methods for Achieving Cognitive Objectives

Methods that are commonly used to achieve cognitive objectives include the following:

- Readings
- Lecture
- Audiovisual materials
- Programmed learning
- Discussion
- Problem-based learning

The use of targeted *readings* can be an efficient method of presenting information and addressing cognitive objectives. The completion of readings, however, depends on the presence of sufficient opportunity for the learner to read and on the motivation of individual learners. Before they are assigned, existing publications should be assessed to ensure that they efficiently target a curriculum's objectives. Learners can be directed to use readings more effectively if they are given explicit objectives and content for individual readings. A written syllabus can target specific educational objectives but requires faculty resources to construct it. Readings are also commonly used to supplement other educational methods.

> **EXAMPLE:** *Syllabus Materials.* To teach medical students how to critically appraise the literature, a curriculum was designed that introduced problem-based educational materials into the weekly clerkship tutorial, including 1) a set of objectives and guidelines for how to use the package, 2) a patient scenario presenting a clinical dilemma, 3) a relevant journal article, and 4) an essay defining and discussing quality standards that should be met by the article. A worksheet was provided for each journal article (6).

> **EXAMPLE:** *Specifically Prepared Readings with Questions and Patient Case Scenarios.* The American College of Physicians' Medical Knowledge Self-Assessment Program consists of annotated syllabi in different Internal Medicine subspecialties, self-assessment questions, and patient case scenarios. Participants can review the information, self-test at their own pace, and receive feedback on their performance at regular intervals. Regional courses are offered to supplement the program. References are provided for further reading.

Perhaps the most universally applied method for addressing cognitive objectives is the *lecture*, which has as its advantages structure, low technology, and the ability to teach many learners in a short period of time. Successful lecturers develop skills that promote the learners' interest and acquisition of knowledge, such as control of the physical environment, assessing and engaging their audience, organizing their material, making transitional and summary statements, presenting examples, using emphasis and selected repetition, effectively using audiovisual aids, and facilitating an effective question-and-answer period (7–10). Medical lectures are often topic-based, with the learners serving as passive recipients of information. The inclusion of problem-solving exercises or case discussions can engage the learners in a more active process that

Table 5.3.   Summary of Advantages and Limitations of Different Educational Methods

Educational Method	Advantages	Disadvantages
Readings	Low cost Cover fund of knowledge Little preparation time	Passive learning Learners must be motivated to complete
Lectures	Low cost Accommodate large numbers of learners Structured presentation of complicated topics	Passive learning Teacher-centered Quality depends on speaker/audiovisual material
Programmed learning	Active learning Do not need clinical material at hand Safe simulations for learners Immediate feedback on knowledge, sequencing, efficiency, clinical decision making Learner applies new knowledge	Developmental costs if not commercially available
Discussion	Active learning Permits assessment of learner needs Allows learner to apply newly acquired knowledge Suitable for higher order cognitive objectives: problem solving and clinical decision making; can address affective objectives Exposes students to different perspectives	More faculty intensive than readings or lectures Cognitive/experience base required of learners Group dependent Usually facilitator dependent
Reflection on experience	Promotes learning from experience Promotes self-awareness/mindfulness Can be built into discussion/group learning activities Can be done individually through assigned writings/portfolios	Requires protected time Usually requires scheduled interaction time with another/others. Often facilitator dependent
Feedback on performance	Promotes learning from experience Can be used with role-play, artificial models/simulation, standardized patients, clinical experience, and audio/video review	Requires observer who is a skilled provider of feedback

Table 5.3.   *(continued)*

Educational Method	Advantages	Disadvantages
Small group learning	Active learning Resources usually available Allows multidisciplinary approaches Suitable for team-based and problem-based learning, clinical decision making, community-based projects Encourages cooperation, teamwork among learners Incorporates discussion	Group should have some training in group process skills, conflict management, etc. May require faculty facilitators with training in above Time required for successful functioning
Problem-based learning (PBL)	Active learning Facilitates higher cognitive objectives: problem solving and clinical decision making; can incorporate objectives that cross domains: ethics, humanism, cost-efficiency	Developmental costs Requires faculty facilitators and small groups Less efficient for transferring factual information
Team-based learning (TBL)	Active learning Facilitates higher cognitive objectives; constructive knowledge Students take responsibility for learning Collaborative Uses less faculty than PBL/ other small group learning methods	Developmental costs for Readiness Assurance Test (RATs) and application exercises Students need to be self-directed Requires orientation of students to process of teamwork and peer evaluation
Learning projects	Active learning Promote, teach self-directed learning Learners sets individual learning objectives Suitable for higher order cognitive objectives	Learners need motivation Learners need basic skills to access and optimally use learning resources Requires effective faculty mentor
Role models	Faculty often available Impact often seems profound	Require valid evaluation process to identify effective role models Specific interventions usually unclear Impact depends on interaction between specific faculty member and learner Outcomes multifactorial and difficult to assess

Table 5.3.   *(continued)*

Educational Method	Advantages	Disadvantages
Demonstration	Efficient method for demonstrating skills/ procedures	Passive learning Teacher-centered Quality depends on teacher/ audiovisual material
Role-plays	Suitable for objectives that cross domains: knowledge, attitudes, and skill Efficient Low cost Can be structured to be learner- centered Safe environment for skills practice	Require trained faculty facilitators Learners need some basic knowledge or skills Can be resource intensive if large numbers of learners
Artificial models and simulation	Safe environments to practice skills Learners can use at own pace; less faculty supervision required	May not be available for specific curriculum Can be expensive
Standardized patients	Ensure appropriate clinical material Approximate "real life" more closely than role-plays Safe environment for skills practice Can give feedback to learners on performance Can be reused for ongoing curricula	Cost Expertise required to develop and train standardized patients
Clinical experience	"Real life" Promotes learner motivation and responsibility Promotes higher level cognitive, attitudinal, skill, and performance learning	Requires clinical material when learner is ready Requires faculty to supervise and to provide feedback Learner needs basic knowledge or skill Needs to be monitored for case mix, appropriateness Requires reflection, follow-up
Audio or video reviews of learner	Provides accurate feedback on performance Provides opportunity for self- observation	Requires trained faculty/facilitators Recording can be awkward or intrusive and can pose logistic problems Requires patient permission
Behavioral/ environmental interventions*	Influence performance	Assume competence Require control over learners' real- life environment

*Removal of barriers to performance; provision of resources that promote performance; reinforcements that promote performance.

helps them to recognize what they may not know (i.e., set learning objectives) and to apply new knowledge as it is learned.

> **EXAMPLE:** *Lecture Combined with Cases and Testing.* Endocrinology lectures in a year 1 physiology course begin with a brief overview of one to three simplified cases, followed by the didactic lecture. At the end of the lecture, the cases are reviewed in detail and the whole class is invited to respond to a series of questions (11).

The use of audience response systems has also increased the interactivity of the lecture, allowing faculty to pose questions and solicit commitments (answers) from the learners.

Audiovisual materials are frequently used within the context of lectures, but they can also be used in other contexts to reinforce content presented as readings or lecture. Clinic wall charts, wallet-sized flash cards, or computer reminders can reinforce items discussed previously in greater depth, such as preventive practice guidelines. *Videotapes and video files* can be used to present a lecture when a lecturer is unavailable or to provide online resource for review by learners at an unscheduled time. Video can also be used to demonstrate techniques such as taking a sexual history, performing a pelvic exam, or doing a surgical procedure. Some schools have included video files of lectures in software that increases interaction when viewed online, with the addition of questions to check for understanding, supplements of notes, and opportunities to query the lecturer.

Programmed learning refers to the use of programmed textbooks or software that present material in organized sequential fashion, such as the self-assessment exercises developed by the National Board of Medical Examiners (NBME®). Learners using these systems can proceed at their own pace, identify their own knowledge deficiencies, and set their own objectives, as well as receive immediate feedback, not only on their knowledge base but also on efficiency and cost-effectiveness. There are a number of initiatives to develop programmed learning available through computer technology. If not previously developed, the start-up costs for an individual curriculum may be high.

> **EXAMPLE:** *Internet-based Curriculum, Programmed Learning.* An ambulatory curriculum for internal medicine residents was developed and delivered with Web-based software. The curriculum covered 16 topics with a programmed pretest-didactics-posttest. The didactics included immediate feedback to answers and links to abstracts or full text articles. Comparison of pre- and posttests of knowledge showed improved knowledge of curricular content (12).

Discussion moves the learner from a passive to an active role that facilitates the acquisition of new knowledge. Much of the learning that occurs in a discussion format depends on the skills of the instructor to create a supportive learning climate, to assess learners' needs, and to effectively use a variety of interventions such as maintaining focus, questioning, generalizing, and summarizing for the learner (13). *Group discussion* of cases as in attending rounds or morning report is a popular method that allows learners to process new knowledge with faculty and peers and to identify specific knowledge deficiencies. Group discussions are most successful when facilitated by teachers trained in the techniques of small group teaching (13–16) and when participants have some background knowledge or experience. Preparatory readings can help. The *combination of lecture and small group discussion* can be extremely effective in imparting knowledge, as well as in practicing the higher order cognitive skills of assessment and integration of medical facts. *Individual instruction, or one-on-one teaching,* has the ability to be the most learner-centered technique, as well as to require active participation on the part of the learner. However, it is faculty intensive and does not provide an opportunity for peer interaction.

Problem-Based Learning (PBL) is a particular use of small groups that was designed to promote vital learning principles of being constructive (in the cognitive psychology sense), collaborative, self-directed, and contextual (17). In PBL, learner groups are presented with a case and set their own learning objectives, often dividing the work and teaching each other, guided by a tutor-facilitator. In a case of renal failure in a child, for instance, the learning objectives may include genitourinary anatomy, renal physiology, calcium metabolism in renal failure, and genetic disorders of renal function. Students bring new knowledge back to the PBL group and the group problem-solves the case together. PBL is highly dependent on the tutor-facilitators and requires intensive faculty and case development. After 30 years of use in medical education, the efficacy of PBL compared with conventional approaches in achieving cognitive objectives is still debated, although learners report higher levels of satisfaction with this method (18, 19).

Team-Based Learning (TBL) is a relatively new application of small groups that requires fewer faculty than PBL (20, 21). It combines reading, testing, discussion, and collaboration to achieve both knowledge and higher order cognitive learning objectives.

EXAMPLE: *Team-Based Learning.* The process of TBL is as follows:

Phase I:
1. Students are assigned readings or self-directed learning before class.

Phase II:
2. On arrival to class, students take a brief knowledge test, the *Readiness Assurance Test* (RAT), and are individually scored.
3. Students work in teams of six to seven to retake the RAT and turn in consensus answers for immediate scoring and feedback (Group or GRAT).

Phase III (may last several class periods):
4. Groups work on problem-solving or application exercises that require use of knowledge objectives.
5. Groups eventually share responses to exercise with entire class, and discussion is facilitated by instructor.

Methods for Achieving Affective Objectives

Methods that are commonly used to achieve affective objectives include the following:

-   Exposure (readings, discussions, experiences)
-   Facilitation of openness, introspection, and reflection
-   Role models

Attitudes can be difficult to measure, let alone change (22). Some undesirable attitudes are based on insufficient knowledge and will change as knowledge is expanded in a particular area. Others, such as "this is not my responsibility," may be based in insufficient skill or lack of confidence. Attitudinal change requires exposure to knowledge, experiences, or the views of respected others that contradict undesired and confirm desired attitudes (23). Targeted readings may be helpful adjuncts to other methods for developing desirable attitudes. Probably more than any other learning objective, attitudinal change is helped by the use of *facilitation techniques with individuals and with groups that promote openness, introspection, and reflection* (24–26). These facilitation methods can be incorporated into skill-building methods, such as role-plays or simulated patient exercises, where the learner may be encouraged by the group process to explore barriers to performance. Properly facilitated small group discussions can also promote changes in attitudes, by bringing into awareness the interests, attitudes, values, and feelings of learners and making them available for discussion. Finally, *role-model* health professionals can help change attitudes by demonstrating successful approaches to a particular problem. Interestingly, the professional attitudes that educators often aim to instill in students, such as competency, excellence, sensitivity, enthusiasm, and genuineness, are those attributes most valued by students in their teachers (27, 28).

> **EXAMPLE:** *Attitude toward Role, Role Modeling Combined with Reflection and Discussion.* A geriatrics curriculum has as an objective that primary care residents will believe that it is their role to document advance directive wishes of their elderly outpatients. A needs assessment instrument discovered that most residents believed that their patients did not want these discussions or had no biases about advance directives. A videotape interview of a respected geriatrician with several of his patients was used to model the technique of the advance directive interview, as well as the reaction of patients to the discussion. The videotape was used as a trigger tape in small group discussions of residents to discuss patient reactions to advance directives.

> **EXAMPLE:** *Attitude toward Socioeconomic Class, Experience Combined with Reflection and Discussion.* Medical students and nursing students participated in a one-day *Poverty Simulation* (29). During the simulation, the students were divided into families with specific roles. The goal was to ensure that the family had shelter and services for a month. Volunteers served as grocery store clerks, immigration officials, and other community roles. By the end of the day, some families were successful, and others were homeless. Students debriefed the exercise and the impact of making difficult decisions such as deciding between food and medicine, or between work and staying home with a sick child.

> **EXAMPLE:** *Awareness and Management of Negative Feelings, Trigger Tape Combined with Reflection and Discussion, Role-modeling Success.* In a substance abuse and HIV curriculum, residents watch a trigger tape of a difficult interaction between a substance-abusing HIV-infected patient and a physician. They identify and discuss the emotions and attitudes evoked by the tape and reflect on how these might influence their management of such patients. Subsequently, residents work with a highly respected role-model physician in a practice that successfully manages such patients.

Methods for Achieving Psychomotor Objectives

Skill or Competency Objectives   Methods commonly used to achieve skill or competency objectives include the following:

- Supervised clinical experience
- Simulations
  Artificial models
  Role-plays

Standardized patients
- Audio or visual review of skills

Rarely is knowledge the sole prerequisite to a learner's achievement of competence in a health-related area. In medicine, learners need to develop a variety of skills, including basic auditory and visual skills of the physical examination, manual skills for procedures and techniques, and communication skills in the medical interview. The learning of skills can be facilitated when learners 1) are *introduced* to the skills by didactic presentations, demonstration, and discussion; 2) are given the opportunity to *practice* the skill; 3) are given the opportunity to *reflect* on their performance; 4) receive *feedback* on their performance; and then 5) *repeat the cycle* of discussion, practice, reflection, and feedback until mastery is achieved.

The development of experiential learning methods can be a creative process for curriculum developers, one that provides an opportunity for innovation in medical education. Experiential learning can be challenging for the learner and teacher alike. Experiential learning requires learners to expose their strengths and weaknesses to themselves and others. Interpersonal skills, feelings, biases, psychological defenses, and previous experiences may affect performance and need to be discussed. Creation of a *safe and supportive learning environment* is, therefore, helpful. Methods include the development of faculty-learner rapport, disclosure by faculty of their own experiences and difficulties with the material, explicit recognition and reinforcement of the learner's strengths, and provision of feedback about deficiencies in a factual, nonjudgmental, helpful, and positive manner.

The classic experiential method of medical training is the *"see one–do one–teach one"* approach, which occurs daily in clinical settings. Inherent in the success of this method is modeling of the ideal behavior or skill by an experienced clinician, the availability of clinical opportunities for the learner to practice the skill under observation, time to reflect and receive feedback on performance (30), and, last, the opportunity to teach the skill to another generation of learners. Effective clinical teachers can facilitate this type of experience (see General References).

EXAMPLE: *Supervised Clinical Experience.* To train internal medicine residents in adequate performance of the pelvic examination, faculty for an ambulatory gynecology curriculum created a checklist of tasks and behaviors to be executed during the examination, including attention to patient comfort, correct order of examination, and proper technique for the Pap smear. Residents attended a family planning clinic, observed the demonstration of pelvic examination technique by a faculty member, and performed pelvic exams observed by faculty, after which they received oral feedback on their performance and written feedback through the checklist instrument. These residents are likely, in the future, to demonstrate the procedure to another group of medical students or interns and supervise them in their performance of pelvic examinations.

A number of difficulties have been noted with this approach to skills training, however, especially in an era of patient safety and patient-centeredness. The shortened length of stay in inpatient settings and the reduced work hours for resident and student trainees have decreased the opportunities to acquire sufficient practice in real-life settings to achieve competence. When expert clinicians are not readily available for demonstration or the appropriate clinical situations are not available for practice, supplementary methods should be considered. *Videos* can be used to demonstrate a skill before the learner practices in another situation. *Simulations* of clinical situations provide the opportunity for learners to practice skills in a "safe" learning environment in which risks can be taken and mistakes made without harm (31). Simulation has been defined as "a person, device, or set of conditions which attempts to present evaluation problems authentically. The student . . . is required to respond to the problems as he or she would under natural circumstances" (32). Simulations include the use of standardized patients, artificial models, manikins with computer technology to reproduce physiology (anesthesia simulators), and virtual reality high-fidelity simulators (laprascopic surgery simulators).

> **EXAMPLES:** *Cardiac Patient Simulator.* Medical students enrolled in a cardiology elective were randomized to a two-week multimedia educational intervention including the "Harvey" patient simulator plus 2 weeks of ward work versus 4 weeks of ward work. In posttest analysis, intervention students acquired nearly twice the core bedside cardiology skills in half the time as the control group (33).

Role-playing, during which the learner plays one role (e.g., physician) and another learner or faculty member plays another role (e.g., patient), provides the opportunity for learners to experience different roles (34, 35). It is most useful for teaching interviewing skills, physical examination techniques, and the recognition of normal physical examination findings. It permits the learner to try, observe, and discuss alternative techniques until a satisfactory performance has been achieved. It is efficient, inexpensive, portable, and able to be used spontaneously in any setting. It may be as effective as the use of simulated patients (36). Role-plays can be constructed on the spot to address individual learner needs as they are identified. Limitations include variable degrees of artificiality and learner and faculty discomfort with the technique. Students are often initially uncomfortable with this method. Facilitators can alleviate this discomfort by discussing it at the outset, by establishing ground rules for the role-play, and by attending to the creation of a safe and supportive learning environment (see above).

> **EXAMPLE:** *Role-play, Video Review.* A group of medical school faculty sought additional training in the skills of the medical interview, as part of a faculty development program. Participants were videotaped in a role-play of giving bad news to a patient. The participants reflected on their performance, received feedback from the other participants in the role-play and from the group at large, and defined areas for continued improvement.

> **EXAMPLE:** *Ground Rules for Role-play.* The following ground rules are used for setting up and debriefing role-plays:
>
> Preparation:
> - Choose a situation that is relevant and readily conceptualized by the learners.
> - Describe the situation and critical issues for each role-player.
> - Choose/assign roles and give learners time to assimilate and add details.
> - Identify observers and clarify their functions.
> - Establish expectations for time-outs by the learner and interruptions by others (e.g., time limits).
>
> Execution:
> - Ensure compliance with agreed-upon ground rules.
> - Ensure that learners emerge comfortably from their roles.
>
> Debriefing:
> - First give the principal learner the opportunity to self-assess what they did well, what they would want to do differently, and what they would like help with.

- Assess the feelings and experiences of other participants in the role-play.
- Elicit feedback from all observers on what seemed to go well.
- Elicit suggestions regarding alternative approaches that might have been more effective.

Replay:
- Give the principal learner the opportunity to repeat the role-play using alternative approaches.

Standardized (simulated) patients are actors or real patients trained to play the roles of patients with specific problems. As with role-play, the use of standardized patients ensures that important content areas will be covered and allows learners to try new techniques, make mistakes, and repeat their performance until a skill is achieved. In addition to basic communication and physical diagnosis skills, professionalism and ethics teaching cases have been developed using standardized patients (37). Standardized patients can be trained to provide feedback and instruction, even in the absence of a faculty member. The method has proven efficacy, both for teaching and for evaluating learners (36, 38). The major limitation is the need to recruit, train, schedule, and pay standardized patients (39). Following the introduction of USMLE Step 2 Clinical Skills in 2004–5, most medical schools in the United States now have active standardized patient programs or access to partner institutions with standardized patient programs (40).

Review of recorded (audio or video) performances of role-play, standardized patient, or real patient encounters can serve as helpful adjuncts to experiential learning (41–43). The tapes can provide information on learner and patient behaviors, which may not have been noticed or remembered by the participants. They provide learners with the rare opportunity to observe their own performance from outside of themselves. Properly facilitated audio or video reviews promote helpful reflection on and discussion of a learner's performance.

> **EXAMPLE:** *Review of Observed Performance.* An interdisciplinary team runs a mock code using a human simulator that is videotaped in the simulation center. After receiving performance evaluation on the appropriateness and timeliness of interventions during the code, the group reviews the videotape and is guided in facilitated reflection. The group concludes that the major errors occurred in failed communications between team members.

Behavioral or Performance Objectives.   Methods commonly used to achieve behavioral or performance objectives include the following:

- Removal of barriers to performance
- Provision of resources that facilitate performance
- Provision of reinforcements for performance

Changing learners' behaviors can be one of the more challenging aspects of a curriculum. There is no guarantee that helping learners develop new skills and even improved attitudes will result in the desired performance when learners are in actual clinical situations. Skill training is necessary but not sufficient to ensure performance in real settings. To promote desired performance, curriculum developers may need to address *barriers to performance* in the learners' environment, provide *resources that promote performance*, and design *reinforcements* that will encourage the continued use of the newly acquired skills. Attention to the learner's subsequent environment can reduce or eliminate the decay of performance that often occurs after an educational intervention.

> **EXAMPLE:** *Systems Improvements and Feedback of Audit Results.* A curriculum in assessing fall risk was introduced to geriatric fellows after a chart audit indicated neglect in this area in their geriatric outpatient practice. In addition to lecture discussion, the curriculum developers placed fall-risk questions on the previsit questionnaire completed by patients and added a trigger question on the problem list face sheets of patients' charts. The assessment of fall risk was included in the annual chart audit, and results were given to each fellow.

> **EXAMPLE:** *Self-audit, Patient and Systems Surveys, Expert Consultation, and Systems Improvement.* Fourteen practicing internists completed a practice improvement project that included a self-audit of medical records for diabetes practice indicators, a practice system survey, and a patient survey. Following data analysis, a consultant advised quality improvement methods and tools for the practice. In follow-up, the participating physicians felt that the audit significantly improved their practice behaviors (44).

Methods for Promoting Learner-Centeredness

Methods for promoting learner-centeredness include the following:

- Formal or informal assessment of learner needs
- Tailoring of educational content and methods to meet learners' needs

A curriculum is learner-centered to the extent that it is tailored to meet the specific needs of its individual learners and its targeted group of learners. This could mean 1) adapting methods to specific learning styles or preferences; 2) addressing specific learner needs in the cognitive, affective, or psychomotor areas related to established curricular objectives; 3) allowing flexibility in both the timing of the method and the time required to achieve objectives; or 4) accommodating specific learner objectives not included in the curriculum.

The *needs assessment of targeted learners* discussed previously is the first step in tailoring a curriculum to a specific group of learners. *Formal evaluations of individual learners*, such as pretests, and *informal observations of individual learners*, which can occur during small group and one-on-one teaching sessions, can help the faculty identify the needs of individual learners, as can *discussion with individual learners*, during which learners are asked about their learning-style preferences and perceived needs. This discovery process is more likely to occur when the faculty use observational, listening, and question-asking skills.

Once the faculty are aware of these specific needs, they may be able to modify or add to the curriculum's educational strategies to address the specific needs. Such accommodation is more likely to be possible in *one-on-one and small group teaching* than in lecture situations, although online lectures allow flexibility in timing for learners.

Generally speaking, learner-centered approaches to education require more time and effort on the part of educators than teacher-centered approaches. They are more likely, however, to engage the learner and succeed in helping the learner achieve agreed-on objectives. The curriculum developer will need to decide to what extent learner-centered approaches are critical for the achievement of curricular objectives, desirable but not critical, and feasible within resource constraints.

EXAMPLE: *Use of Self-assessments.* At the beginning of a rotation in communication skills and the psychosocial domain of medical practice, PGY–1 residents assess their competencies and learning needs. The self-assessments are shared with course faculty. Most of the learning in the course occurs in small group or one-on-one sessions that employ experiential methods (e.g., role-play, standardized patients, video review of actual patient encounters). The faculty use information from the self-assessments and from their own observations of learner performance to tailor their approaches to address individual learner needs (43).

EXAMPLE: *Curriculum with Built-in Flexibility in Terms of Depth and Pace, and Remedial Instruction for Those Who Do Not Achieve Competency.* Students studying biochemistry receive a set of objectives that outlines both the minimum requirement of the course and those areas that they can study in more depth. Students study the subject individually from printed material or programmed tape/slide presentations at their own pace. They may also choose those materials that best suit their learning styles. When the students feel that they have mastered a phase of the course, they arrange for an assessment. If they have not achieved an acceptable level of competency, a remedial program of instruction is developed by the staff and student (45).

Methods for Promoting New Competencies

As noted in Chapter 4, six core competencies were introduced into graduate medical education in 1999 by the U.S. Accreditation Council for Graduate Medical Education (ACGME) (46) and have influenced the approach to learning outcomes in all phases of medical training. While some of these competencies relate directly to previous types of objectives, such as medical knowledge as a cognitive objective and patient care and interpersonal/communication skills as psychomotor objectives, two (Practice-Based Learning and Improvement and Systems-Based Practice) are new, complex, and require integrative approaches.

Practice-Based Learning and Improvement (PBLI).   The Practice-Based Learning and Improvement competency requires that trainees examine, evaluate, and improve the care they provide, appraising and assimilating scientific evidence in the process (46). The habits of lifelong learning and self-directed learning are included in this competency.

Methods for promoting PBLI and self-directed learning (47, 48) include the following:

- Training in skills relevant to self-directed learning
    Self-assessment, including audits of one's own patient care/clinical practice
    Information searching
    Critical appraisal
    Clinical decision making
- Independent learning projects
- Personal learning plans or contracts
- Use of learning portfolios (49, 50)
- Encouraging learners to formulate and answer their own questions
- Role modeling
- Training in teaching skills

In an era of burgeoning information and ever-evolving advances in medical care, it is important for curriculum developers to consider how learners will continue to develop in relevant cognitive, affective, and psychomotor areas after completion of the curriculum. Most overall educational programs have as a stated or unstated goal that their learners, by the end of the program, will be effective self-directed learners. *Effective self-directed learners* take primary responsibility for their own learning, accurately identify their own learning needs, clarify their learning goals and objectives, successfully identify and use resources and educational strategies that can help them achieve their goals and objectives, accurately assess their achievements, and repeat the learning cycle if necessary. By its very nature, self-directed learning is learner-centered. An advantage of self-directed learning is that active learners are said to learn more things more efficiently, to retain that knowledge better, and to use it more effectively than passive learners (48).

A self-directed learning approach is most applicable when the learner already has some relevant knowledge and experience. It is easiest when the learner already possesses *skills that facilitate self-directed learning*, such as self-assessment skills, library and informatics skills for searching the health care literature and other databases, skills in reading and critically appraising the medical literature, and clinical decision making skills.

Curriculum developers must decide how their curriculum will fit into an educational program's overall approach to promoting the development of self-directed learners. If a focused curriculum is toward the beginning of a multifaceted educational program, it may need to take responsibility for teaching learners skills relevant to a self-directed learning approach (see above). If learners have already developed these fundamental skills but are relatively inexperienced in self-directed learning, they may benefit from a special orientation to self-directed learning and from an intensive mentoring process. If an effective self-directed learning approach has already been established in the overall program, a curriculum can simply include methods with which the learners are already familiar.

Required *independent learning projects and reports* are the method that is most commonly used to promote self-directed learning. Curricula can also require that learners develop a *personal learning plan or contract* (51), usually in combination with a preceptor or mentor, that specifies learning objectives, learning methods, resources, and evaluation methods. Faculty can promote self-directed learning by encouraging *targeted independent reading or consultation* related to clinical or other problems that are encountered, by *encouraging and helping learners to answer some of their own questions*, and by *modeling* self-directed learning themselves.

A curriculum is most likely to be successful in promoting self-directed learning if it schedules sufficient protected time for the activity, clearly communicates expectations to the learner, requires products (e.g., formal or informal presentations or reports), provides ongoing mentoring and supervision throughout the process, and provides training for learners in skills that facilitate self-directed learning, if they are lacking.

EXAMPLE: *Training in Skills Relevant to Self-directed Learning.* All PGY–1 residents are assigned to a one-month rotation in which they learn informatics, critical appraisal, and clinical decision making skills. Each resident is required to apply these skills by critically assessing a clinical practice of their choice. At the end of the month, they formally present their findings to an invited audience. Time is provided within the curriculum for residents to work on their projects.

EXAMPLE: *Identifying, Answering, and Reporting on Clinical Questions Identified in the Course of Patient Care.* PGY–2 and PGY–3 residents are required to identify a question related to the care of one of their clinic patients each week, look up the answer, and briefly report the sources used, the search time required, and the answer to their question during the next clinic session.

EXAMPLE: *Self-audit, Reflection, and Goal Development.* All residents perform a self-audit of three to four of the clinic charts of their continuity patients once yearly, using rating forms and agreed-on standards of record keeping and preventive care. They review their rating forms with their clinic preceptor, identify strengths and deficits, and develop written goals for the following year.

Systems-Based Practice and Teamwork.   The Systems-Based Practice competency is demonstrated by "an awareness of and responsiveness to the larger context and system of health care and the ability to effectively call on system resources to provide care that is of optimal value" (46). Competence in this area includes knowledge of health care delivery systems and costs of care, as well as the skills to work with other health care team members within a system to improve care outcomes. In this respect, this competency overlaps with the *Interpersonal and Communications Skill* competency, which includes effective teamwork with other health care professionals.

Methods that can be used to help develop knowledge of health care systems include the following:

- Inclusion of other health professionals on health care teams
- Providing feedback on costs of care
- Case conferences focused on cost-effectiveness and quality of care
- Opportunities to work in disease management programs
- Redesigning teaching services toward multidisciplinary integration
- Participation in quality improvement and safety teams

EXAMPLE: *Quality-improvement Project.* A quality-improvement project was designed to reduce drug-prescribing errors in a teaching hospital intensive care unit. Inclusion of a senior pharmacist on daily rounds who was available for consultation significantly decreased adverse drug events when compared to a control unit (52).

EXAMPLE: *Revised Morbidity and Mortality Conference, Use of a Health Care Matrix.* A residency program revised its Morbidity and Mortality conference to include the use of a health care matrix, which linked the Institute of Medicine aims for quality improvement and the knowledge, skills, and attitudes necessary to affect patient outcomes. The discussant was charged with completing the matrix as it related to the case under discussion (53).

As medical knowledge has increased, and as societal expectations for customer-friendly, high-quality, cost-effective care have risen, the mechanisms for providing the best health care have become more complex. It is becoming unlikely that an independent practitioner will be able to provide the best care to individual patients, a panel of patients, or the community. Rather, health care professionals will have to work effectively in teams to accomplish desired goals (54, 55).

Medical curricula that have traditionally fostered a competitive approach to learning and an autocratic approach to providing care now need to foster collaborative approaches to learning and to prepare learners to be effective team members. Health care professionals need to become knowledgeable about and skilled in facilitating group process, in running and participating in meetings, in being appropriately assertive, in managing conflict, in facilitating organizational change, in motivating others, in delegating and supervising others, and in feedback and general communication skills. Baker elucidated (56), and others corroborated (57, 58), a framework of principles that characterize effective teamwork, including leadership skills, elucidation of shared goals and objectives, effective communication, trust, task sharing and backup behavior, adaptability, and performance monitoring/feedback.

Methods for promoting and reinforcing team skills include the following:

- Focused curricula on team functioning and related skills
- Involvement of trainees in collaborative versus competitive approaches to learning
- Learner participation in multidisciplinary teams and in work environments that model effective teamwork
- Having learners assess and discuss the functioning of the teams in which they are involved

EXAMPLE: *Team-Based Learning.* Team-Based Learning (TBL) is a relatively new educational method discussed above under Methods for Achieving Cognitive Objectives. It combines individual and collaborative learning approaches. In addition to addressing cognitive objectives, it promotes self-directed learning, professionalism, and teamwork (20, 21). Peer evaluation is done within teams at designated times in the course (21).

EXAMPLE: *Longitudinal Task-focused Small Groups, with Training and Reflection on Group Process and Team Functioning.* In a longitudinal faculty development program for curriculum development, groups of two to five faculty work over 9 months to develop and pilot medical curricula. At the beginning of the program, a facilitator guides participants in a discussion of effective group behaviors and provides participants with a group process rating sheet by which to evaluate their own groups. With this background, program participants throughout the year are asked to reflect on the functioning of their groups and the impact of group process on their curricular projects.

Methods for Promoting Professionalism

Professionalism, while not new, has been given increased emphasis by the ACGME and others (46, 59–61). Professionalism includes respect for others; compassion; cross-cultural sensitivity; effective communication; shared decision making; honesty and integrity; self-awareness; responsiveness to the needs of patients and society that supersedes self-interest; accountability; sense of duty; a commitment to ethical principles; confidentiality; appropriate management of conflicts of interest; and a commitment to excellence, scientific knowledge, and ongoing professional development (46, 59–62). It is a challenging domain to practice and teach (62–63). Unfortunately, there is evidence that some elements of professionalism deteriorate with training and that lapses of professionalism are common in medical settings (63). Methods for promoting professionalism include the following:

- Faculty role modeling (63)
- Facilitated reflection on and discussion of experiences embodying professionalism (63)
- Participation in writing professionalism goals (64)
- Ethics consultation rounds
- Peer evaluations

- Participation in Honor Boards
- Participation in patient advocacy groups
- Service learning and volunteerism
- Attention of institutional and program leaders to the policies and culture of the training institution, as well as to the hidden and informal curricula that influence trainees (63, 65–67).

EXAMPLE: *Summer Internship with Seminars and Community Experience.* A summer internship for medical students included seminars related to professionalism and clinical experience in community-based organizations with community mentors. Students reported that the internship taught them about influences on professionalism, especially pharmaceutical companies, the role of physician advocacy for patients, and the experience of vulnerable populations with the health care system (68).

CONCLUSION

The challenge of Step 4 is to devise educational strategies that achieve the curricular objectives set out in Step 3, within the resource constraints of available time, space, money, clinical material, and faculty. The need to promote learner-centeredness, professionalism, and the newly defined competencies of Practice-Based Learning and Improvement (PBLI) and Systems-Based Practice may be additional considerations that are consistent with initiatives in the overall training program or school, or the educational philosophy of the curriculum developers themselves. Creativity in the development of educational strategies is an opportunity for facilitating meaningful, enduring learning and for scholarship, particularly if the curriculum is carefully evaluated, as we shall see in a subsequent chapter.

QUESTIONS

For the curriculum you are coordinating, planning, or would like to be planning, please answer or think about the following questions:

1. In the table below write one important, specific measurable objective in each of the following domains: cognitive, affective, and psychomotor.

2. Choose educational methods from Table 5.3 to achieve each of your educational objectives.

3. Is each educational method congruent with the domain of its objective?

4. Are you concerned that there will be decay over time in the achievement of any of your objectives?

5. From Tables 5.1 and 5.3, choose an additional method for each objective that would most likely prevent decay after its achievement.

6. Identify the resources that you will need to implement your educational methods. Consider available teachers in your institution, costs for simulations or clinical experiences, time in the training program or elective, and space. Are your methods feasible?

Domain of the Objective

	Cognitive (Knowledge)	Affective (Attitudinal)	Psychomotor (Skill or Performance)
Specific measurable objectives			
Educational method to achieve			
Educational method to prevent decay			
Resources required			

7. Have you included any methods that are learner-centered or that promote self-directed learning? If yes, what are they?

8. Will your curriculum include educational strategies that promote Practice-Based Learning and Improvement or Systems-Based Practice? Why or why not? If yes, what are they?

9. Will your curriculum include educational strategies that promote professionalism? Why or why not? If yes, what are they?

10. Have the methods you suggested in your answers to questions 7–9 affected your need for resources? How? Are your methods feasible?

GENERAL REFERENCES

Brookfield S. Adult learning: an overview. In Tuinjman A, ed. *International Encyclopedia of Education*, 2nd ed. Oxford: Pergamon Press; 1996.
    A short but comprehensive summary that covers four major research areas underlying adult learning (self-directed learning, critical reflection, experiential learning, and learning to learn) and three emerging trends (cross-cultural adult learning, practical theorizing, and distance learning) and identifies 10 areas for further research. Available at www.fsu.edu/~elps/ae/download/ade5385/Brookfield.pdf. Accessed March 7, 2009.

Clark RC, Mayer RE. *e-Learning and the Science of Instruction: Proven Guidelines for Consumers and Designers of Multimedia Learning*, 2nd ed. San Francisco: Pfeiffer; 2007.
    An introductory text on Web-based instruction for the adult learner. The book reviews adult learning theory and concepts relevant to multimedia formats, basing recommendations on proven strategies. Many examples are given throughout the book, and while these are mainly geared toward corporate human resources training, they are helpful for the medical educator interested in e-learning applications. 496 pages.

Cross KP. *Adults as Learners: Increasing Participation and Facilitating Learning*. San Francisco: Jossey-Bass; 1981.
    Classic text, written for educators and trainers of adult learners in any discipline or profession. The

author describes and synthesizes research findings into two explanatory models: one for under-standing motivations of adult learners and the other for organizing knowledge about their charac-teristics. There is also a chapter on facilitation. 300 pages.

Dick W, Carey L, Carey JO. *The Systematic Design of Instruction*, 6th ed. Boston: Pearson Allyn & Bacon; 2005.
   The authors present a framework for instructional design similar to that proposed in this chapter. The book places particular emphasis on behavioral objectives, pre-instructional activities, student participation, and testing. Chapters 8 and 9 address the development of instructional strategy and selection of instructional materials. Specific (non-health-related) examples are detailed in the text. 376 pages.

Ende J, Atkins E. Conceptualizing curriculum for graduate medical education. *Acad Med.* 1992;67:528–34.
   Discusses limitations of objective-driven curricula and how to structure educational programs to maximize learning from experience. (See also discussion at end of Chapter 5, Step 4: Goals and Objectives.)

Green LW, Kreuter MW, Deeds SG, Partridge KB. Selection of educational strategies. In: *Health Education Planning: A Diagnostic Approach*. Palo Alto, Calif.: Mayfield Publishing; 1980. Pp. 86–115.
   Classic text that uses a conceptual framework for planning and implementing health programs. The framework includes epidemiologic diagnosis/health problem definition, behavioral and edu-cational diagnosis, social/community/target group factors, and administrative diagnosis. Chapter 6 discusses the selection of educational strategies in the context of this framework. The book is oriented to educational interventions for communities and patient populations, but the concepts are also applicable to educational programs targeted at health professionals. 306 pages.

Grunwald T, Corsbie-Massey C. Guidelines for cognitively efficient multimedia learning tools: educational strategies, cognitive load, and interface design. *Acad Med.* 2006;81:213–23.
   This narrative review summarizes existing research in the use of multimedia, including how edu-cational theories and design should be considered in crafting effective multimedia.

Harden RM, Sowden S, Dunn WR. Educational strategies in curriculum development: the SPICES model. *Med Educ.* 1984;18:284–97.
   This paper provides a concise summary of six strategies in medical education, which are repre-sented as a continuum of dichotomous approaches: 1) student (learner)-centered/teacher-cen-tered, 2) problem-based/information-gathering, 3) integrated/discipline-based, 4) community-based/hospital-based, 5) elective/uniform program, and 6) systematic/apprenticeship-opportunis-tic. Each approach is defined and its strengths and weaknesses noted. The paper provides anoth-er set of criteria by which to classify curricular strategies.

Knowles MS, Holton EF, Swanson RA. *The Adult Learner: The Definitive Classic in Adult Education and Human Resource Development*, 6th ed. Burlington, Mass.: Elsevier; 2005.
   Classic work by Malcolm Knowles, updated posthumously by two professors of education, Elwood Holton II and Richard Swanson. The book covers adult learning theory, recent advances, and application. 378 pages.

Mezirow J. *Transformative Dimensions of Adult Learning*. San Francisco: Jossey-Bass; 1991.
   Classic book that describes transformational learning as learning that affects how learners inter-pret or construct meaning out of experience and their beliefs, attitudes, and emotions. Such learn-ing is influenced by past and new experiences, culture, communication with others, and critical reflection. The interpretive lens through which a person views experiences influences one's behav-ior. The book integrates perspectives on learning from many disciplines, including education, psychology, sociology, and philosophy, to develop this theory of transformative learning. 247 pages.

Michaelsen LK, Knight AB, Fink LD. *Team-Based Learning: A Transformative Use of Small Groups in College Teaching*. Sterling, Va.: Stylus Publishing; 2004.

Detailed guide for implementing team-based learning teaching strategies written by the originator. 286 pages.

Michaelsen LK, Parmelee DX, McMahon KK, Levine RE. *Team-Based Learning for Health Professions Education: A Guide to Using Small Groups for Improving Learning*. Sterling, Va.: Stylus Publishing; 2007.
This book provides an introduction to team-based learning for health educators; it covers theory, structure, models, and detail of implementation, including performance feedback and evaluation. 256 pages.

Rogers CR. Significant learning in therapy and education. In: *On Becoming a Person: A Therapist's View of Psychotherapy*. Boston: Houghton Mifflin; 1961. Pp. 279–96.
Chapter in a classic book by Carl Rogers that describes conditions that promote transformational learning: genuineness and congruence of the teacher; empathetic understanding and acceptance of the learner; contact with problems; provision of resources; and a safe, supportive learning environment.

Rubenstein W, Talbot Y. *Medical Teaching in Ambulatory Care: A Practical Guide*. New York: Springer Publishing Co.; 2003.
A short, practical, useful text on office-based precepting that includes a section on challenging learning situations. 152 pages.

Schon DA. *Educating the Reflective Practitioner*. San Francisco: Jossey-Bass; 1987.
Classic book on the critical role of reflection, in as well as on action, in professional education. 355 pages.

Whitman N, Schwenk TL. *The Physician as Teacher*, 2nd ed. Salt Lake City, Utah: Whitman Associates; 1997.
This book discusses teaching as a form of communication and relationship, as well as specific teaching responsibilities: lectures, group discussions, teaching rounds and morning report, bedside teaching, and teaching in the ambulatory setting. 275 pages.

Whitman NA, Schwenk TL. *Preceptors as Teachers: A Guide to Clinical Teaching*, 2nd ed. Salt Lake City, Utah: University of Utah School of Medicine; 1995.
An excellent practical, pithy text that covers the essentials of clinical teaching. 30 pages.

SPECIFIC REFERENCES

1. Grunwald T, Corsbie-Massay C. Guidelines for cognitively efficient multimedia learning tools: educational strategies, cognitive load, and interface design. *Acad Med.* 2006;81:213–23.
2. Watkins RS, Moran WP. Competency-based learning: the impact of targeted resident education and feedback on Pap smear adequacy rates. *J Gen Intern Med.* 2004;19:545–48.
3. Price GE. Diagnosing learning styles. In: Smith RM. *Helping Adults Learn How to Learn*. San Francisco: Jossey-Bass; 1983. Pp. 49–55.
4. Felder RM, Sparlin J. Applications, reliability and validity of the Index of Learning Styles. *Int J Engng Ed.* 2005;21:103–12.
5. Soloman BA, Felder RM. Index of learning styles questionnaire. Available at www.engr.ncsu .edu/learningstyles/ilsweb.html. Accessed March 1, 2009.
6. Bennett CJ, Sackett KD, Haynes RB, Neufeld VR, Tugwell P, Roberts R. A controlled trial of teaching critical appraisal of the clinical literature to medical students. *JAMA.* 1987;257:2451–54.
7. Fairman RP, Robichaud AM, Glauser FL. Is anyone out there listening? The art and science of lecturing. *Medical Times.* 1989;117:124–30.

8. Whitman N, Schwenk TL. *The Physician as Teacher,* 2nd ed. Salt Lake City, Utah: Whitman Associates; 1997. Pp. 103–29.
9. Westberg J, Jason H. *Making Presentations: A Guide Book for Health Professions Teachers.* Boulder, Colo.: Center for Instructional Support; 1991. Pp. 1–89.
10. Whitman NA. *There is No Gene for Good Teaching: A Handbook on Lecturing for Medical Teachers.* Salt Lake City, Utah: University of Utah School of Medicine; 1982.
11. Walters MR. Problem based learning within endocrine physiology lectures. *Adv Physiol Educ.* 2001;25:225–27.
12. Sisson SD, Hughes MT, Levine D, Brancati FL. Effect of an Internet-based curriculum on postgraduate education: a multicenter intervention. *J Gen Intern Med.* 2004;19:505–9.
13. Whitman NE, Schwenk TL. *A Handbook for Group Discussion Leaders: Alternatives to Lecturing Medical Students to Death.* Salt Lake City, Utah: University of Utah School of Medicine; 1983. Pp. 1–38.
14. Whitman N, Schwenk TL. *The Physician as Teacher,* 2nd ed. Salt Lake City, Utah: Whitman Associates; 1997. Pp. 131–46.
15. Tiberius RG. *Small Group Teaching: A Trouble-Shooting Guide.* Toronto, Ont.: Ontario Institute for Studies in Education Press; 1990. Pp. 1–194.
16. Westburg J, Jason H. *Fostering Learning in Small Groups: A Practical Guide.* New York: Springer Publishing; 1996. Pp. 1–267.
17. Dolmans DH, DeGrave W, Wolfhagen IH, van der Vleuten CP. Problem-based learning: future challenges for educational practice and research. *Med Educ.* 2005;39(7):732–41.
18. Distlehorst LH, Dawson E, Robbs RS, Barrows HS. Problem-based learning outcomes: the glass half-full. *Acad Med.* 2005;80(3):294–99.
19. Mamede S, Schmidt HG, Norman GR. Innovations in problem-based learning: what can we learn from recent studies? *Adv Health Sci Educ.* 2006;11:403–22.
20. Michaelsen LK, Knight AB, Fink LD, eds. *Team-Based Learning: A Transformative Use of Small Groups in College Teaching.* Sterling, Va.: Stylus Publishing; 2004.
21. Michaelsen LK, Parmelee DX, McMahon KK, Levine RE, eds. *Team-Based Learning for Health Professions Education: A Guide to Using Small Groups for Improving Learning.* Herndon, Va.: Stylus Publishing; 2007.
22. Henerson ME, Morris LL, Fitz-Gibbon CT. *How to Measure Attitudes.* (Book number 6) In: *Program Evaluation Kit.* Newbury Park, Calif.: Sage Publications; 1987. Pp. 9–13.
23. Dick W, Carey L, Carey JO. *The Systematic Design of Instruction,* 6th ed. Boston: Pearson Allyn & Bacon; 2005. Pp. 205–6, 210–11.
24. Bentley TJ. *Facilitation: Providing Opportunities for Learning.* Berkshire, England: McGraw-Hill Publishing; 1994. Pp. 25–60.
25. Brookfield SD. *Understanding and Facilitating Adult Learning.* San Francisco: Jossey-Bass; 1987. Pp. 123–26.
26. Rogers CR. Significant learning in therapy and education. In: Rogers CR. *On Becoming a Person: A Therapist's View of Psychotherapy.* Boston: Houghton Mifflin; 1961. Pp. 279–96.
27. Wright S, Wong A, Newill C. The impact of role models on medical students. *J Gen Intern Med.* 1997;12:53–56.
28. Wright S. Examining what residents look for in their role models. *Acad Med.* 1996;71:290–92.
29. ROWEL. Life in the State of Poverty: the ROWEL Welfare Simulation. St. Louis, Mo.: Reform Organization of Welfare Education Association; 1995.
30. Ende J. Feedback in clinical medical education. *JAMA.* 1983;250(6):777–81.
31. McGaghie WC, Issenberg SB, Petrusa ER, Scalese RJ. Effect of practice on standardized learning outcomes in simulation-based medical education. *Medical Educ.* 2006;40:792–97.

32. McGaghie WC. Simulation in professional competence assessment: basic considerations. In: Tekian A, McGuire CH, McGaghie WC, eds. *Innovative Simulations for Assessing Professional Competence: From Paper and Pencil to Virtual Reality*. Chicago: University of Illinois at Chicago; 1999.

33. Issenberg SB, Petrusa ER, McGaghie WC, et al. Effectiveness of a computer-based system to teach bedside cardiology. *Acad Med.* 1999;74:S93–95.

34. Simpson MA. How to use role play in medical teaching. *Medical Teacher.* 1985;7:75–82.

35. Nestel D, Tierney T. Role-play for medical students learning about communication: guidelines for maximising benefits. *BMC Med Educ.* 2007;7:3.

36. Lane C, Rollnick S. The use of simulated patients and role-play in communication skills training: a review of the literature to August, 2005. *Patient Educ Couns.* 2007;67:13–20.

37. Singer PA, Robb A, Cohen R, Norman G, Turnbull J. Performance-based assessment of clinical ethics using an objective structured clinical examination. *Acad Med.* 1996;71: 495–98.

38. Stillman PL, Swanson D, Regan B, et al. Assessment of clinical skills of residents utilizing standardized patients. *Ann Intern Med.* 1991;114:393–401.

39. King AM, Perkowski-Roberts LC, Pohl HS. Planning standardized patient programs: case development, patient training, and costs. *Teaching and Learning in Medicine.* 1994;6:6–14.

40. Barzansky B, Etzel SI. Education programs in US medical schools, 2003–2004. *JAMA.* 2004;292:1025–31.

41. Edwards A, Tzelepis A, Klingbeil C, et al. Fifteen years of a videotape review program for internal medicine and medicine-pediatrics residents. *Acad Med.* 1996;71:744–48.

42. Guerlain S, Adams RB, Turentine FB, Shin T, Guo H, Collinis SR, Calland JF. Assessing team performance in the operating room: development and use of a "black-box" recorder and other tools for the intraoperative environment. *J Am Coll Surg.* 2005;200:29–37.

43. Kern DE, Grayson M, Barker LR, Roca RP, Cole KA, Roter D, Golden AS. Residency training in interviewing skills and the psychosocial domain of medical practice. *J Gen Intern Med.* 1989;4:421–31.

44. Holmboe ES, Meehan TP, Lynn L, et.al. Promoting physicians' self-improvement and quality improvement: the ABIM diabetes improvement module. *J Contin Educ Health Prof.* 2006;26:109–19.

45. Harden RM, Snowden S, Dunn WR. Educational strategies in curriculum development: the SPICES model. *Med Educ.* 1984;18:284–97.

46. Accreditation Council of Graduate Medical Education. ACGME Outcome Project. Competencies. Available at www.acgme.org/Outcome/. Accessed March 1, 2009.

47. Brookfield S, ed. *Self-Directed Learning: From Theory to Practice*. San Francisco: Jossey-Bass; 1985.

48. Knowles MS. *Self-Directed Learning: A Guide for Learners and Teachers*. New York: Cambridge (The Adult Education Co.); 1975.

49. Challis M. AMEE medical education guide no. 11 (revised): Portfolio-based learning and assessment in medical education. *Med Teach.* 1999;4:370–86.

50. Kjaer NK, Maagaard R, Wied S. Using an online portfolio in postgraduate training. *Med Teach.* 2006;28:708–12.

51. Knowles MS. *Using Learning Contracts*. San Francisco: Jossey-Bass; 1986. Pp. 3–8.

52. Leape LL, Cullen DJ, Clapp MD, Burdick E, Demonaco HJ, Erickson JI, Bates DW. Pharmacist participation on physician rounds and adverse drug events in the intensive care unit. *JAMA.* 1999;282:267–70.

53. Bingham JW, Quinn DC, Richardson MG, Miles PV, Gabbe SG. Using a healthcare matrix to assess patient care in terms of aims for improvement and core competencies. *Jt. Comm J Qual Patient Saf.* 2005;31:98–105.

54. Manion J, Lorimer W, Leander WJ. *Team-Based Health Care Organizations: Blueprint for Success*. Gaithersburg, Md.: Aspen Publications; 1996.

55. Pritchard P, Pritchard J. *Teamwork for Primary and Shared Care: A Practical Workbook,* 2nd ed. Oxford, England: Oxford University Press; 1994.

56. Baker DP, Salas E, King H, Battles J, Barach P. The role of teamwork in the professional education of physicians: current status and assessment recommendations. *Jt Comm J Qual Patient Saf.* 2005;31(4):185–202.

57. Salas E, Sims DE, Burke CS. Is there a "big five" in teamwork? *Small Group Research.* 2005;36(5):555.

58. Wilson KA, Burke CS, Priest HA, Salas E. Promoting health care safety through training high reliability teams. *Qual Saf Health Care.* 2005;14(4):303–9.

59. ABIM Foundation. American Board of Internal Medicine, ACP-ASIM Foundation. American College of Physicians-American Society of Internal Medicine, European Federation of Internal Medicine. Medical professionalism in the new millennium: a physician charter. *Ann Intern Med.* 2002;136:243–46.

60. Blank L, Kimball HABIM Foundation, ACP Foundation, et al. Medical professionalism in the new millennium: a physician charter 15 months later. *Ann Intern Med.* 2003;138:839–41.

61. Inui TS. *A Flag in the Wind: Educating for Professionalism in Medicine.* Washington, D.C.: Association of American Medical Colleges; 2003.

62. Ratanawongsa N, Bolen S, Howell EE, Kern DE, Sisson SD, Larriviere D. Resident's perceptions of professionalism in training and practice: barriers, promoters, and duty hour requirements. *J Gen Intern Med.* 2006;21:758–63.

63. Branch WT, Kern D, Haidet P, Weissmann P, Gracey CF, Mitchell G, Inui T. Teaching the human dimensions of care in clinical settings. *JAMA.* 2001;286:1067–74.

64. Goldstein EA, Maestas RR, Fryer-Edwards K, et al. Professionalism in medical education: an institutional challenge. *Acad Med.* 2006;81:871–76.

65. Suchman AT, Williamson PR, Litzelman DK, Frankel RM, Mossbarger DL, Inui TS, et al. Toward an informal curriculum that teaches professionalism: transforming the social environment of a medical school. *J Gen Intern Med.* 2004;19:501–4.

66. Hafferty FW. Beyond curriculum reform: confronting medicine's hidden curriculum. *Acad Med.* 1998;73:403–7.

67. Hundert EM, Hafferty FW, Christakis D. Characteristics of the informal curriculum and trainees' ethical choices. *Acad Med.* 1996;71:624–33.

68. O'Toole, TP, Kathuria N, Mishra M, Schukart D. Teaching professionalism within a community context: perspectives from a national demonstration project. *Acad Med.* 2005;80:339–43.

CHAPTER SIX

Step 5
Implementation

. . . making the curriculum a reality

Mark T. Hughes, M.D., M.A.

IMPORTANCE

For a curriculum to achieve its potential, careful attention must be paid to issues of implementation. The curriculum developer must ensure that sufficient resources, political and financial support, and administrative structures have been developed to successfully implement the curriculum (Table 6.1).

Implementation can be viewed as a developmental process with four stages, as put forth in a model by Lemon (1). The first stage is establishing the need for change by

Table 6.1. Checklist for Implementation

___ Identify resources
    ___ Personnel: faculty, audiovisual, computing, information technology, secretarial and other support staff, patients
    ___ Time: faculty, support staff, learners
    ___ Facilities: space, equipment, clinical sites, virtual space (servers, content management software)
    ___ Funding/costs: direct financial costs, hidden or opportunity costs

___ Obtain support
    ___ Internal
        from: those with administrative authority (dean's office, hospital administration, department chair, program director, division director, etc.), faculty, learners, other stakeholders
        for: personnel, resources, political support
    ___ External
        from: government, professional societies, philanthropic organizations or foundations, accreditation bodies, other entities (e.g., managed care organizations), individual donors
        for: funding, political support, external requirements, curricular or faculty development resources

___ Develop administrative mechanisms to support the curriculum
    ___ Administrative structure: to delineate responsibilities and decision making
    ___ Communication:
        content: rationale; goals and objectives; information about the curriculum, learners, faculty, facilities and equipment, scheduling; changes in the curriculum; evaluation results; etc.
        mechanisms: Web sites, memos, meetings, syllabus materials, site visits, reports, etc.
    ___ Operations: preparation and distribution of schedules and curricular materials; collection, collation, and distribution of evaluation data; curricular revisions and changes; etc.
    ___ Scholarship: plans for presenting and publishing about curriculum; human subjects protection considerations; IRB approval, if necessary

___ Anticipate and address barriers
    ___ Financial and other resources
    ___ Competing demands
    ___ People: attitudes, job/role security, power and authority, etc.

___ Plan to introduce the curriculum
    ___ Pilot
    ___ Phase-in
    ___ Full implementation

developing leadership for the program and generating support. The second stage is to plan for change, such that curricular and clinical site issues are well thought out and curricular goals are clearly conveyed to stakeholders. The third stage involves promptly responding to operational problems as they arise. If concerns are not readily addressed, then faculty or clinical site personnel may become disillusioned with the curriculum. The fourth stage of curricular implementation is securing the viability of the curriculum by establishing ongoing financial support and procedures for evaluation (1). These four stages correspond to the six steps of curriculum development. Stages 1 and 2 address problem identification, general and targeted needs assessments, and creation of clearly articulated goals, objectives, and educational strategies (Chapters 2–5). Stages 3 and 4 are addressed in this and the following two chapters: Implementation, Evaluation and Feedback, and Curriculum Maintenance and Enhancement.

IDENTIFICATION OF RESOURCES

In many respects, Step 5 requires that the curriculum developer become a project manager, overseeing the people and operations that will successfully implement the curriculum. The curriculum developer must realistically assess the resources that will be required to implement the educational strategies (Chapter 5) and the evaluation (Chapter 7) planned for the curriculum. Resources include personnel, time, facilities, and funding.

Personnel

Personnel includes curriculum directors, curriculum faculty, instructors, and support staff. The curriculum developers often become the *curriculum directors* and need to have sufficient time blocked in their schedules to oversee the implementation of the curriculum. Ideally *faculty* and *instructors* will be available and skilled in both teaching and content. If there are insufficient numbers of skilled faculty, one must contemplate hiring new faculty or developing existing faculty.

> **EXAMPLE:** *Faculty Development before the Start of the Curriculum.* A curriculum was developed with small group learning as its main educational method. The faculty were relatively inexperienced in this method of teaching. A targeted two-session faculty development program on small group facilitation techniques was held, as well as periodic faculty meetings, to promote faculty acquisition, discussion, and continued development of these skills.

> **EXAMPLE:** *Faculty Development in Response to Evaluation.* Evaluations from an existing clinical skills course for second-year medical students revealed some deficiencies in preceptors' provision of feedback. The course director asked other faculty from the same institution, who were experts in faculty development, to develop a 2 1/2 hour workshop on feedback skills that could be integrated into the orientation session for course preceptors. After 2 years of workshops, evaluations reflected an improved performance in this area.

For large curricula involving many learners or extending over a long period of time, curriculum developers may need to hire a dedicated *curriculum administrator. Administrative assistants and other support staff* are usually needed to prepare budgets, curricular materials, and evaluation reports; coordinate and communicate schedules; collect evaluation data; and support learning activities. Institutional curricular support such as scheduling rooms, academic computing assistance, or audiovisual support must be planned. Sometimes *additional personnel,* such as standardized patients, will be required. A suitable mix of real *patients* is a "personnel" need that may be required to provide learners with critical clinical experience, and it should not be overlooked.

Time

Curriculum directors need time to coordinate management of the curriculum, which includes working with support staff to be sure that faculty are teaching, learners are participating, and process objectives are being met. Faculty require time to prepare and teach, as well as time to give feedback to learners. Time should also be budgeted for faculty to provide summative evaluations of the learners and of the curriculum back to curriculum developers. For curriculum directors and faculty who have other responsibilities (e.g., meeting clinical productivity expectations), the implementation plan must include ways to compensate, reward, and/or accommodate faculty for the time they devote to the curriculum.

Learners require time not only to attend scheduled learning activities but also to read, reflect, do independent learning, and apply what they have learned. As part of the targeted needs assessment (Chapter 3), curriculum developers should become familiar with the learners' schedule and understand what barriers exist for participation in the curriculum. For instance, postgraduate medical trainees may have to meet expectations on regulatory work hour limits.

Support staff members need time to perform their functions. Clearly delineating their responsibilities can help to budget the amount of time they require for curriculum implementation.

If educational research is to be performed as part of the targeted needs assessment (see Chapter 3) or curriculum evaluation (see Chapter 7), curriculum developers may need to budget time for review and approval of the research plans by an institutional review board (IRB). Thinking early about this in the Implementation phase can prevent delays in the development and delivery of the curriculum (see below).

Facilities

Curricula require facilities, such as space and equipment. The simplest curriculum may require only a room in which to meet or lecture. Clinical curricula often require access to patients and must provide learners with clinical equipment.

> **EXAMPLE:** *Access to Patients and Clinical Equipment.* The curriculum developers of a home care curriculum wanted residents to have the experience of making home visits as part of their ambulatory rotation. The support of key stakeholders needed to be garnered in order to ensure that residents could visit housebound elderly patients in an existing home care program and discuss their visits with their faculty preceptors. A "travel kit" that served as the "doctor's black bag" was created to guarantee that the resident had the supplies and equipment necessary to evaluate the patient in his or her home.

Other curricula may need special educational equipment, such as audio or video equipment, computers, or artificial models to teach clinical skills.

> **EXAMPLE:** *Use of Simulation.* A curriculum was developed to teach surgical residents basic laparoscopic skills. In addition to watching video clips reviewing proper technique in maneuvering a laparoscope, a skills lab using a laparoscopic simulator was established. Faculty preceptors observed the residents' technique and provided feedback and guidance on use of the instrument.

A curriculum that addresses acquisition of clinical knowledge or skills may need a clinical site that can accommodate learners and provide the appropriate volume and mix of patients to ensure a valuable clinical experience.

EXAMPLE: *Case-Mix.* A musculoskeletal curriculum was developed for internal medicine residents. In a rheumatology rotation, the case-mix was concentrated on patients with inflammatory arthritis and connective tissue disease. Experiences in an orthopedic clinic involved a case-mix that included many postoperative patients. The targeted needs assessment identified that residents needed to learn about musculoskeletal conditions commonly encountered in a primary care practice (e.g., shoulder pain, back pain, knee pain). In addition, learners wanted to practice exam maneuvers and diagnostic/therapeutic skills (e.g., arthrocentesis) that did not require specialist training. Therefore, curriculum developers created a weekly musculoskeletal clinic for primary care patients with common joint and muscle complaints. The musculoskeletal clinic was staffed by attending general internists who precepted residents as they saw patients referred by their usual GIM provider (2).

Funding/Costs

Sometimes curricula can be accomplished by redeploying existing resources. If this appears to be the case, one should ask, what will be given up in redeploying the resources, i.e., what is the hidden or opportunity cost of the curriculum? When additional resources are required, they must be provided from somewhere. If additional funding is requested, it is necessary to develop and justify a budget.

Whether or not additional funding is requested, it is often useful to determine how a curriculum is funded and what it really costs.

EXAMPLE: *Financial Support and Opportunity Costs of a New Curriculum.* The Johns Hopkins Hospital Center for Innovation and Safety financially supported a two-day Patient Safety course offered to second-year medical students as preparation for their clinical clerkships. The curriculum included discussions of hospital patient safety initiatives, the strengths of high-reliability teamwork, and effective team communications. Simulation Center activities included stations dedicated to basic cardiac life support, sterile technique, infection control procedures, and isolation practices. In addition to obtaining financial support, curriculum developers had to obtain permission from faculty leaders in the medical students' pathophysiology course to block time from their course to allow students to attend the clerkship preparation course.

Curriculum developers must also be cognizant of the financial costs of conducting educational scholarship. In addition to whatever funds are needed to deliver the curriculum, funds may also be necessary to perform robust curriculum evaluation with a view toward dissemination of the curriculum. It has been shown that manuscripts reporting on well-funded curricula are of better quality and have higher rates of acceptance for publication in a peer-reviewed journal (3, 4).

OBTAINING SUPPORT FOR THE CURRICULUM

A curriculum is more likely to be successful in achieving its goals and objectives if it has broad support.

Internal Support

It is important that curriculum developers and coordinators recognize who are the stakeholders in a curriculum and foster their support. Stakeholders are those individuals who directly affect or are directly affected by a curriculum. For most curricula, stakeholders include the learners, the faculty who will deliver the curriculum, and individuals with administrative power within the institution. Having the support of *learners* when implementing the curriculum can make or break the curriculum. Adult learners, in particular, need to be convinced that the goals and objectives are important to them and that the curriculum has the means to achieve their personal goals (Chapter 5) (5, 6). Learners' opinions can also influence those with administrative power.

> **EXAMPLE:** *Support of Learners.* Evaluations and example videotapes from a curriculum in interviewing skills and the psychosocial domain of medical practice (7), which was developed in 1979 for general internal medicine residents, were shared with the department chair. As a result, the curriculum was expanded in 1983 to include traditional track as well as primary care track residents. When the primary care track temporarily lost its federal funding in 1987, consideration was given to eliminating the one-month "med-psych" rotation. On learning about this possibility, residents communicated their strong support for continuation of the training to the program director and department chair. This support was influential in the decision to maintain the curriculum and its associated faculty.

> **EXAMPLE:** *Support of Learners.* At an annual resident retreat residents proposed a restructuring of a required outpatient selective from a focus on gastroenterology to a "teaching resident rotation," which they saw as better use of their elective time. General goals of the two-week rotation were developed by the residents. The program director then charged an associate program director to further develop content and communicate with rotating residents and the medicine clerkship director to ensure that teaching sessions were scheduled with medical students.

Curricular faculty can devote varying amounts of their time, enthusiasm, and energy to the curriculum. Gaining broad faculty support may be important for some innovative curricula; for example, creating roles for subspecialists may foster their commitment to success of a generalist training program (1). *Other faculty* who have administrative influence or who may be competitors for curricular space or time can facilitate or create barriers for a curriculum.

> **EXAMPLE:** *Barriers from Other Faculty.* A new curriculum for a geriatrics elective in an internal medicine residency program was developed by junior faculty. Although the curriculum developers had met with key stakeholders along the way, they had not secured commitment from the director of the elective. When it came time to implement the curriculum, the director of the elective, an influential faculty member in the division, decided to continue to teach the old curriculum, rather than incorporate the new curriculum. The curriculum developers then modified the curriculum to make it suitable for fourth-year medical students and implemented it later that year.

Those with administrative authority (e.g., dean, hospital administrators, department chair, program director, division director) can allocate or deny the funds, space, faculty time, curricular time, and political support that are critical to a curriculum.

Individuals who feel that a curriculum is important, effective, and popular, who believe that a curriculum positively affects them or their institution, and who have had input into that curriculum are more likely to support it. It is, therefore, helpful to *encourage input* from stakeholders as the curriculum is being planned, as well as to *provide* stakeholders with the appropriate *rationale* (see Chapters 2 and 3) *and evaluation data* (Chapter 7) to address their concerns.

> **EXAMPLE:** *Early Success of Curriculum Convincing Stakeholder to Expand Program.* A one-month evidence-based medicine rotation was developed in the primary care track of a resi-

dency training program. Collation of resident evaluations of the curriculum, which were exceptionally positive, was shared with all stakeholders. Because the curriculum was so popular with the residents and so consistent with the values of internal medicine and the goals of the overall training program, the department chair asked that it be expanded during its second year to include all residents. To accommodate the curriculum, he created a second ambulatory block rotation without inpatient service requirements for the traditional (categorical) track residents.

Curriculum developers may need to *negotiate* with key stakeholders to obtain the political support and resources required to implement their curriculum successfully. Developing skills related to negotiation can therefore be useful. There are five generally recognized modes for conflict management (8–10). A *collaborative* or principled negotiation style that focuses on interests, not positions, is most frequently useful (11). When negotiating with those who have power or influence, this model would advise the curriculum developer to find areas of common ground, to understand the needs of the other party, and to focus on mutual interests, rather than negotiating from fixed positions. Most of the examples provided in this section have ingredients of a collaborative approach, in which the goal is a win-win solution. Sometimes one must settle for a *compromise* (less than ideal, better than nothing) solution. Occasionally, the curriculum developer may need to *compete* for resources and support, which creates the possibility of either winning or losing. At other times, *avoidance* or *accommodation* (see "barriers from other faculty" example above) may be the most reasonable approach, at least for certain aspects of the curriculum implementation. By engaging stakeholders, addressing their needs, providing a strong rationale, providing needs assessment and evaluation data, and building broad-based political support, curriculum developers put themselves in an advantageous bargaining position.

In some situations, the curriculum developer must be a change agent to champion curricular innovation at an institution. It helps if a new curriculum is consistent with the institution's mission, goals, and culture and if the institution is open to educational innovation (12). When these factors are not in place, it is necessary for the curriculum developer to become an agent of change (13–17).

EXAMPLE: *Becoming an Organizational Change Agent.* A junior faculty member identified as his academic focus improving the systems of care within health care organizations through quality improvement and educational interventions. Over several years he assumed increasing responsibility in positions of clinical care leadership, quality improvement, and patient safety at his academic medical center. In 1995 he introduced into the internal medicine residency training program a novel, collaborative multidisciplinary conference on patient care that examined systems issues, including use of resources (18). In 2001, he introduced a multidisciplinary Patient Safety and Quality of Care Conference into the residency training program. Two years later, because of the conference's popularity and unique approach, it replaced the traditional monthly morbidity and mortality conferences during Grand Rounds (19). This innovative morbidity and mortality conference used both systems and individual perspectives in a problem-solving manner without assigning blame. It has evolved to include a matrix to examine cases from both quality-of-care and core competencies perspectives (20–22). The conference has stimulated systems improvements in areas such as triage of patients into intensive care units, the placement and maintenance of intravenous lines, and management of patients with acute abdominal pain and vascular compromise. Organizational change has occurred, as evidenced by the promotion of a collaborative, multidisciplinary, system-based approach to the clinical and educational programs at the institution.

Organizational change can occur when the curriculum developer is intentional about creating a vision but also flexible in how the vision comes to fruition (13, 14).

External Support

Sometimes there are insufficient institutional resources to support part or all of a curriculum or to support its further development or expansion. In these situations, developing a sound budget and seeking a source of external support are critical.

Potential sources of *external funding* (see Appendix B) include government agencies, professional societies, philanthropic organizations or foundations, corporate entities, and individual donors. Research and development grants may be available from one's own institution, and the competition may be less intense than for truly external funds. External funds are more likely to be obtained when there has been a request for proposals by a funding source, when support is requested for an innovative or particularly needed curriculum, and when the funding is legitimately not available from internal sources. Funding for student summer jobs (usually by universities, professional schools, or professional societies) is another resource that may be available to support needed curricular or evaluation activities. A period of external funding can be used to build a level of internal support that may sustain the curriculum after cessation of external funding.

> **EXAMPLE:** *External Funding Leading to Institutional Support.* Federal funding was obtained in 1978 to develop a primary care track within an existing traditional internal medicine training program. From 1978 to 1987, a program was developed that included a much-expanded ambulatory primary care experience, training in interviewing skills and the psychosocial domain of medical practice (med-psych), and ambulatory training in a number of non-internal-medicine specialties. Grant requirements and the provision of funding led to initial political acceptance of these program components by internal stakeholders. Additional residents were hired to decrease inpatient service requirements, new faculty were hired to teach the med-psych curriculum, and existing general internal medicine (GIM) faculty increased their administrative and teaching time. The GIM track became a recruiting tool for the residency and developed national recognition and internal support independent of the external support. When federal funding ended temporarily from 1987 to 1990, and permanently after 1999, the hospital and faculty group funded the additional residents, faculty, and other curricular expenses.

Government, professional societies, and other entities may have *influence,* through their political or funding power, that can affect the degree of internal support for a curriculum. The curriculum developer may want to bring guidelines or requirements of such bodies to the attention of stakeholders within one's own institution.

> **EXAMPLE:** *Accreditation Standards.* ACGME (Accreditation Council for Graduate Medical Education) requirements (22) can have a major influence on a curriculum developer's institution. For example, ACGME requirements for written curricula with clearly articulated learning objectives have resulted in support by many institutions for the development of curricula in the six core competencies (patient care, medical knowledge, practice-based learning and improvement, interpersonal and communication skills, professionalism, and systems-based practice). The ACGME Outcome Project requires an assessment of a program's accomplishment in achieving learning objectives across the residency training experience (22).

Finally, professional societies or other institutions may have *curricular or faculty development resources* that can be used by curriculum developers (see Appendix B).

ADMINISTRATION OF THE CURRICULUM

Administrative Structure

A curriculum does not operate by itself. It requires an administrative structure to assume responsibility, to maintain communication, and to make operational and policy decisions (e.g., Who should one talk to about a problem with the curriculum? When should syllabus material be distributed? When and where will evaluation data be collected? Should there be a midpoint change in curricular content? Should a learner be assigned to a different faculty member?). Often these functions are those of the curriculum director. Some types of decisions can be delegated to a curriculum administrator for segments of the curriculum. Major policy changes may best be made with the help of a core faculty group or after even broader input. In any case, a structure for efficient communication and decision making should be established and made clear to faculty, learners, and support staff.

Communication

As implied above, the rationale, goals, and objectives of the curriculum, evaluation results, and changes in the curriculum need to be communicated in appropriate detail to all involved stakeholders. Lines of communication need to be open to and from the stakeholders. Therefore, the curriculum coordinator needs to establish *mechanisms for communication*, such as a Web site, periodic meetings, memos, syllabi, presentations, site visits or observations, and a policy regarding one's accessibility.

Operations

Mechanisms need to be developed to ensure that important functions that support the curriculum are performed. Such functions include preparing and distributing schedules and curricular materials, collecting and collating evaluation data, and supporting the communication function of the curriculum director. Large curricula usually have support staff to whom these functions can be delegated and who need to be supervised in their performance.

EXAMPLE: *Operation of a School-wide Curriculum.* A one-day course on research ethics for principal investigators and members of the research team in a medical school is coordinated through the combined efforts of the Office of Research Administration and the Office of Continuing Medical Education. An overall course director delegates operational functions to support staff from both offices, while serving as a point person for learners and faculty. Support staff in the Office of Research Administration administer the online curricular materials, while a course administrator in the Office of Continuing Medical Education communicates with learners and coordinates the logistics (registration of learners, printing and distribution of syllabus materials, scheduling classroom space, collection and analysis of evaluations, etc.).

Scholarship

As discussed in Chapter 9, curriculum developers may wish to disseminate, through presentation or publication, information related to their curricula, such as the needs assessment, curricular methods, or curricular evaluations. When dissemination is a goal, additional resources and administration may be required for more rigorous needs assessments, educational methodology, evaluation designs, data collection and analysis, and/or assessment instruments.

Curriculum developers also have to address ethical issues related to research (Chapter 7). Issues such as informed consent of learners, confidentiality, and the use of incentives to encourage participation in a curriculum all need to be considered (23). An increasingly important consideration is whether learners are to be classified as human research subjects. Federal regulations governing research in the United States categorize many educational research projects as exempt from the regulations if the research involves the study of normal educational practices or records information about learners in such a way that they cannot be identified (24). However, IRBs may differ in their interpretation of what is exempt under the regulations. Or some IRBs may want to ensure additional safeguards for learners than what the regulations require. It is, therefore, prudent for curriculum developers to seek guidance from their IRBs about how best to protect the rights and interests of the learners who are also research subjects (25, 26). Failure to consult one's IRB before implementation of the curriculum can have adverse consequences for the curriculum developer who later tries to publish research about the curriculum (27).

ANTICIPATING BARRIERS

Before initiating a new curriculum or making changes in an old curriculum, it is helpful to anticipate and address any potential barriers to their accomplishment. Barriers can relate to finances, other resources, or people (e.g., competing demands for resources; nonsupportive attitudes; issues of job or role security, credit, and political power) (28).

> **EXAMPLE:** *Competition.* In planning the ambulatory component of the internal medicine clerkship for third-year medical students, the curriculum developer anticipated resistance from the inpatient clerkship director, based on loss of curricular time and responsibility/power. The curriculum developer built a well-reasoned argument for the ambulatory component based on external recommendations and current needs. She ensured student support for the change and the support of critical faculty. She gained support from the dean's office and was granted additional curricular time for the ambulatory component, which addressed some of the inpatient director's concerns about loss of curricular time for training on the inpatient services. She invited the inpatient coordinator to be on the planning committee for the ambulatory component, to increase his understanding of needs, to promote his sense of ownership and responsibility for the ambulatory component, and to promote coordination of learning and educational methodology between the inpatient and ambulatory components.

> **EXAMPLE:** *Resistance.* The developers of a tool to evaluate the surgical skills of residents anticipated resistance from faculty in completing an evaluation after each surgery. They therefore had to make the evaluation tool user-friendly and readily accessible. Knowing that collection and collation of paper-based forms would be cumbersome and difficult, the curriculum developers created an online instrument. Because the evaluation would be completed postoperatively, when there were still patient care issues to address, the developers also anticipated the need to make the instrument brief enough to be completed in a couple of minutes.

INTRODUCING THE CURRICULUM

Piloting

It is important to pilot critical segments of a new curriculum on friendly or convenient audiences before formally introducing it. Critical segments might include needs assessment and evaluation instruments, as well as educational methods. Piloting enables curriculum developers to receive critical feedback and to make important revisions that increase the likelihood of successful implementation.

> **EXAMPLE:** *Piloting.* For a new course on research ethics for all faculty conducting human subjects research in the school of medicine, course developers first piloted the curriculum in an abbreviated fashion during the orientation for new faculty. The pilot mainly involved the use of small group workshops in which participants commented on the ethical issues involved in a mock research protocol. Piloting the curriculum on new faculty allowed curriculum developers to get a fresh perspective from learners not yet familiar with institutional culture. Feedback was obtained from learners and course faculty to aid in shaping the eventual curriculum that was rolled out to the entire faculty the subsequent year.

Phasing in

Phasing in a complex curriculum one part at a time or the entire curriculum on a segment of the targeted learners permits a focusing of initial efforts, as faculty and staff learn new procedures. When the curriculum represents a cultural shift in an institution or requires attitudinal changes in the stakeholders, introducing the curriculum one step at a time, rather than all at once, can lessen resistance and increase acceptance, particularly if the stakeholders are involved in the process (13). Like piloting, phasing in affords the opportunity to have a cycle of experience, feedback, evaluation, and response before full implementation.

> **EXAMPLE:** *Prolonged Phase-in.* When the previously described med-psych curriculum was first introduced in 1979, interviewing skills and the psychosocial domain of medical practice were not widely accepted components of internal medicine training. It was required and funded, however, by the primary care training grant the department had received. During the first few years, the curriculum was co-taught by behavioral science faculty experienced in the teaching of communication skills and psychiatry but not in the practice of internal medicine and by internal medicine faculty interested but inexperienced in teaching the content of the curriculum. The learners were residents who had been recruited specifically for the primary care track and who were generally receptive to the material. The program evolved, based on development of both the behavioral science and internal medicine faculty, feedback from an interested group of residents, and frequent faculty interaction and observation of residents. Early feedback from residents, for example, led to the abandonment of lectures on interviewing skills and to an increase in the number of sessions devoted to role-playing, simulated patient exercises, and videotape reviews. By 1983, the curriculum was considered so successful that the department contributed additional resources to expand it to include all residents. This is an example of a prolonged phase-in period that permitted time not only for revisions in the curriculum but also for faculty development and some cultural shifts in the internal medicine department.

Both the piloting and phasing-in approaches to implementing a curriculum advertise it as a curriculum in development, increase participant tolerance and desire to help, decrease faculty resistance to negative feedback, and increase the chance for success on full implementation.

Full Implementation

In general, full implementation should follow a piloting and/or phasing-in experience. Sometimes, however, the demand for a full curriculum for all learners is so pressing, or a curriculum is so limited in scope, that immediate full implementation is preferable. In this case, the first cycle of the curriculum can be considered a "pilot" cycle. Evaluation data on educational outcomes (i.e., achievement of goals and objectives) and processes (i.e., milestones of curriculum delivery) from initial cycles of a curriculum can then be used to refine the implementation of subsequent cycles (29, 30). (See Chapter 7.) Of course, a successful curriculum should always be in a stage of continuous improvement, as described in Chapter 8.

INTERACTION WITH OTHER STEPS

As one thinks through what is required to implement a curriculum as it has initially been conceived, one often discovers that there are insufficient resources and administrative structures to support such a curriculum. The curriculum developer should not become discouraged. With insight about the targeted learners and their learning environment, further prioritization and focusing of curricular objectives, educational strategies, and/or evaluation are required. For this reason it is usually wise to be thinking of Step 5 (Implementation) in conjunction with Step 2 (Targeted Needs Assessment), Step 3 (Goals and Objectives), Step 4 (Educational Strategies), and Step 6 (Evaluation).

It is better to anticipate problems than to discover them too late. Curriculum development is an interactive cyclical process, and each step affects the others. It may be more prudent to start small and build on a curriculum's success than to aim too high and watch the curriculum fail due to unachievable goals, insufficient resources, or inadequate support. *Implementation is the step that converts a mental exercise to reality.*

QUESTIONS

For the curriculum you are coordinating, planning, or would like to be planning, please answer or think about the questions below. If your thoughts about a curriculum are just beginning, you may wish to answer these questions in the context of a few educational strategies, such as the ones you identified in your answers to the questions at the end of Chapter 5.

1. What *resources* are required for the curriculum you envision, in terms of personnel, time, and facilities? Will your faculty need specialized training before implementation? Did you remember to think of patients as well as faculty and support staff? What are the internal costs of this curriculum? Is there need for external resources or funding? If there is a need for external funding, construct a budget. Finally, are your curricular plans feasible in terms of the required resources?

2. What is the degree of *support* within your institution for the curriculum? Where will the resistance come from? How could you increase support and decrease resistance? How likely is it that you will get the support necessary? Will external support be necessary? If so, what are possible sources and what is the nature of the support that is required (e.g., funds, resource materials, political support)?

3. What sort of *administration,* in terms of *administrative structure, communications, operations, and scholarship,* is necessary to implement and maintain the curriculum? Think of how decisions will be made, how communication will take place, and what operations are necessary for the smooth functioning of the curriculum (e.g., preparation and distribution of schedules, curricular and evaluation materials, evaluation reports). Are IRB review and approval of an educational research project needed?

4. What *barriers* do you anticipate to implementing the curriculum? Develop plans for addressing them.

5. Develop plans to *introduce* the curriculum. What are the most critical segments of the curriculum that would be a priority for *piloting*? On whom would you pilot it? Can the curriculum be *phased in*, or must it be implemented all at once on all learners? How will you learn from piloting and phasing in the curriculum and apply this learning to the curriculum? If you are planning on full implementation, what structures are in place to provide feedback to the curriculum for further improvements?

6. Given your answers to questions 1 through 5, is your curriculum likely to be feasible and successful? Do you need to go back to the drawing board and alter your approach to some of the steps?

GENERAL REFERENCES

Glanz K, Rimer BK, Lewis FM, eds. *Health Behavior and Health Education: Theory, Research and Practice,* 3rd ed. San Francisco: Jossey-Bass; 2002.
> This book reviews theories and models for behavioral change important in delivering health education. Health education involves an awareness of the impact of communication, interpersonal relationships, and community on those who are targeted for behavioral change. For the curriculum developer, the chapters on diffusion of innovations and organizational change are particularly relevant. Chapter 14 (pp. 312–34) describes diffusion as a multilevel change process, with success achieved not just by demonstrating efficacy and effectiveness but also by actively implementing strategies to ensure sustainability. Chapter 15 (pp. 335–60) advances the idea that establishment of an education program often involves some degree of organizational change. The chapter reviews the history and characteristics of organizational development theory and includes two health care application examples. 583 pages.

Gray CF, Larson EW. *Project Management: The Managerial Process,* 4th ed. New York: McGraw-Hill/Irwin; 2008.
> A book written for the professional or student business manager but of interest to anyone overseeing the planning and implementation of a project. The book guides the reader through 16 steps in project management, from defining the problem and planning an intervention to executing the project and overseeing its impact. 589 pages.

King JA, Morris LY, Fitz-Gibbon CT. *How to Assess Program Implementation.* Newbury Park, Calif.: Sage Publications; 1987.
> The focus of this book is on planning and executing an evaluation of how well a program has been implemented. Especially useful is the appendix, which contains more than 300 questions to consider when doing an implementation evaluation on all aspects of a program, which in turn are important areas to consider when initially planning and implementing a program. 143 pages.

Knowles MS, Holton EF, Swanson RA. *The Adult Learner: the Definitive Classic in Adult Education and Human Resource Development.* 6th ed. Burlington, Mass.: Elsevier; 2005.

The classic text that reviews learning theory, with emphasis on andragogy and the key principles in adult learning, including the learner's need to know, the learner's self-concept of autonomy, the importance of prior experience, the learner's readiness to learn, the learner's problem-based orientation to learning, and the learner's motivation to learn derived from the intrinsic value and personal payoff from learning. Includes suggestions on how to put andragogy into practice. 390 pages.

Kolbe LJ, Iverson DC. Implementing comprehensive school health education: educational innovation and social change. *Health Education Quarterly.* 1981;8:57–80.
Well-written article about school health education programs with high applicability to curricula in the medical school and hospital teaching environment. Included are sections on five approaches to analyzing program implementation, characteristics of programs that influence their diffusion, four approaches to implementing educational innovations, four levels or stages of implementation, and maintenance or continuation of a health program.

Kotter JP. *Leading Change.* Boston: Harvard Business School Press; 1996.
An excellent book on leadership, differentiating leadership and management, and outlining the qualities of a good leader. The author discusses eight steps critical to creating major change in an organization: 1) establishing a sense of urgency, 2) creating a guiding coalition, 3) developing a vision and strategy, 4) communicating the change vision, 5) empowering broad-based action, 6) generating short-term wins, 7) consolidating gains and producing more change, and 8) anchoring new approaches in the culture. 187 pages.

Lewis JP. *The Project Manager's Desk Reference,* 3rd ed. New York: McGraw-Hill; 2007.
A comprehensive text on project management applying systems-based thinking to the process. Some of the material is directed more at the business professional, but overarching concepts will be helpful to the curriculum developer. Includes a glossary of terms, as well as a description of the life cycle of a project, with checklists for each stage in the management of a project. 584 pages.

Meyerson D. *Tempered Radicals: How People Use Differences to Inspire Change at Work.* Boston: Harvard Business School Press; 2001.
Describes individuals who work within an organization, balancing organizational views with other perspectives and their own values, to achieve fundamental change. 240 pages.

Rogers EM. *Diffusion of Innovations,* 5th ed. New York: Free Press; 2003.
Classic text describing all aspects and stages of the process whereby new phenomena are adopted and diffused throughout social systems. The book contains a discussion of the elements of diffusion, the history and status of diffusion research, the generation of innovations, the innovation-decision process, attributes of innovations and their rate of adoption, innovativeness and adopter categories, opinion leadership and diffusion networks, the change agent, innovations in organizations, and consequences of innovations. Among many other disciplines, education, public health, and medical sociology have made practical use of the theory with empirical research of Rogers's work. Implementation is addressed specifically in several pages (pp. 179–88, 430–32), highlighting the great importance of implementation to the diffusion process. 551 pages.

Romiszowski AJ. Why projects fail (Chapter 30). In: *Designing Instructional Systems: Decision Making in Course Planning and Curriculum Design.* New York: Nichols Publishing; 1981.
This chapter details the stages of implementing an educational program, sources of potential failure in those stages, and how to avoid failure. The author reviews the concept of scale effect, pointing out factors in small, medium, and large instructional designs where problems can arise. The chapter includes several "information maps" for addressing sources of failure in implementation, dissemination, and/or reproduction of an educational program. Pp. 380–97.

Westley F, Zimmerman B, Patton MQ. *Getting to Maybe: How the World Is Changed.* Toronto: Random House Canada; 2006.
Richly illustrated with real-world examples, this book focuses on complex organizations and social change. Change can come from the bottom up as well as the top down. The authors contend that an agent of change needs to have intentionality and flexibility, must recognize that achieving success can have peaks and valleys, should understand that relationships are key to engaging in

social intervention, and must have a mind-set framed by inquiry rather than certitude. With this framework, the book outlines the steps necessary to achieve change for complex problems. 258 pages.

Whitman N, Weiss E. *Executive Skills for Medical Faculty,* 3rd ed. Pacific Grove, Calif.: Whitman Associates; 2006.
Many of the skills needed by health care leaders are also important for successful development and implementation of curricula, such as improving communication skills, becoming a leader, working through others, negotiating, implementing change, strategic planning, getting things done, team building and coaching, and planning a career strategy. 195 pages.

SPECIFIC REFERENCES

1. Lemon M, Greer T, Siegel B. Implementation issues in generalist education. *J Gen Intern Med.* 1994;9(Suppl 1):S98–104.
2. Houston TK, Connors RL, Cutler N, Nidiry MA. A primary care musculoskeletal clinic for residents: success and sustainability. *J Gen Intern Med.* 2004;19(5 Pt 2):524–29.
3. Reed DA, Cook DA, Beckman TJ, Levine RB, Kern DE, Wright SM. Association between funding and quality of published medical education research. *JAMA.* 2007;298:1002–9.
4. Reed DA, Beckman TJ, Wright SM, Levine RB, Kern DE, Cook DA. Predictive validity evidence for medical education research study quality instrument scores: quality of submissions to JGIM's Medical Education Special Issue. *J Gen Intern Med.* 2008 Jul;23(7):903–7.
5. Knowles MS, Holton EF, Swanson RA. *The Adult Learner: the Definitive Classic in Adult Education and Human Resource Development,* 6th ed. Burlington, Mass.: Elsevier; 2005.
6. Brookfield S. *Understanding and Facilitating Adult Learning.* San Francisco: Jossey-Bass; 1986.
7. Kern DE, Grayson M, Barker LR, Roca RP, Cole KA, Roter D, Golden A. Residency training in interviewing skills and the psychosocial domain of medical practice. *J Gen Intern Med.* 1989;4:421–31.
8. Thomas KW. *Introduction to Conflict Management: Improving Performance Using the TKI.* Mountain View, Calif.: CPP; 2002.
9. Thomas KW, Thomas GF. *Introduction to Conflict and Teams: Enhancing Team Performance Using the TKI.* Mountain View, Calif.: CPP; 2004.
10. Womack DF. Assessing the Thomas-Kilmann Conflict Mode Survey. *Management Communication Quarterly.* 1988;1:321–49.
11. Fisher R, Ury W. *Getting to Yes: Negotiating Agreement without Giving In,* 2nd ed. New York: Penguin Books; 1991.
12. Bland CJ, Starnaman S, Wersal L, Moorehead-Rosenberg L, Zonia S, Henry R. Curricular change in medical schools: how to succeed. *Acad Med.* 2000;75(6):575–94.
13. Kotter JP. *Leading Change.* Boston: Harvard Business School Press; 1996.
14. Westley F, Zimmerman B, Patton MQ. *Getting to Maybe: How the World Is Changed..* Toronto: Random House Canada; 2006.
15. Cameron KS, Quinn RE. *Diagnosing and Changing Organizational Culture: Based on the Competing Values Framework.* San Francisco: Jossey-Bass; 2006.
16. de Caluwé L, Vermaak H. *Learning to Change: A Guide for Organization Change Agents.* Thousand Oaks, Calif.: Sage Publications; 2003.
17. Meyerson D. *Tempered Radicals: How People Use Differences to Inspire Change at Work.* Boston: Harvard Business School Press; 2001.
18. Kravet SJ, Wright, SW, Carrese JA. Teaching resource and information management using an innovative case-based conference. *J Gen Intern Med.* 2001;16(6):399–403.

19. Kravet SJ, Wright SM. Morbidity and mortality conference, grand rounds, and the ACGME's core competencies. *J Gen Intern Med.* 2006;21(11):1192–94.

20. Report of The Committee on Quality of Health Care in America. Institute of Medicine. *Crossing the Quality Chasm: A New Health System for the 21st Century.* Washington, D.C.: National Academies Press; 2001.

21. Quinn DC, Bingham JW, Shourbaji NA, Jarquin-valdivia AA. Medical students learn to assess care using the healthcare matrix. *Med Teach.* 2007;29(7):660–65.

22. Accreditation Council for Graduate Medical Education. See Review Committees/Program Requirements, and Outcome Project. Available at www.acgme.org. Accessed March 11, 2009.

23. Roberts LW, Geppert C, Connor R, Nguyen K, Warner TD. An invitation for medical educators to focus on ethical and policy issues in research and scholarly practice. *Acad Med.* 2001;76(9):876–85.

24. Miser WF. Educational research—to IRB, or not to IRB? *Fam Med.* 2005;37(3):168–73.

25. Henry RC, Wright DE. When do medical students become human subjects of research? The case of program evaluation. *Acad Med.* 2001 Sep;76(9):871–75.

26. Dyrbye LN, Thomas MR, Papp KK, Durning SJ. Clinician educators' experiences with institutional review boards: results of a national survey. *Acad Med.* 2008 Jun;83(6):590–95.

27. Tomkowiak JM, Gunderson AJ. To IRB or not to IRB? *Acad Med.* 2004 Jul;79(7):628–32.

28. Whitman N. Implementing change. In: Whitman N, Weiss E, eds. *Executive Skills for Medical Faculty.* 3rd ed. Pacific Grove, Calif.: Whitman Associates; 2006. Pp. 71–87.

29. Scheirer MA, Shediac MC, Cassady CE. Measuring the implementation of health promotion programs: the case of the Breast and Cervical Cancer Program in Maryland. *Health Education Research.* 1995;10(1):11–25.

30. Cassady CE, Orth DA, Guyer B, Goggin ML. Measuring the implementation of injury prevention programs in state health agencies. *Injury Prevention.* 1997;3:94–99.

CHAPTER SEVEN

Step 6
Evaluation and Feedback

. . . assessing the achievement of objectives and stimulating continuous improvement

Pamela A Lipsett, M.D., and David E. Kern, M.D., M.P.H.

DEFINITIONS

Evaluation, for the purposes of this book, is defined as the identification, clarification, and application of criteria to determine the merit or worth of what is being evaluated (1). While often used interchangeably, assessment is sometimes used to connote characterizations and measurements while evaluation is used to connote appraisal or judgment. In education, assessment is often of an individual student, while evaluation is of a program; for the most part, we follow this convention in this chapter. Feedback is defined as the provision of information on an individual's or curriculum's performance to learners, faculty, and other stakeholders in the curriculum.

IMPORTANCE

Step 6, Evaluation and Feedback, closes the loop in the curriculum development cycle. The evaluation process helps those who have a stake in the curriculum make a decision or judgment about the curriculum. The evaluation step helps curriculum developers ask and answer the critical question, "Were the goals and objectives of the curriculum met?" Evaluation provides information that can be used to guide individuals and the curriculum in cycles of ongoing improvement. Evaluation results can also be used to maintain and garner support for a curriculum, to assess student achievement, to satisfy external requirements, to document the accomplishments of curriculum developers, and to serve as a basis for presentations and publications.

It is helpful to be methodical in designing the evaluation for a curriculum, to ensure that important questions are answered and relevant needs met. This chapter outlines a 10-task approach that begins with consideration of the potential users and uses of an evaluation, moves to the identification of evaluation questions and methods, proceeds to the collection of data, and ends with data analysis and reporting of results.

TASK I: IDENTIFY USERS

The first step in planning the evaluation for a curriculum is to identify the likely users of the evaluation. *Participants* in the curriculum have an interest in the assessment of their own performance and the performance of the curriculum. Evaluation can provide feedback and motivation for continued improvement for *learners*, *faculty,* and *curriculum developers*.

Other stakeholders who have administrative responsibility for, allocate resources to, or are otherwise affected by the curriculum will also be interested in evaluation results. These might include individuals in the *dean's office, hospital administrators,* the *department chair,* the *program director* for the residency program or medical student education, the *division director, other faculty* who have contributed political support or who might be in competition for limited resources, and *individuals, granting agencies, or other organizations that have contributed funds or other resources* to the curriculum. Individuals who need to make decisions about whether or not to participate in the curriculum, such as *future learners or faculty*, may also be interested in evaluation results.

To the extent that a curriculum innovatively addresses an important need or tests new educational strategies, evaluation results may also be of interest to *educators from other institutions* and serve as a basis for publications/presentations. As society is often the intended beneficiary of a medical care curriculum, society members are also stake-holders in this process.

Finally, evaluation results can document the achievements of *curriculum develop-ers*. Promotion committees and department chairs assign a high degree of importance to clinician-educators' accomplishments in curriculum development (2, 3), and these accomplishments can be included in the educational portfolios that are increasingly being used to support applications for promotion (4–6).

TASK II: IDENTIFY USES

Generic Uses

In designing an evaluation strategy for a curriculum, the curriculum developer should be aware of the generic uses of an evaluation. These generic uses can be clas-sified along two axes, as shown in Table 7.1. The first axis refers to whether the evalu-ation is used to appraise the performance of *individuals*, the performance of the entire *program,* or both. The assessment of an individual usually involves determining wheth-er he/she has achieved the cognitive, affective, or psychomotor objectives of a curricu-lum (see Chapter 4). Program evaluation usually determines the aggregate achieve-ments of all individuals, clinical or other outcomes, the actual processes of a curricu-lum, or the perceptions of learners and faculty. The second axis in Table 7.1 refers to whether an evaluation is used for *formative* purposes (to improve performance) (7), for *summative* purposes (to judge performance and make decisions about its future or adoption) (8), or for both purposes.

From the discussion and examples below, the reader may surmise that *some eval-uations can be used for both summative and formative purposes.* The evaluation of specific curricular components, for example, can be used not only to judge their effec-tiveness but also to target areas for revision.

Specific Uses

Having identified the likely users of the evaluation and understood the generic uses of curriculum evaluation, the curriculum developer should consider the specific needs of different users and the specific ways in which they will put the evaluation to use (9, 10). Specific uses for evaluation results might include the following:

- *Feedback on and improvement of individual performance:* Both learners and faculty can use the results of timely feedback (formative individual assessment) to direct improvements in their own performances. This type of assessment identifies areas for improvement and provides specific suggestions for improvement (feedback). It, therefore, also serves as an educational method (see Chapter 5).

  EXAMPLE: *Formative Individual Assessment.* During an ambulatory medicine clerkship, stu-dents perform a history and physical examination on a standardized patient with low back pain and are given specific oral feedback about both history taking and performance of the physical examination to improve their performance.

- *Judgments regarding individual performance:* The accomplishments of individual learners may need to be documented (summative individual assessment) to assign grades, to demonstrate mastery in a particular area or achievement of certain

Table 7.1.   Evaluation Types: Levels and Uses

Use	Level	
	Individual	Program
Formative	Evaluation of an individual learner or faculty member that is used to help the individual improve performance: - identification of areas for improvement - specific suggestions for improvement	Evaluation of a program that is used to improve program performance: - identification of areas for improvement - specific suggestions for improvement
Summative	Evaluation of an individual learner or faculty member that is used for judgments or decisions about the individual: - verification of achievement for individual - motivation of individual to maintain or improve performance - certification of performance for others - grades - promotion	Evaluation of a program that is used for judgments or decisions about the program or program developers: - judgments regarding success, efficacy - decisions regarding allocation of resources - motivation/recruitment of learners and faculty - influencing attitudes regarding value of curriculum - satisfying external requirements - prestige, power, influence, promotion - dissemination: presentations, publications

curricular objectives, or to satisfy the demands of external bodies, such as specialty boards. In these instances, it is important to clarify criteria for the achievement of objectives or competency before the evaluation. Assessment of individual faculty can be used to make decisions about their continuation as curriculum faculty, as material for their promotion portfolios, and as data for teaching awards. Used in this manner, assessments become evaluations.

EXAMPLE: *Summative Individual Assessment.* At the conclusion of the ambulatory medicine clerkship in a multistation Objective Structured Clinical Examination (OSCE), each student conducts a focused history and physical examination on a standardized patient with back pain and is assessed using a checklist form, from which a passing score in each station determines mastery of both the history and physical examination.

- *Feedback on and improvement of program performance:* Curriculum coordinators can use evaluation results (formative program evaluation) to identify parts of the curriculum that are effective and parts that are in need of improvement. Evaluation results may also provide suggestions about how parts of the curriculum could be improved.

Such formative program evaluation usually takes the form of surveys (see Chapter 3) of learners to obtain feedback about and suggestions for improving a curriculum. Quantitative information, such as ratings of various aspects of the curriculum, can help identify areas that need revision. Qualitative information, such as responses to open-ended questions about program strengths, program weaknesses, and suggestions for change, provides feedback in areas that may not have been anticipated and ideas for improvement. Information can also be obtained from faculty or other observers, such as nurses and patients. Aggregates of formative and summative individual assessments can be used for formative program evaluation as well, to identify specific areas of the curriculum in need of revision.

EXAMPLE: *Formative Program Evaluation.* At the midpoint of a neurology clinical clerkship, students met with the clerkship director for a discussion of experiences to date. Several students wanted additional patient responsibilities while on ward rounds. The clerkship director reviewed this information with neurology faculty and team leaders, who implemented measures to encourage more active participation of students in ward rounds.

EXAMPLE: *Formative Program Evaluation.* After each didactic lecture of the surgery residency curriculum, residents were asked to complete an evaluation form, which asked them to rate the effectiveness of the speaker and the usefulness of the talk. The residents did not find an introductory lecture on postoperative respiratory complications as useful as they had previously because it now followed a lecture on mechanical ventilation, which covered the most severe complications. The sequence of didactic experiences was reordered, and the content of the lecture on mechanical ventilation was adjusted to reinforce and extend learning on complications from the introductory lecture.

- *Judgments regarding program success:* Summative program evaluation provides information on the degree to which a curriculum has met its various objectives and expectations under what specific conditions and at what cost. It can also document the curriculum's success in engaging, motivating, and pleasing its learners and faculty. In addition to quantitative data, summative program evaluation may include qualitative information about unintended barriers, unanticipated factors encountered in the program implementation, or unintended consequences of the curriculum. It may identify aspects of the hidden curriculum (11, 12). The results of summative program evaluations are often reported to others to obtain or maintain curricular time, funding, and other resources.

EXAMPLE: *Summative Program Evaluation.* At the conclusion of an ambulatory clinical clerkship, 90% of students received a passing grade in the performance of a standardized patient examination, which assessed five cognitive and nine skill objectives in the areas of history, physical examination, diagnosis, management, and counseling.

EXAMPLE: *Summative Program Evaluation Leading to Further Investigation and Change.* One curricular objective of an intensive care unit (ICU) rotation stated that surgery residents would correctly prescribe and use noninvasive positive pressure ventilation (NIPPV) in lieu of intubation and mechanical ventilation in eligible patients. During the residents' second ICU rotation later that year, the use of NIPPV was examined and compared with the use of mechanical ventilation. NIPPV was not used in spite of residents correctly prescribing respiratory support. Examination of the reasons why NIPPV had not been used revealed a shortage of NIPPV devices. Review of this information with department administrators led to leasing of NIPPV devices as need was determined.

EXAMPLE: *Summative Program Evaluation Leading to Curricular Expansion.* Summative evaluation results of a curriculum directed at improving interpersonal skills, teamwork, and communication in first-year residents revealed a high level of learner, staff, and patient satisfaction and decreases in both patient/staff complaints and adverse events. As a result of the success with the first-year residents, the curriculum was expanded as additional resources became available, first to all resident levels and later to faculty.

- *Justification for the allocation of resources:* Those with administrative authority can use evaluation results (summative program evaluation) to guide and justify decisions about the allocation of resources for a curriculum, and they may be more likely to allocate limited resources to a curriculum if the evaluation provides evidence of success. In the above example, program success led to an expanded allocation of resources.

- *Motivation and recruitment:* Feedback on individual and program success and the identification of areas for future improvement can be motivational to faculty (formative and summative individual assessment and program evaluation). Evidence of program success can also help in the recruitment of future faculty and learners (summative program evaluation), as well as recruitment of a specialized patient population.

- *Attitude change:* Evidence that significant change has occurred in learners (summative program evaluation) with the use of an unfamiliar method, such as participation in quality improvement projects, or in a previously unaccepted content area, such as systems-based practice, can significantly alter attitudes about the importance of such methods and content.

- *Satisfaction of external and internal requirements:* Summative individual and program evaluation results can be used to satisfy the requirements of regulatory bodies, such as Residency Review and Graduate Medical Education Committees, and therefore will be welcomed by those who have administrative responsibility for an overall program.

- *Demonstration of popularity:* Evidence that learners and faculty truly enjoyed and valued their experience (summative program evaluation) and evidence of other stakeholder support (patients, benefactors) may be important to educational and other administrative leaders, who want to satisfy their existing trainees, faculty, and other stakeholders and recruit new ones. A high degree of learner, faculty, and stakeholder support provides strong political support for a curriculum.

- *Prestige, power, promotion, and influence:* A successful program (summative program evaluation) reflects positively on its institution, department chair, division chief, overall program director, curriculum coordinator, and faculty, thereby conveying a certain degree of prestige, power, and influence. Summative program and individual assessment data can be used as evidence of accomplishment in one's promotion portfolio.

- *Presentations, publications, and adoption of curricular components by others:* To the degree that an evaluation (summative program evaluation) provides evidence of the success (or failure) of an innovative or insufficiently studied educational program or method, it will be of interest to educators at other institutions and to publishers (see Chapter 9).

TASK III: IDENTIFY RESOURCES

The most carefully planned evaluation will fail if the resources are not available to accomplish it (13). Limits in resources may require prioritization of evaluation questions and changes in evaluation methods. For this reason, curriculum developers should *consider resource needs early in the planning of the evaluation process*, including *time, personnel, equipment, facilities,* and *funds.* Appropriate *time* should be allocated for the collection, analysis, and reporting of evaluation results. *Personnel* needs often include staff to help in the collection and collation of data and distribution of reports, as well as people with statistical or computer expertise to help verify and analyze the data. *Equipment and facilities* might include the appropriate computer hardware and software. *Funding* from internal or external sources is required for resources that are not otherwise available, in which case a budget and budget justification may have to be developed.

Often formal funding is not available, but informal networking will reveal potential assistance locally, such as computer programmers or biostatisticians interested in measurements pertinent to the curriculum, or quality improvement personnel in a hospital interested in measuring patient outcomes. Survey instruments can be adopted from other residency programs or clerkships within an institution or can be shared among institutions. Medical schools and residency programs often have summative assessments in place for students and residents, in the form of subject, specialty board, and in-service training examinations. Specific information on learner performance in the knowledge areas addressed by these tests can be readily accessed through the department chair with little cost to the curriculum.

> **EXAMPLE:** *Use of an Existing Resource for Curricular Evaluation.* An objective of an infection prevention curriculum for anesthesia residents is the prevention of surgical site infections and the appropriate administration of prophylactic antibiotics within 60 minutes of an operative incision. The evaluation plan included the need for a follow-up audit of this practice, but resources were not available for this independent audit. The information was then added to the comprehensive electronic intraoperative record collected by the operating room staff, which provided both measures of individual resident performance and overall program success in the timely administration of antibiotics.

TASK IV: IDENTIFY EVALUATION QUESTIONS

Most evaluation questions (14–16) should relate to the specific measurable learner, process, or clinical outcome objectives of a curriculum (see Chapter 4). As described in Chapter 4, specific measurable objectives should state who will do how much (how well) of what by when. The "who" may refer to learners or instructors, or to the program itself, if one is evaluating program activities. "How much (how well) of what by when" provides a standard of acceptability that is measurable. Often, in the process of writing evaluation questions and thinking through what designs and methods might be able to answer a question, it becomes clear that a curricular objective needs further clarification.

> **EXAMPLE:** *Clarifying an Objective for the Purpose of Evaluation.* An objective, as initially drafted, stated, "By the end of the curriculum, all residents will be proficient in smoking cessation counseling." In formulating the evaluation question and thinking through the evaluation methodology, it became clear to the curriculum developers that "proficient" needed to be defined operationally. Also, they decided that they would consider the curriculum a success if 90% or more of the residents were proficient by the end of the curriculum, and if there was a statistically and quantitatively significant (>25%) increase in the number of residents who were proficient by the end of the curriculum. After appropriate revisions in the objective, the evaluation questions became "By the end of the curriculum, what percent of residents

have achieved a passing score on the curriculum's proficiency checklist for smoking cessation counseling, as assessed using standardized patients?" and "Has there been a statistically and quantitatively (>25%) significant increase in the number of proficient residents, as defined above, from the beginning to the end of the curriculum?"

The curriculum developer should also make sure that the evaluation question is *congruent* with the related curricular objective.

EXAMPLE: *Congruency between an Objective and the Evaluation Question.* An objective of the interpersonal skills and communication workshop is that residents will become proficient in obtaining informed consent for invasive procedures that includes six identified critical elements (a skill or competence objective). The evaluation question "In what percentage of eligible patients do residents obtain appropriate informed consent?" is not congruent with the objective because the evaluation question addressed a behavioral or performance objective and not a skill objective (see Chapter 4). A congruent evaluation question would be "By the end of the workshop, what percentage of residents are able to obtain informed consent that includes all six critical elements during an observed patient encounter?" Curriculum developers may ask themselves whether they want to include a behavioral objective. If so, educational methods would be required in an expanded curriculum that addresses attitudes (such as discussions and experiences that reinforce residents' sense of the importance of and their responsibility for appropriately obtaining informed consent), the hidden curriculum (e.g., staff development to ensure that faculty demonstrate obtaining informed consent appropriately and faculty and nurses reinforce doing so when they observe residents), and environmental factors (e.g., making available general and procedure-specific forms that enable informed consent).

Often resources will limit the number of objectives for which accomplishment can be assessed. In this situation it is necessary to *prioritize and select key evaluation questions*, based on the needs of the users and the feasibility of the related evaluation methodology. Sometimes several objectives can be grouped efficiently into a single evaluation question.

EXAMPLE: *Prioritizing Which Objective to Evaluate.* A curriculum has cognitive, attitudinal, skill, and behavioral objectives related to the prevention of central venous catheter bloodstream infections. The curriculum coordinators decided that what mattered most was postcurricular behavior or performance, and that effective performance required achievement of the appropriate cognitive, attitudinal, and skill objectives. Central venous catheters must be placed, used, and maintained under specific conditions in order to prevent infection. Their evaluation question and evaluation methodology, therefore, assessed postcurricular behaviors, rather than knowledge, attitudes, or technical skill mastery. It was assumed that if the performance objectives were met, there would be sufficient accomplishment of the knowledge, attitude, and skill objectives.

Not all evaluation questions need to relate to explicit, written curricular objectives. Some curricular objectives are implicitly understood, but not written down, to prevent a curriculum document from becoming unwieldy. Most curriculum developers, for example, will want to *include evaluation questions that relate to the effectiveness of specific curricular components or faculty,* even when the related objectives are implicit rather than explicit.

EXAMPLE: *Evaluation Question Directed toward Curricular Processes.* What was the perceived effectiveness of the curriculum's small group discussions, simulated patients, clinical experiences, and required case presentations?

Sometimes there are unexpected strengths and weaknesses in a curriculum. Sometimes the curriculum on paper may differ from the curriculum as delivered (17). Therefore, it is almost always helpful to *include some evaluation questions that do not relate to specific curricular objectives and that are open ended in nature*.

> **EXAMPLES:** *Use of Open-ended Questions Related to Curricular Processes.* What actually happens during the learning sessions? What issues are most frequently raised, and how are they addressed? What do learners perceive as the major strengths and weaknesses of the curriculum? Did the sessions proceed as planned? How could the curriculum be improved?

TASK V: CHOOSE EVALUATION DESIGNS

Once the evaluation questions have been identified and prioritized, the curriculum developer should *consider which evaluation designs* (18–25) *are most appropriate to answer the evaluation questions and most feasible in terms of resources*.

An evaluation is said to possess *internal validity* (22) if it accurately assesses the impact of a specific intervention on specific subjects in a specific setting. An internally valid evaluation that is generalizable to other populations and other settings is said to possess *external validity* (22). Usually a curriculum's targeted learners and setting are predetermined for the curriculum developer. To the extent that their uniqueness can be minimized and their representativeness maximized, the external validity of the evaluation will be strengthened.

The choice of evaluation design directly affects the internal validity and indirectly affects the external validity of an evaluation (an evaluation cannot have external validity if it does not have internal validity). In choosing an evaluation design, one must be aware of each design's strengths and limitations with respect to *factors that could threaten the internal validity of the evaluation*. These factors include subject characteristics (selection bias), loss of subjects (mortality), location, instrumentation, testing, history, maturation, attitude of subjects, statistical regression, and implementation (18–19, 22–25). The term *subject characteristics* refers to the differences between individuals or groups and is also known as *selection bias*. *Selection bias* occurs when subjects in an intervention or comparison group possess characteristics that affect the results of the evaluation, by affecting the measurements of interest or the response of subjects to the intervention. If subjects are lost from or fail to complete an evaluation process, this can be a *mortality* threat. This is common because many evaluations occur over time. When subjects who drop out are different from those who complete the evaluation, the evaluation will not represent all subjects. *Location* refers to the fact that the particular place where data are collected or where an intervention has occurred may affect results. For example, an intervention in one intensive care unit that is modern and well resourced with a large amount of technology may provide different effects from the same intervention in another intensive care unit with fewer resources. *Instrumentation* refers to the effects that changes in raters or measurement methods, or lack of precision in the measurement instrument, might have on obtained measurements. *Testing* refers to the effects of an initial test on subjects' performance on subsequent tests. *History* refers to events or other interventions that affect subjects during the period of an evaluation. *Maturation* refers to changes within subjects that occur as a result of the passage of time, rather than as a result of discrete external interventions. The *attitude of the subjects* or the manner in which evaluation subjects view an intervention and their participation can affect the evaluation outcome. This is also known as the Hawthorne effect. *Statistical regression* can occur when subjects have been selected on the basis of low or high pre-intervention performance. Because of temporal variations in the performance of individuals, and because of characteristics of the test itself that result in imperfect test-retest reliability (see Task VI), subsequent scores on the performance assessment are likely to be less extreme, whether or not an educational intervention takes place. An *implementation threat* occurs when the results of an evaluation differ because the people who administer the evaluation differ in ways that are related to the outcome. It may not be possible or feasible, in the choice of evaluation design, to prevent all of the above factors from affecting a given evaluation. However, the curriculum developer should be aware of the potential effects of these factors when choosing an evaluation design and when interpreting the results.

The most commonly used *evaluation designs* are posttest only, pretest-posttest, nonrandomized controlled pretest-posttest, randomized controlled posttest only, and randomized controlled pretest-posttest (18–24). *As the designs increase in methodological rigor, they also increase in the amount of resources required to execute them.*

A *single-group, posttest-only* design can be diagrammed as follows:

$$X - - - O$$

where X represents the curriculum or educational intervention and O represents observations or measurements. This design permits assessment of what learners have achieved after the educational intervention, but the achievements could have been present before the intervention (selection bias), occurred as part of a natural maturation process during the period of the evaluation (maturation), or resulted from other interventions that took place during the evaluation period (history). Because of these limitations, the conclusions of single-group, posttest-only studies are nearly always tentative. The design is acceptable when the most important evaluation question is the certification of proficiency. The design is also well suited to assess participant perceptions of the curriculum, to solicit suggestions for improvement in the curriculum, and to solicit feedback on and ratings of student or faculty performance.

A *single-group, pretest-posttest* design can be diagrammed as

$$O_1 - - - X - - - O_2$$

where O_1 represents the first observations or measurements, in this case before the educational intervention, and O_2 the second observations or measurements, in this case after the educational intervention. This design can demonstrate that changes in proficiency have occurred in learners during the course of the curriculum. However, the changes could have occurred because of factors other than the curriculum (e.g., history, maturation, testing, instrumentation).

The addition of a *control group* helps confirm that an observed change occurred because of the curriculum, particularly if the control group was *randomized*. A *pretest-posttest controlled evaluation design* can be diagrammed as

$$R \quad \begin{array}{ll} E & O_1 - - - X - - - O_2 \\ C & O_1 - - - - - - - O_2 \end{array}$$

where E represents the experimental or intervention group, C represents the control or comparison group, and R (if present) indicates that subjects were randomized between the intervention and control groups. A *posttest-only randomized controlled design* requires fewer resources, especially when the observations or measurements are difficult and resource intensive. It cannot, however, demonstrate changes in learners. Furthermore, the success of the randomization process in achieving comparability between the intervention and control group before the curriculum cannot be assessed. This design can be diagrammed as follows:

$$E \quad X - - - O_1$$
$$R$$
$$C \quad \quad - - - O_1$$

Evaluation designs are sometimes classified as pre-experimental, quasi-experimental, and true experimental (19, 22–25). *Pre-experimental designs* usually lack controls. *Quasi-experimental designs* usually include controls but lack random assignment. *True experimental designs* include both random assignment to experimental and control groups and concurrent observations or measurements in the experimental and control groups.

The advantages and disadvantages of each of the discussed evaluation designs are displayed in Table 7.2. Additional designs are possible (see General References).

Political or ethical considerations may prohibit withholding a curriculum from some learners. This obstacle to a controlled evaluation can sometimes be overcome by delaying administration of the curriculum to the control group until after data collection has been completed for a randomized controlled evaluation. This can be accomplished without interference when, for other reasons, the curriculum can be administered to only a portion of targeted learners at the same time.

EXAMPLE: *Controlled Evaluation without Denying the Curriculum to the Control Group.* The design for such an evaluation might be diagrammed as follows:

$$E \quad O_1 - - -X - - - O_2 \quad \quad \quad (- - - O_3)$$
$$R$$
$$C \quad O_1 - - - - - - - O_2 - - - - - X \quad (- - - O_3)$$

When one uses this evaluation design, a randomized controlled evaluation is accomplished without denying the curriculum to any learner. Inclusion of additional observation points, as indicated in the parentheses, is more resource intensive but permits inclusion of all (not just half) of the learners in a noncontrolled pretest-posttest evaluation.

It is important to realize that formative assessment and feedback may occur in an ongoing fashion during a curriculum and could be diagrammed as follows:

$$O_1 - - - X - - - O_2 - - - X - - - O_3 - - - X - - - O_4$$

In this situation, a formative assessment and feedback strategy is also an educational strategy for the curriculum.

Table 7.2.   Advantages and Disadvantages of Commonly Used Evaluation Designs

Design	Diagram	Advantages	Disadvantages
Single group, posttest only (preexperimental)	X - - - O	Simple Economical Can document proficiency Can document process (what happened) Can ascertain learner and faculty perceptions of efficacy and value Can elicit suggestions for improvement	Accomplishments may have been preexisting Accomplishments may be the result of natural maturation Accomplishments may be due to factors other than the curriculum
Single group, pretest-posttest (pre-experimental)	O_1 - - - X - - - O_2	Intermediate in complexity and cost Can demonstrate pre-post changes in cognitive, affective, and psychomotor attributes, performance, and perceptions	Accomplishments may be the result of natural maturation Accomplishments may be due to factors other than the curriculum Accomplishments could result from learning from the first test or evaluation rather than from the curriculum
Controlled pretest-posttest (quasi-experimental)	E O_1 - - - X - - O_2 C O_1 - - - - - O_2	Controls for maturation, if control group equivalent Controls for the effects of measured factors, other than the curriculum Controls for learning from the test or evaluation	Complex Resource intensive Control group may not be equivalent to the experimental group and changes could be due to differences in unmeasured factors Curriculum denied to some (see text)
Randomized controlled posttest only (true-experimental)	E X - - - O_1 R C - - - O_1	Controls for maturation Controls for effects of measured and unmeasured factors Less resource intensive than a randomized controlled pretest-posttest design, while preserving the benefits of randomization	Complex Resource intensive Does not demonstrate changes in learners Totally dependent on the success of the randomization process in eliminating pretest differences in independent and dependent variables Curriculum denied to some (see text)

Table 7.2.   *(continued)*

Design	Diagram	Advantages	Disadvantages
Randomized controlled pretest-posttest (true-experimental)	E O_1 - - X - - O_2 R C O_1 - - - - - O_2	Controls for maturation Controls for effects of measured and unmeasured factors Controls for the effects of testing	Most complex Most resource intensive Curriculum denied to some (see text) Depends on success of the randomization process in eliminating pretest differences in unmeasured independent and dependent variables

Note: O = observation or measurement; X = curriculum or educational intervention; E = experimental or intervention group; C = control or comparison group; R = random allocation to experimental and control groups.

TASK VI: CHOOSE MEASUREMENT METHODS AND CONSTRUCT INSTRUMENTS

The choice of assessment or measurement methods and construction of measurement instruments are critical steps in the evaluation process because they determine the data that will be collected, determine how they will be collected (Task VIII), and make certain implications about how the data will be analyzed (Task IX). Formal measurement methods are discussed in this section. Table 8.2 lists additional, often informal, methods for determining how a curriculum is functioning (see Chapter 8).

Choice of Measurement Methods

Measurement methods commonly used to evaluate individuals and programs include rating forms, self-assessment forms, essays, written or computer-interactive tests, oral examinations, questionnaires (see Chapter 3), individual interviews (see Chapter 3), group interviews/discussions (see Chapter 3, focus groups), direct observation, and performance audits (26–30). The uses, strengths, and limitations of each of these measurement methods are displayed in Table 7.3.

As with the choice of evaluation design, it is important to *choose a measurement method that is congruent with the evaluation question* (29, 30). A written test is an appropriate method for assessing knowledge acquisition. Direct observation using agreed-on standards is an appropriate method for assessing skill attainment. Chart audit and unobtrusive observations are appropriate methods for assessing real-life performance.

It is desirable to choose measurement methods that have *optimal accuracy (reliability and validity), credibility,* and *importance.* Generally speaking, patient/health care outcomes are considered most important, followed by behaviors/performance, skills, knowledge or attitudes, and satisfaction or perceptions, in that order (31). Objective measurements are preferred to subjective ratings. Curricular evaluations that incorpo-

Table 7.3.   Uses, Strengths, and Limitations of Commonly Used Evaluation Methods

Method	Uses	Strengths	Limitations
Global rating forms (separated in time from observation)	Cognitive, affective, or psychomotor attributes; real-life performance	Economical Can evaluate anything Open-ended questions can provide information for formative purposes	Subjective Rater biases Inter- and intra-rater reliability Raters frequently have insufficient data on which to base ratings
Self-assessment forms	Cognitive, affective, psychomotor attributes; real-life performance	Economical Can evaluate anything Promotes self-assessment Useful for formative evaluation	Subjective Rater biases Agreement with objective measurements often low Limited acceptance as method of summative evaluation
Essays on respondent's experience	Attitudes, feelings, description of respondent experiences, perceived impact	Rich in texture Provides unanticipated as well as anticipated information Respondent-centered	Subjective Rater biases Requires qualitative evaluation methods to analyze Focus varies from respondent to respondent
Written or computer-interactive tests	Knowledge; higher level cognitive ability	Often economical Objective Multiple choice exams can achieve high internal consistency reliability, broad sampling Good psychometric properties, low cost, low faculty time, easy to score Widely accepted Essay-type questions or computer-interactive tests can assess higher level cognitive ability, encourage students to integrate knowledge, reflect problem solving	Constructing tests of higher level cognitive ability, or computer-interactive tests, can be resource intensive Reliability and validity vary with quality of test (e.g., questions that are not carefully constructed can be interpreted differently by different respondents, there may be an insufficient number of questions to validly test a domain)

Table 7.3.   *(continued)*

Method	Uses	Strengths	Limitations
Oral examinations	Knowledge; higher level cognitive ability; indirect measure of affective attributes	Flexible, can follow-up and explore understanding Learner-centered Can be integrated into case discussions	Subjective scoring Inter- and intra-rater reliability Reliability and validity vary with quality of test (e.g., questions that are not carefully constructed can be interpreted differently by different respondents, there may be an insufficient number of questions to validly test a domain) Faculty intensive Can be costly
Questionnaires	Attitudes; perceptions; suggestions for improvement	Economical	Subjective Constructing reliable and valid measures of attitudes requires time and skill
Individual interviews	Attitudes; perceptions; suggestions for improvement	Flexible, can follow-up and clarify responses Respondent-centered	Subjective Rater biases Constructing reliable and valid measures of attitudes requires time and skill Requires interviewers
Group interviews/ discussions	Attitudes; perceptions; suggestions for improvement	Flexible, can follow-up and develop/ explore responses Respondent-centered Efficient means of interviewing several at once Group interaction can enrich or deepen information Can be integrated into teaching sessions	Subjective Requires skilled interviewer or facilitator to control group interaction and minimize facilitator influence on responses Does not yield quantitative information Information may not be representative of all participants

Table 7.3.   *(continued)*

Method	Uses	Strengths	Limitations
Direct observation	Skills; performance	First-hand data Can provide immediate feedback to observed Development of standards, use of observation checklists, and training of observers can increase reliability and validity. The Objective Structured Clinical Examination (OSCE) (62, 63) and Objective Structured Assessment of Technical Skills (OSATS) (64–66) combine direct observation with structured checklists to increase reliability and validity.	Rater biases Inter- and intra-rater reliability Personnel intensive Unless observation covert, assesses capability rather than real-life performance
Performance audits	Record keeping; provision of recorded care (e.g., tests ordered, provision of preventive care measures, prescribed treatments)	Objective Reliability and accuracy can be measured and enhanced by the use of standards and the training of raters Unobtrusive	Dependent on what is reliably recorded; much care is not documented Dependent on available, organized records or data sources

rate measurement methods at the higher end of this hierarchy are more likely to be disseminated or published. However, it is more important for what is measured to be congruent with the program or learning objectives than to aspire to measure the "highest" level in the outcome hierarchy.

It is also necessary to choose measurement methods that are *feasible in terms of available resources.* Curriculum developers usually have to make difficult decisions regarding how to spread limited resources among the problem identification, needs assessment, educational intervention, and assessment and evaluation. Global rating forms for use by faculty supervisors and self-assessment questionnaires for completion by learners provide indirect, inexpensive measures of skill attainment and real-life performance. However, they are subject to numerous rating biases. Direct observation or audits using trained raters and agreed-on standards are more reliable and have more validity evidence for measuring skills and performance than global rating forms, but they also require more resources. There is little point in using the latter measurement methods, however, if their use would drain resources that are critically important for achieving a well-conceived educational intervention.

Construction of Measurement Instruments

Most evaluations will require the construction of curriculum-specific measurement instruments such as tests, rating forms, interview schedules, or questionnaires.

The *methodological rigor* with which the instruments are constructed and administered affects the reliability and validity of the scores and, unfortunately, the cost of the evaluation. Formative individual assessments and program evaluations generally require the least rigor, summative individual assessments and program evaluations for internal use an intermediate level of rigor, and summative individual assessments and program evaluations for external use (e.g., certification of mastery or publication of evaluation results) the most rigor. When a high degree of methodological rigor is required, it is worth exploring whether there is an *already existing measurement instrument* (32–36) that is appropriate in terms of content, reliability, validity, feasibility, and cost. When a methodologically rigorous instrument must be constructed specifically for a curriculum, it is wise to seek *advice or mentorship from individuals with expertise in designing such instruments.*

A useful first step in constructing measurement instruments is to determine the desired *content.* For assessments of curricular impact, this involves the identification of independent variables and dependent variables. *Independent variables* are factors that could explain or predict the curriculum's outcomes (e.g., the curriculum itself, previous or concurrent training, environmental factors). *Dependent variables* are program outcomes (e.g., knowledge or skill attainment, real-life performance, clinical outcomes). To keep the measurement instruments from becoming unwieldy, it is prudent to focus on a few dependent variables that are most relevant to the main evaluation questions and, similarly, to focus on the independent variables that are most likely to be related to the curriculum's outcomes.

Next, attention must be devoted to the *format* of the instruments. In determining the acceptable *length* for a measurement instrument, methodological concerns and the desire to be comprehensive must be balanced against constraints in the amount of curricular time allotted for evaluation, imposition on respondents, and concerns about response rate. Individual items should be worded and displayed in a manner that is *clear and unambiguous. Response scales* (e.g., true-false; strongly disagree, disagree, neither agree nor disagree, agree, strongly agree) should make sense relative to the question asked. There is no consensus about whether it is preferable for response scales to have middle points or not (e.g., neither agree nor disagree) or to have an even or odd number of response categories. In general, four to seven response categories permit greater flexibility in data analysis than two or three. It is important for the instrument as a whole to be *user-friendly* and attractive. This is done by organizing the instrument in a manner that facilitates quick understanding and efficient recording of responses. It is desirable for the instrument to *engage* the interest of respondents. In general, response categories should be *precoded* to facilitate data entry and analysis. Today, *online questionnaires* can provide an easy mode of delivery and facilitate collation of data for different reports (37). Some institutions have created secure Internet Web sites for this purpose and have noted improved compliance in response rates, a decrease in administrative time, and an improvement in quality (37).

Before using an instrument for evaluation purposes, it is almost always important to *pilot* it on a convenient audience. Audience feedback can provide important information about the instrument: how it is likely to be perceived by respondents, acceptable length, clarity of individual items, user-friendliness of the overall format, and specific ways in which the instrument could be improved.

Reliability, Validity, and Bias

Because measurement instruments are never perfect, the data they produce are never absolutely accurate. An understanding of potential threats to accuracy is helpful to the curriculum coordinator in planning the evaluation and reporting results and to the users of evaluation reports in interpreting results. In recent years, there has been an emerging consensus in the educational literature about the meaning of the terms validity and reliability (38–40). Validity is now considered a unitary concept that encompasses both reliability and validity. All validity relates to the construct that is being measured and is now considered construct validity.

The emphasis on construct validity has emerged from the growing realization that an instrument's scores are usually meaningful only inasmuch as they accurately reflect an abstract concept (or construct) such as knowledge, skill, or patient satisfaction. Validity is best viewed as a hypothesis regarding the link between the instrument's scores and the intended construct. Evidence is collected from a variety of sources (see below) to support or refute this hypothesis. Validity can never be "proven" just as a scientific hypothesis can never be proven; it can be supported (or refuted) only as evidence accrues.

It is also important to note that validity and reliability refer to an instrument's scores and not the instrument itself. The scores may have high validity (or reliability) in one context or for one purpose but be ill-suited for another context (see examples in reference 40).

The construct validity of an instrument's scores can be supported by various types of evidence. One well-accepted system identifies five discrete evidence sources:

1. *Internal structure evidence*, which relates to the psychometric characteristics of the measurement instrument; it includes categories previously considered reliability: inter-rater and intra-rater reliability, stability or test-retest reliability, equivalence or alternate-form reliability, homogeneity or internal consistency; and other psychometric properties such as scale development and scoring, item analysis for difficulty and discrimination, and response characteristics in different settings and by different populations.
2. *Content evidence*, which includes the old terms face, surface, and content validity.
3. *Relation to other variables evidence,* which includes criterion-related validity (concurrent and predictive) and the old more narrowly conceived construct validity.

4. *Response process evidence*, which includes evidence of data integrity, related to the instrument itself, its administration, and the data collection process.
5. *Consequences evidence*, which relates to the impact or consequences of the assessments on examinees, faculty, patients, and society. Does the use of the instrument have intended/useful or unintended/harmful consequences?

Because for some readers these new terms will replace more familiar terms, we will use both the old and new terminology in this book and relate the two to each other (Table 7.4).

Internal Structure Evidence.   Internal structure validity relates to the psychometric characteristics of the measurement scores and, as such, includes all forms of reliability assessment, as well as other psychometrics of the test. As noted above, it includes the concepts of inter-rater and intra-rater reliability, stability or test-retest reliability, equivalence or alternate-form reliability, and homogeneity or internal consistency. Reliability refers to the consistency or reproducibility of measurements (35, 36, 38–40). As such it is a necessary but not sufficient determinant of validity evidence. There are several different methods for assessing reliability of a measurement. Reliability is usually reported as a coefficient between 0 and 1. The reliability coefficient can also be thought of as the proportion of score variance explained by differences between subjects, with the remaining due to error (random and systematic). For high-stakes examinations (licensure), reliability should be greater than 0.9. For many testing situations a reliability of 0.7-0.8 may be acceptable. Ideally, measurements should be the same when repeated by the same person (*intra-rater reliability*) or made by different people (*inter-rater reliability*). Intra- or inter-rater reliability can be assessed by the percentage agreement between raters or by statistics such as kappa (41), which corrects for chance agreement. A commonly used method of estimating inter-rater reliability is the intraclass correlation coefficient, accessible in commonly available computer software, which uses analysis of variance to estimate the variance of different factors. It permits estimation of the inter-rater reliability of the *n* raters used, as well as the reliability of a single rater. It can also manage missing data (39). A sophisticated method for estimating inter-rater agreement often used in performance examinations uses generalizability theory analysis, where variance for each of the variables in the evaluation can be estimated (i.e., subjects or true variance vs. raters and measurements or error variance). Changes can be made in the number of measurements or raters dependent on the variance seen in an individual variable (42).

> **EXAMPLE:** *Generalizability Theory Analysis.* Resident performance is assessed at the end of the month by asking for four items to be rated by three different faculty members. Generalizability theory analysis demonstrated that the reliability (true variance/total variance) of this assessment was only 0.5, that is, that only 50% of the total variance was due to the difference between subjects (true variance) and the rest of the variance was due to difference between raters, items, and interactions among the three sources of variation. The reliability was improved to 0.8 by adding six items and five raters.

Other forms of internal structure validity include stability, equivalence, and homogeneity or internal consistency. *Stability or test-retest reliability* is the degree to which the same test produces the same results when repeated under the same conditions. This is not commonly done because of time, cost, and the possibility of contamination by intervening variables when the second test is separated in time. *Equivalence or*

Table 7.4. Reliability and Validity: Terminology and Definitions

New Terminology (All validity is construct validity)	Old Terminology	Definition	Comments/Example
Internal structure validity		Psychometric characteristics of the measurement	
	Item analysis measures	Item difficulty, other measures of item/test characteristics	
	Intra-rater reliability	Consistency of measurement results when repeated by same individual	
	Inter-rater reliability	Consistency of measurement results when performed by different individuals	Can be assessed by statistical methods such as kappa or phi coefficient, intraclass correlation coefficient, generalizability theory analysis. See text.
	Stability/test-retest reliability	Degree to which same test produces same results when repeated under same conditions	
	Equivalence/alternate-form reliability	Degree to which alternate forms of the same measurement instrument produce the same result	Of relevance in pretest-posttest evaluation, when each test encompasses only part of the domain being taught, and when learning, related to test taking, could be limited to the items being tested. In such situations, it is desirable to have equivalent but different tests.
	Homogeneity/internal consistency	Extent to which same items legitimately team together to measure a single characteristic	Can be assessed with statistical methods such as Cronbach's alpha. Uni- versus multidimensionality can be assessed by factor analysis. See text.

Table 7.4.   *(continued)*

New Terminology (All validity is construct validity)	Old Terminology	Definition	Comments/Example
Content validity		Degree to which a measurement instrument accurately represents the skill or characteristic it is designed to measure.	
	Face, surface, content validity	The term "face" or "surface" implies informal or subjective ways of assessing this, whereas the term "content" implies more formal ways, such as literature review, work sampling, and formal methods for consensus building (see text). The new terminology only acknowledges formal methods.	Formal processes such as focus groups, nominal group technique, Delphi technique, daily diaries, work sampling, time and motion studies, critical incident reviews, and reviews of ideal performance cases are discussed in Chapter 2.
Relationship to other variables		How the instrument under consideration relates to other instruments or theory	
	Criterion-related validity Concurrent validity	Degree to which a measurement instrument produces the same results as another accepted or proven instrument that measures the same characteristics	E.g., comparison to a previously validated but more resource-intensive measurement instrument

Table 7.4.   *(continued)*

New Terminology (All validity is construct validity)	Old Terminology	Definition	Comments/Example
	Predictive validity	Degree to which a measurement instrument accurately predicts theoretically expected outcomes	E.g., higher scores on an instrument that assesses communication skills should predict higher patient satisfaction scores
	Construct validity (narrowly conceived)	Whether an instrument performs as would theoretically be expected in groups that are known to possess or not possess the attribute being measured, or in comparison to tests that are known to measure the same attribute (high correlation) or a different attribute (low correlation)	E.g., an instrument that assesses clinical reasoning would be expected to distinguish novice from experienced clinicians. Scores on an instrument designed to measure communication skills would not be expected to correlate with scores on an instrument designed to measure technical proficiency in a procedure.
Response process validity		Evidence of data integrity, related to test administration and data collection	E.g., documentation of data collection, entry, and cleaning procedures
Consequences		Degree to which the instrument has intended/ useful vs. unintended/ harmful consequences, the impact of its use	E.g., it would be a problem if results from a measurement method of limited reliability and validity were being used to make decisions about career advancement, when the intent was to use the results as feedback to stimulate and direct trainee improvement

alternate-form reliability is the degree to which alternate forms of the same measure-ment instrument produce the same result. This form of internal structure validity is of particular relevance in pre-post test evaluations, when the test is a sample (only part) of what should have been learned and when specific learning could occur related to test taking, independent of the curricular intervention. In such circumstances, it is desirable to use equivalent but different tests or alternative forms of the same test. *Homogeneity/ internal consistency* is the extent to which various items legitimately team together to measure a single characteristic, such as a desired attitude. Internal consistency can be assessed using the statistic Cronbach's (or coefficient) alpha (41, 43), which is basi-cally the average of the correlations of each item in a scale to the total score. A complex characteristic, however, could have several dimensions. In this situation, the technique of factor analysis (44) can be used to help separate out the different dimensions. When there is a need to assess the reliability of an important measure but a lack of statistical expertise among curricular faculty, statistical consultation is advisable.

> **EXAMPLE:** *Internal Structure Validity: Homogeneity/Internal Consistency.* A group of educa-tors from several institutions worked together to develop a computer-interactive case-based test to assess three cognitive areas: 1) knowledge of facts necessary for the appropriate management of two common medical disorders; 2) clinical decision making that incorpo-rated the use of sensitivity, specificity, predictive values for diagnostic strategies, known efficacy and complications for treatment options, and patient preferences; and 3) cost-effec-tiveness of decisions in relation to outcomes. Factor analysis was able to identify separate generic clinical decision making and cost-effectiveness dimensions. However, there was not a single knowledge dimension. Knowledge split into two separate factors, each of which was specific to one of the two medical disorders. So did disease-specific clinical decision mak-ing, which required knowledge that was not provided in the test. Cronbach's alpha was used to assess homogeneity among items that contributed to each of the six dimensions or fac-tors. There were a large number of items for each dimension. Those items that had low cor-relation with the overall score for each dimension were considered for elimination.

> **EXAMPLE:** *Internal Structure Validity: Psychometrics.* Many residency programs use in-train-ing examinations to assess the knowledge base of their residents. The results of the in-training examinations typically contain a detailed item analysis, which includes an analysis of item difficulty (what percentage of individuals select the correct answer), item discrimination (how well the item distinguishes between those who scored in the upper tier and those who scored in the lower tier), and an analysis of who answered which options. For a high-stakes examination such as an in-training examination, the reliability coefficient determined by any means should be 0.8 or greater, that is, the reproducibility of the score must be very high.

Content Evidence.   Content validity evidence is the degree to which an instrument's scores accurately represent the skill or characteristic the instrument is designed to measure, based on people's experience and available knowledge. It has sometimes been called face or surface validity evidence (terms that have fallen from favor) when the evidence is based on the appearance of the measurement rather than on a formal content analysis. Content validity can be enhanced by conducting an appropriate lit-erature review to identify the most relevant content, using topic experts, and revising the instrument until a reasonable degree of consensus about its content is achieved among knowledgeable reviewers. Formal processes such as focus groups, nominal group technique, Delphi technique, use of daily diaries, observation by work sampling, time and motion studies, critical incident reviews, and reviews of ideal performance cases can also contribute (see Chapter 2).

> **EXAMPLE:** *Content Validity.* At the end of an ambulatory medicine clerkship for medical students a 12 station OSCE designed to assess skills is reviewed by faculty and other expert clinicians as to whether the cases are representative of the domains of primary ambulatory medicine, all of the clinical information is accurate, and the checklists and rating scales are appropriate.

Relationship to Other Variables Evidence.   This form of validity refers to how the instrument under consideration relates to other instruments or theory. As noted above, it encompasses the concepts of criterion-related validity and the old, more narrowly conceived construct validity. *Criterion-related validity* includes concurrent validity and predictive validity. *Concurrent validity* is the degree to which a measurement instrument produces the same results as another accepted or proven instrument that measures the same parameters. *Predictive validity* is the degree to which an instrument's scores accurately predict theoretically expected outcomes (e.g., scores from a measure of attitudes toward preventive care should correlate significantly with preventive care behaviors).

> **EXAMPLE:** *Relationship to Other Variables: Concurrent Validity.* The clinical skills of residents can be assessed by using self-ratings, faculty ratings, or an examination that includes a standardized patient. The faculty agree that the standardized patient examination is likely to yield the most valid scores, but if possible they would like to substitute one of the less costly methods. On literature review, however, scores from the first two measures were found to correlate poorly with scores on a standardized patient examination (45).

> **EXAMPLE:** *Relationship to Other Variables: Concurrent Validity.* As part of the comprehensive assessment of senior medical students, a 10 station OSCE was developed to assess clinical skills. The validity evidence supporting this examination included the scores on an earlier OSCE during clinical skills, clerkship grades, and performance on the clinical skills examination of the United States Medical Licensing Examination (USMLE), Step II.

> **EXAMPLE:** *Relationship to Other Variables: Predictive Validity.* Many residency programs use in-training examinations to assess the knowledge base of their residents. The results of the in-training examinations should be predictive of how well individuals will perform on their certifying examinations. Program directors rely on the predictive validity of the in-training examinations when they counsel residents with low scores on specific subsections.

Construct validity, as narrowly construed, was a term sometimes formerly used to refer to whether a measurement instrument performed as would theoretically be expected in groups that are known to possess or not possess the attribute being measured, or in comparison to tests that are known to measure the same attribute (high correlation) or different attributes (low correlation).

> **EXAMPLE:** *Relationship to Other Variables: Old Construct Validity.* Scores from an instrument that measures clinical reasoning ability would be expected to distinguish between individuals rated by faculty as high and low in clinical reasoning and judgment. Scores on the instrument would be expected to correlate significantly with grades on an evidence-based case presentation, but not with measures of compassion.

Response Process Evidence.   Response process validity includes evidence about the integrity of instrument administration and data collection so that sources of error are controlled or eliminated. It could include information about quality control processes, use of properly trained raters, documentation of procedures used to ensure accuracy and data collection, evidence that students are familiar with test formats, or evidence that a test of clinical reasoning actually invokes higher order thinking in test takers.

> **EXAMPLE:** *Response Process Evidence.* Use of a rigorous process for data collection from a standardized patient performance examination is a form of response process validity evidence. Evidence about how scores are calculated and combined is also an example of response process validity evidence.

Consequences Evidence.   This is a new concept and may be the most controversial area of validity. It refers to the consequences of an assessment on examinees, faculty, patients, and society. It answers the question, what outcomes (good and bad) have occurred as a result of the assessment and related decisions? If the consequences are intended or useful, this evidence supports the ongoing use of the instrument. If the consequences are unintended and harmful, educators may think twice before using the instrument for the same purpose in the future. Consequence validity could also include the method or process to determine the cut scores, as well as the statistical properties of passing scores.

> **EXAMPLE:** *Consequences Validity Evidence.* Following residency training, many specialty boards require a high-stakes examination for certification. Validity evidence related to the consequences of this examination would include the method by which cut score or pass/fail decisions have been made, the percentage of examinees that pass, and how this compares with other examinations.

> **EXAMPLE:** *Consequences Evidence.* Suppose that in a hypothetical medical school a mandatory comprehensive assessment was implemented at the end of the first year. Students who scored below a certain mark were provided one-on-one counseling and remediation. If board scores improve and the number of students failing to graduate drops, this would provide consequences evidence in support of the mandatory assessment (i.e., the assessment had a positive impact on students). If, however, students identified for remediation dropped out at a higher than normal rate, this might suggest an unintended harm from the assessment (negative consequences evidence).

Threats to Validity.   Another way to look at validity, complementary to the above perspective, is to consider the potential threats to validity (i.e., negative validity evidence). Bias related to insufficient sampling of trainee attributes or cases, variations in testing environment, and inadequately trained raters can threaten validity (46). Threats to validity have been classified into two general categories: construct underrepresentation and construct-irrelevant variance (47). These errors interfere with the interpretation of the assessment. *Construct underrepresentation* represents inadequate sampling of the domain to be assessed, biased sampling, or a mismatch of the testing sample to the domain (47).

> **EXAMPLE:** *Construct Underrepresentation Variance.* An instructor has just begun to design a structured clinical examination for students at the end of their clerkship. She developed four cases representative of core material and plans on basing most of the student grade on this examination. This example is likely to represent construct underrepresentation variance because the number of stations is too few to represent the entire domain of the clerkship skills expected. Typically 7–11 cases are required. In addition, the cases must be representative.

Construct-irrelevant variance refers to systematic, as opposed to random, error that is introduced into the assessment and does not have a relationship to the construct being measured. It includes flawed or biased test items, inappropriately easy or difficult test items, indefensible passing scores, poorly trained standardized patients, and rater bias. Rating biases are particularly likely to occur when global rating forms are being used by untrained raters to assess learner or faculty performance. Rating biases can affect both an instrument's reliability and validity (46). *Errors of leniency or harshness* occur when raters consistently rate higher than is accurate (e.g., Garrison Keillor's Lake Wobegon, where "all the women are strong, all the men are good looking, and all the children are above average") or lower than is accurate (e.g., judging junior generalist physicians against standards appropriate to senior specialist physicians). The *error of central tendency* refers to the tendency of raters to avoid extremes. The *halo effect* occurs when individuals who perform well in one area or relate particularly well to others are rated inappropriately high in other, often unobserved, areas of performance. *Attribution error* occurs when raters make inferences about why individuals behave as they do and then rate them in areas that are unobserved based on these inferences.

> **EXAMPLE:** *Construct-irrelevant Variance: Attribution Error.* An individual who consistently arrives late and does not contribute actively to group discussions is assumed to be lazy and unreliable. She is rated low on motivation. The individual has a problem with child care and is quiet, but she has done all the required reading, has been active in defining her own learning needs, and has independently pursued learning resources beyond those provided in the course syllabus.

Rater biases may be reduced and inter- and intra-rater reliability improved by training those who are performing the ratings. Because not all training is effective, it is important to confirm the efficacy of training by assessing the reliability of raters and the accuracy of their ratings.

Internal and external validity is discussed above in reference to evaluation designs (Task V). It is worth noting here that the reliability and validity of the scores for each instrument used in an evaluation affect the internal validity of the overall evaluation.

It is also worth noting here that the reliability and validity of an instrument's scores affect the utility, feasibility, and propriety of the overall evaluation. Many of the threats to validity can be minimized once considered. Thus, open discussion of these issues should occur in the planning stages of the evaluation.

Reliability and Validity in Qualitative Measurement.   The above discussion of reliability and validity pertains to quantitative measurements. Frequently *qualitative information* is also gathered to enrich and help explain the quantitative data that have been obtained. *Qualitative evaluation methods* are also used to explore in depth the processes and impact of a curriculum and to develop hypotheses about how a curriculum works and its effects.

> **EXAMPLE:** *Qualitative Evaluation Methods.* Questionnaires may ask for comments next to quantitative ratings. Respondents may be asked to list strengths, weaknesses, and suggestions for improving components of or an entire curriculum. Essays or open-ended interviews may be used to assess how a curriculum has affected participants.

When qualitative measurements are used as methods of evaluating a curriculum, there may be concern about their accuracy and about the interpretation of conclusions that are drawn from the data. Many of the above methods for assessing reliability and validity pertain to quantitative measurements. However, the above concepts of internal structure evidence, content evidence, relation to other variables, response process evidence, and consequences also pertain to qualitative measurements. While a detailed discussion of the accuracy of qualitative measurement methods is beyond the scope of this book, it is worth noting that there are concepts in qualitative research that parallel the quantitative research concepts of reliability and validity (48–51). *Objectivity* refers to investigators revealing their theoretical perspectives and background characteristics/experiences that may influence their interpretation of observations. *Reflexivity* refers to investigators reflecting on and accounting for these factors (i.e., attempting to remain as free from biases as possible when interpreting data). *Confirmability* provides assurances that the conclusions that are drawn about what is studied would be reached if another investigator undertook the same analysis of the same data or used a different measurement method. Frequently, in qualitative analysis of the same data set, two or more investigators review and abstract themes and then have a process for reaching consensus. Investigators may use more than one method to study a phenomenon (*triangulation* of methods) or point out how their results match or differ from those of other studies (*triangulation* of results). *Dependability* refers to consistency and reproducibility of the research method over time and across research subjects and contexts. There may be quality checks on how questions are asked or the data are coded. There should be an *audit trail* or record of the study's methods and procedures, so that others can replicate what was done. *Internal validity/credibility/authenticity* refers to how much the results of the qualitative inquiry ring true to reality. Study subjects can be asked to confirm, refute, or otherwise comment on the themes and explanations that emerge from qualitative data analysis (*respondent validation* or *member checks*). The investigators should study/account for *exceptions* to the themes that emerge from the qualitative data analysis. They should consider and discuss alternative explanations. There should be a representative, rich or *thick* description of the data, including examples, sufficient to support the investigators' interpretations. The data collection methods should be adequate to address the evaluation question. *All* of the above contribute to the *trustworthiness* of the evaluation/research. *External validity/transferability* deals with the generalizability of findings. Can the results be generalized to other cases or settings? Did the investigators describe their study subjects and setting in sufficient detail? Did they compare their results to those from other studies and to empirically derived theory (*triangulation* of findings)? The reader is referred to General References, Qualitative Evaluation, for a more detailed discussion of these concepts.

Conclusions

Because all measurement instruments are subject to threats to their reliability and validity, the ideal evaluation strategy will employ *multiple measurements using several different measurement methods and several different raters.* When all results are similar, the findings are said to be *robust* and one can feel reasonably comfortable about their validity. This point cannot be overemphasized, as multiple concordant pieces of evidence, each individually weak, can collectively provide strong evidence to inform a program evaluation.

TASK VII: ADDRESS ETHICAL CONCERNS

Propriety Standards

More than any other step in the curriculum development process, evaluation is likely to raise ethical and what are formally called propriety concerns (16, 52). This can be broken down into nine categories (Table 7.5). Major concerns usually fall into the following categories: concern for human rights and human interactions, which usually involve issues of confidentiality, access, and consent; resource allocation; and potential impact of the evaluation. It is wise for curriculum developers to anticipate these ethical concerns and address them in planning the evaluation. In addressing important ethical concerns, it can be helpful to obtain input both from the involved parties, such as learners and faculty, and from those with administrative oversight for the overall program. Institutional policies and procedures, external guidelines, and consultation with uninvolved parties, including those in the community, can also provide assistance.

Confidentiality, Access, and Consent

Concerns about confidentiality, access, and consent usually relate to those being evaluated. Decisions about confidentiality must be made regarding who should have access to an individual's assessments, especially in areas of particular sensitivity such as attitudes, interpersonal skills, and teaching ability. Concerns are magnified when feasibility considerations have resulted in the use of measurement methods of limited reliability and validity, and when there is a need for those reviewing the assessments to understand these limitations.

The decision also has to be made about whether any evaluators should be granted confidentiality (evaluator is unknown to the evaluated but can be identified by someone else) or anonymity (evaluator is known to no one). This concern usually pertains to individuals in subordinate positions (e.g., students, employees) who have been asked to evaluate those in authority over them, and who might be subject to retaliation for an unflattering assessment. Anonymous raters may be more open and honest, but they may also be less responsible in criticizing the person being rated.

Finally, it is necessary to decide whether those being assessed need to provide informed consent for the assessment process. Even if a separate formal consent for the evaluation is not required, decisions need to be made regarding the extent to which those being assessed will be informed: about the assessment methods being used; about the strengths and limitations of the assessment methods; about the potential users of the assessments (e.g., deans, program directors, board review committees); about the uses to which assessment results will be put (e.g., formative purposes, grades, certification of proficiency for external bodies); about the location of assessment results, their confidentiality, and methods for ensuring confidentiality; and, finally, about the assessment results themselves. Which assessment results will be shared with whom, and how will that sharing take place? Will collated or individual results be shared? Will individual results be shared by mailings or through facilitated feedback to individuals? Each of these issues should be addressed and answered during the planning stage of the evaluation process. The "need to know" principle should be widely applied. Publication of evaluation results beyond one's institution constitutes educational research. When publication or other forms of dissemination are contemplated

Table 7.5.   Ethical-Propriety Concerns Related to Evaluation

Issue	Recommendation
Service orientation	Place the needs of program customers in the center Give suggestions for program improvement Expose harmful practices

Formal policy	Have a formal policy regarding:
	    the purpose and questions of the evaluation
	    the release of reports, confidentiality and anonymity of data

Rights of human subjects	Clearly establish the protection of the rights of human subjects Clarify intended uses of the evaluation Ensure informed consent Follow due process Respect diversity Keep stakeholders informed Understand participant values Follow stated protocol Honor confidentiality and anonymity agreements Do no harm
Human interactions	Relate to all stakeholders in a professional manner Keep communication open Follow institutional protocol Respect privacy Honor time commitments Be respectful in addressing participants' concerns, diversity, and cultural differences Be evenhanded in addressing different stakeholders Do not cover up any participants' incompetence, unethical behavior, fraud, waste, or abuse
Complete and fair evaluation	Assess and report a balance of the strengths and weaknesses, unintended outcomes Acknowledge limitations of the evaluation
Disclosure of findings	Define right to know audiences Clearly report the findings and the basis for conclusions Disclose limitations Assure that reports reach their intended audiences
Conflict of interest	Identify conflicts of interest Assure protection against conflicts of interest Use independent parties or reporting agencies as needed to avoid conflicts of interest
Fiscal responsibility	Consider and specify budgetary needs Keep some flexibility Be frugal Include a statement of use of funds Consider evaluation process in context of entire program budget

(see Chapter 9), curriculum developers should consult their institutional review board in the planning stages of the evaluation, before data are collected (see Chapters 6 and 9).

Resource Allocation

The use of resources for one purpose may mean that fewer resources are available for other purposes. The curriculum developer may need to ask whether the allocation of resources for a curriculum is fair and whether the allocation is likely to result in the most overall good. A strong evaluation could drain resources from other curriculum development steps. Therefore, it is appropriate to think about the impact of resource allocation on learners, faculty, curriculum coordinators, and other stakeholders in the curriculum.

A controlled evaluation, for example, may deny an educational intervention to some learners. This consequence may be justified if the efficacy of the intervention is widely perceived as questionable and if there is consensus about the need to resolve the question through a controlled evaluation.

On the other hand, allocation of resources to an evaluation effort that is important for a faculty member's academic advancement, but that diverts needed resources from learners or other faculty, is ethically problematic.

There may also be concerns about the allocation of resources for the different evaluation purposes. How much should be allocated for formative purposes to help learners and the curriculum improve, and how much for summative purposes, to ensure trainee competence for the public or to develop evidence of programmatic success for the curriculum developers, one's institution, or those beyond one's institution?

Potential Impact/Consequences

The evaluation may have an impact on learners, faculty, curriculum developers, other stakeholders, and the curriculum itself. It is helpful to think through the potential uses to which an evaluation might be put, and whether the evaluation is likely to result in more good than harm. An evaluation that lacks methodological rigor due to resource limitations could lead to false conclusions, improper interpretation, and harmful use. It is therefore important to ensure that the uses to which an evaluation is put are appropriate for its degree of methodological rigor, to ensure that the necessary degree of methodological rigor is maintained over time, and to inform users of an evaluation's methodological limitations as well as its strengths.

EXAMPLE: *Individual Assessments That Are Insufficiently Accurate for Summative Assessment.* A residency director is interested in using assessments from a curriculum for certification of learner competence. Because the curriculum coordinator does not have the resources to develop individual summative assessments of sufficient accuracy, she decides to use the observational assessments that are feasible for formative purposes. They are discussed in an interactive way with learners during learning sessions to help learners improve their skills. However, because the assessments lack sufficient inter-rater reliability and accuracy, the assessment results are not kept, used for summative assessment purposes, or entered into the residents' records where others would have access to them.

EXAMPLE: *Inability to Conduct a Sufficiently Accurate Summative Program Evaluation.* As a pilot program, a new curriculum was developed and implemented to enhance communication skills of junior medical students. After 2 months, the curricular committee wanted a report about whether or not to plan to continue the course and wanted proof of measurable benefits of the new curriculum on communication skills. However, curriculum developers planned an evaluation after 1 year based on cost of the evaluation, reliability and validity evidence of the assessment tools, and the small number of students who had completed the curriculum. Based on the possibility that a false conclusion could be drawn on the outcome of the curriculum after 2 months, and that more harm than good could result from the evaluation, the curriculum developers offered a formative evaluation measuring student and faculty satisfaction.

EXAMPLE: *Informing Users of Methodological Limitations of an Evaluation Method.* Global rating forms that are placed in individuals' records are accompanied by a listing of their limitations, information on the wide variety of inter-rater reliability in the institution, and advice on how to interpret them.

TASK VIII: COLLECT DATA

Sufficient data must be collected to ensure a useful analysis. Failure to collect important evaluation data that match the evaluation questions or low response rates can seriously compromise the value of an evaluation. Excessive data collection or inefficiencies in data collection can consume valuable resources.

Response Rates and Efficiency

While the evaluation data design dictates when data should be collected relative to an intervention, curriculum coordinators usually have flexibility with respect to the precise time, place, and manner of data collection. Data collection can therefore be planned to maximize response rates, feasibility, and efficiency. Today, secure Web-based Internet assessment and evaluation tools may allow efficiency in the collection and analysis of data (37).

Response rates can be boosted and the need for follow-up reduced when data collection is built into scheduled learner and faculty activities. Response rates can also be increased if completion of an evaluation by a learner is required to achieve needed credit.

EXAMPLE: *Integrating Data Collection into the Curriculum.* Fifteen minutes were scheduled during a curriculum's last learning session for learners to complete a questionnaire evaluating the curriculum. Follow-up was necessary for only two learners who missed the final session, but who needed to complete the questionnaire to obtain credit for the course.

Sometimes an evaluation method can be designed to serve simultaneously as an educational method. This strategy reduces imposition on the learner and uses curriculum personnel efficiently.

EXAMPLE: *A Method Used for both Teaching and Evaluation.* Interactions between faculty participants and a standardized learner were videotaped at the beginning and end of a five-session faculty development workshop. The videotapes were reviewed for educational purposes with participants during the sessions. Later they were reviewed in a blinded fashion by trained raters as part of a pre-post program evaluation.

Occasionally, data collection can be incorporated into already scheduled evaluation activities.

EXAMPLE: *Use of an Existing Evaluation Activity.* A multistation examination was used to assess student accomplishments at the end of a clinical clerkship in emergency medicine. Curriculum developers for a mini-curriculum on universal precautions and follow-up of needle sticks were granted a station for a computer-interactive assessment during the examination.

EXAMPLE: *Use of an Existing Evaluation Activity.* Developers of a geriatric curriculum on advance directives convinced the director of the residents' ambulatory continuity clinic experience to include documentation of discussions about advance directives as an item in the residents' yearly chart audit.

Impact of Data Collection on Instrument Design

What data are collected is determined by the choice of measurement instruments (see Task VI). However, the design of measurement instruments needs to be tempered by the process of data collection. Response rates for mailed questionnaires will fall as their length and complexity increase. The amount of time and resources that has been allocated for data collection cannot be exceeded without affecting learners, faculty, or other priorities.

EXAMPLE: *Impact of Time Constraints on Instrument Length.* If 15 minutes of curricular time are allocated for evaluation, a measurement instrument that requires 30 minutes to complete will intrude on other activities and is likely to reduce participant cooperation.

Assignment of Responsibility

Measurement instruments must be distributed, collected, and safely stored. Nonrespondents require follow-up. While different individuals may distribute or administer measurement instruments within scheduled sessions, it is usually wise to delegate overall responsibility for data collection to one person.

EXAMPLE: *Assignment of Responsibility.* A faculty member with a particular interest in evaluation was named evaluation coordinator for a curriculum. He worked with the curriculum secretary to ensure that measurement instruments were distributed, collected, and stored in a reliable manner. Nonrespondents were consistently pursued by the curriculum secretary.

TASK IX: ANALYZE DATA

After the data have been collected, they need to be analyzed (53–60). *Data analysis, however, should be planned at the same time that evaluation questions are being identified and measurement instruments developed.*

Relation to Evaluation Questions

The nature of evaluation questions will determine, in part, the type of statistical approach required to answer them. Questions related to participant perceptions of a curriculum, or to the percentage of learners who achieved a specific objective, generally require only descriptive statistics. Questions about changes in learners generally require more sophisticated tests of statistical significance.

Statistical considerations may also influence the choice of evaluation questions. A *power analysis* (53–55) is a statistical method for estimating the ability of an evaluation to detect a statistically significant relationship between an outcome measure (dependent variable) and a potential determinant of the outcome (independent variable, such as exposure to a curriculum). The power analysis can be used to determine whether a curriculum has a sufficient number of learners to justify a determination of the statistical significance of its impact.

Sometimes there are limitations in the evaluator's statistical expertise and in the resources available for statistical consultation. Evaluation questions can then be worded in a way that at least ensures *congruence* between the questions and the analytic methods that will be employed.

> **EXAMPLE:** *Congruence between the Evaluation Question and the Analytic Methods Required.* To avoid having to apply tests of statistical significance, an evaluation question was changed from "Does the curriculum result in a statistically significant improvement in the proficiency of its learners in skill X?" to "What percentage of learners improve or achieve proficiency in skill X by the end of the curriculum?"

When the curriculum evaluation involves a large number of learners, analysis could reveal a statistically significant but an educationally meaningless impact on learners. The latter consideration might prompt curriculum evaluators to develop an evaluation question that addresses the magnitude as well as the statistical significance of any impact. *Effect size* is increasingly used to provide a measure of the size of a change, or the degree to which sample results diverge from the null hypothesis (59). Several measurements have been used to give an estimate of effect size: correlation coefficient, r, which is the measure of the relationship between variables, with the value of r^2 indicating the proportion of variance shared by variables; eta-square, η^2, which is reported in analysis of variance and is interpreted as the proportion of the variance of an outcome variable explained by the independent variable; odds ratios; risk ratios; absolute risk reduction; and most commonly Cohen's d, which is the difference between two means (e.g., pre-post scores or experimental vs. control groups) divided by the pooled standard deviation associated with that measurement. The effect size is said to be small if Cohen's $d = 0.20$, medium if equal to 0.50, and large if ≥ 0.80 (60). However, measures of effect size are probably more meaningful when judging the results of several studies with similar designs and directly comparable interventions rather than using these thresholds in absolute terms. For example, it would not be surprising to see a large Cohen's d when comparing a multimodal curriculum against no intervention, whereas the expected Cohen's d for a study comparing two active educational interventions would be much smaller. It is important to remember that educational meaningfulness is still an interpretation that rests not only on the statistical significance and size of a change but also on its nature and the relation of the change to other outcomes deemed important, such as a reduction in morbidity or mortality.

Relation to Measurement Instruments

The measurement instrument determines the type of data that is collected. The *type of data,* in turn, *helps determine the type of statistical test that is appropriate to analyze the data* (56–58) (Table 7.6). *Categorical* data are data that fit into discrete categories. *Numerical* data are data that have meaning on a numerical scale. Numerical data can be continuous (e.g., age, weight, height) or discrete (e.g., number of procedures performed, number of sessions attended). *Nominal* data are categorical data that fit into discrete nonordered categories (e.g., sex, race, eye color, exposure or not to an intervention). *Ordinal data* are categorical data that fit into discrete but inherently ordered or hierarchical categories (e.g., grades A, B, C, D, F; highest educational level completed: grade school, high school, college, postcollege degree program; condition: worse, same, better). *Interval data* are numerical data with equal intervals, distances, or differences between categories, but no zero point (e.g., dates on a calendar). *Ratio data* are interval data with a meaningful zero point (e.g., weight; age).

Data analysis considerations may affect the design of the measurement instrument. When a computer is being used, the first step in data analysis is *data entry.* In this situation, it is helpful to construct one's measurement instruments in a way that facilitates data entry, such as the precoding of responses. If one prefers to use a specific test for statistical significance, one needs to ensure that the appropriate type of data is collected.

Choice of Statistical Methods

The choice of statistical method depends on several factors, including the evaluation question, evaluation design, sample size, number of study groups, whether groups are matched or paired for certain characteristics, number of measures, data distribution, and the type of data collected. *Descriptive statistics* are often sufficient to answer questions about participant perceptions, distribution of characteristics and responses, and percentage change or achievement. For all types of data, a display of the percentages or proportions in each response category is an important first step in analysis. Medians and ranges are sometimes useful in characterizing ordinal as well as numerical data. Means and standard deviations are reserved for describing numerical data. Ordinal data can sometimes be treated as numerical data so that means and standard deviations (or other measures of variance) can be applied.

> **EXAMPLE:** *Conversion of Ordinal to Numerical Data for the Purpose of Statistical Analysis.* Curriculum evaluators found it useful to convert the following response categories to numerical data so that responses could be summarized by means: not at all [0], a little [1], a moderate amount [2], a lot [3], completely [4]; and strongly disagree [1], disagree [2], neither agree nor disagree [3], agree [4], strongly agree [5].

Statistical tests of significance are required to answer questions about the statistical significance of changes in individual learners or groups of learners and of associations between various characteristics. *Parametric statistics,* such as *t*-tests, analysis of variance, regression, and Pearson correlation analysis, are often appropriate for numerical data. Parametric tests assume that the data are "normally" distributed in a bell-shaped curve around the mean, but they are often robust enough to tolerate some deviation from this assumption. Sometimes ordinal data can be treated as numerical data (see example above) to permit the use of parametric statistics. *Nonparametric statistics*, such as chi-square, Wilcoxon rank-sum test, Spearman's correlation statistic, and nonparametric versions of analysis of variance, are often appropriate for small sample sizes, categorical data, and non-normally distributed data. Computer programs are available that can perform parametric and nonparametric tests on the same data. This approach can provide a check of the statistical results, when numerical data do not satisfy all of the assumptions for parametric tests. One can be confident about using parametric statistics on ordinal level data when nonparametric statistics confirm decisions regarding statistical significance obtained using parametric statistics.

Table 7.6. Commonly Used Statistical Methods

Type of Measurement (Dependent Variable)	Tests/Methods Used for Evaluating Statistically Significant Differences or Associations						
	One Sample (observed vs. expected)	Two Samples		N Samples		Correlation	Mulivariate Analysis*
		Independent	Related (pre-post)	Independent	Related (pre-post)		
Nominal	Binomial Test Chi-square	Fisher exact test Chi-square	McNemar's test	Chi-square	Cochran's Q test	Contingency co-efficient	Cumulative logistic regression Discriminant function analysis
Dichotomous	Binomial Test Chi-square	Chi-square Odds ratio Relative risk Prevalence ratio	McNemar's test	Chi-square Logistic regression (odds ratios)	Logistic regression (odds ratios)		Logistic regression (odds ratios) Generalized estimating equations (GEE) Discriminant functional analysis
Ordinal or Ordered	Kolmogorov-Smirnov one sample test One-sample runs test	Median test Mann-Whitney U Kolmogorov-Smirnov test Wald-Wolfowitz runs test	Sign test Wilcoxon matched pairs signed rank test	Kruskal-Wallis ANOVA (one-way ANOVA)	Friedman's two-way ANOVA†	Spearman's r Kendall's τ (tau) Kendall's w	Multiple regression Polychotomous logistic regression Generalized estimating equations (GEE) Hierarchical regression models (mixed regression)

Interval and Ratio	Confidence interval	t-test	Paired t-test	ANOVA	Repeated-measures ANOVA Generalized estimating equations (GEE) Hierarchical regression models (mixed regression)	Pearson r	Linear regression Partial correlation Multiple correlation Multiple regression ANCOVA[‡] Generalized estimating equations (GEE) Hierarchical regression models (mixed regression) Canonical correlation

* Multivariate analysis involves analysis of more than one variable at a time and permits analysis of the relationship between one independent variable (e.g., the curriculum) and a dependent variable of interest (e.g., learner skill or behavior), while controlling for other independent variables (e.g., age, gender, level of training, previous or concurrent experiences).

† ANOVA: Analysis of variance.

‡ ANCOVA: Analysis of covariance.

Curriculum developers have varying degrees of statistical expertise. Those with modest levels of expertise and limited resources (the majority) may choose to keep data analysis simple. They can consult textbooks (see General References, Statistics) on how to perform simple statistical tests, such as *t*-tests, chi-squares, and the Wilcoxon rank-sum test. These tests, especially for small sample sizes, can be performed by hand or with a calculator (online calculators are now available) and do not require access to computer programs. Sometimes, however, the needs of users will require more sophisticated approaches. Often there are individuals within or beyond one's institution who can provide statistical consultation. The curriculum developer will use the statistician's time most efficiently when the evaluation questions are clearly stated and the key independent and dependent variables are clearly defined. Some familiarity with the range and purposes of commonly used statistical methods can also facilitate communication. Table 7.6 displays the situations in which statistical methods are appropriately used, based on the type of data being analyzed, the number and type of samples, and whether correlational or multivariate analysis is desired. One type of situation that is not captured in the table is statistical analysis of time to a desired educational outcome or event, which can be analyzed using various survival analysis techniques such as the log-rank test (bivariate analysis) or Cox regression (bivariate or multivariate analysis). Cox (or proportional hazards) regression has the advantage of providing hazard ratios (akin to odds ratios).

TASK X: REPORT RESULTS

The final step in evaluation is the reporting and distributing of results (61). In planning evaluation reports, it is helpful to think of the *needs of users.*

The *timeliness* of reports can be critical. Individual learners benefit from the immediate feedback of formative assessment results, so that the information can be processed while the learning experience is still fresh and can be used to enhance subsequent learning within the curriculum. Evaluation results are helpful to faculty and curriculum planners when they are received in time to prepare for the next curricular cycle. Important decisions, such as the allocation of educational resources for the coming year, may be influenced by the timely reporting of evaluation results. External bodies, such as funding agencies or specialty boards, may impose deadlines for the receipt of reports.

The *format* of a report should match the needs of its users in content, language, and length. Individual learners, faculty members, and curriculum developers may want detailed evaluation reports pertaining to their particular (or the curriculum's) performance that include all relevant quantitative and qualitative data provided by the measurement instruments. Administrators, deans, and department chairs may prefer brief reports that provide background information on the curriculum and that synthesize the evaluation information relevant to their respective needs. External bodies and publishers (see Chapter 10) may specify the format they expect for a report.

It is always desirable to *display results in a succinct and clear manner and to use plain language; an Executive Summary* can be helpful to the reader. Collated results can be enhanced by the addition of descriptive statistics, such as percentage distributions, means, medians, and standard deviations. Other results can be displayed in a clear and efficient manner in tables, graphs, or figures. Specific examples can help explain and bring to life summaries of qualitative data.

CONCLUSION

Evaluation is not the final step in curriculum planning, but one that affects and should evolve in concert with other steps in the curriculum development process (see also Chapter 1). It provides important information that helps a program and individuals to improve their performances. It provides information that facilitates judgments and decisions about individuals and a curriculum. A stepwise approach can help ensure an evaluation that meets the needs of its users and that balances methodological rigor with feasibility.

ACKNOWLEDGMENTS

We thank David A. Cook, M.D., M.H.P.E., for his thoughtful review and suggestions to the section on Reliability, Validity, and Bias, and Ken Kolodner, Sc.D., for his helpful input to the section Analyze Data and Table 7.6.

QUESTIONS

For the curriculum you are coordinating, planning, or would like to be planning, please answer or think about the following questions:

1. Who will be the *users* of your curriculum?

2. What are their needs? *How will evaluation results be used?*

3. What *resources* are available for evaluation, in terms of *time, personnel, equipment, facilities, funds,* and *existing data*?

4. Identify one to three critical *evaluation questions.* Are they *congruent* with the objectives of your curriculum? Do either the objectives or evaluation questions need to be changed?

5. Name and diagram the most appropriate *evaluation design* for each evaluation question, considering both methodological rigor and feasibility (see Table 7.2 and text).

6. Choose the most appropriate *measurement methods* for the evaluation you are designing above (see Table 7.3). Are the measurement methods *congruent* with the evaluation questions (i.e., are you measuring the correct items)? Would it be *feasible* for you, given available resources, to construct and administer the required measurement instruments? If not, do you need to revise the evaluation questions or choose other evaluation methods? What issues related to reliability and validity pertain to your measurement instrument?

7. What *ethical issues* are likely to be raised by your evaluation in terms of confidentiality, access, consent, resource allocation, potential impact, or other concerns? Should you consult your institutional review board?

8. Consider the *data collection* process. *Who will be responsible* for data collection? How can the data be collected so that *resource use* is minimized and *response rate* is maximized? Are data collection considerations likely to influence the *design of your measurement instruments*?

9. How will the data that are collected be *analyzed*? Given your evaluation questions, are *descriptive statistics* sufficient or are *tests of statistical significance* required? Is a *power analysis* desirable? Will statistical consultation be required?

10. List the goals, content, format, and time frame of the various *evaluation reports* you envision, given the needs of the users (refer to Questions 1 and 2). How will you ensure that the reports are completed?

Congratulations! You have read and thought about six steps critical to curriculum development. At this point rereading Chapter 1 may be worthwhile, to review briefly the six steps and reflect on how they interact.

GENERAL REFERENCES

Comprehensive

Fink A. *Evaluation Fundamentals*: *Insights into the Outcomes, Effectiveness, and Quality of Health Programs.* 2nd ed. Thousand Oaks, Calif.: Sage Publications; 2005.
Reader-friendly, basic comprehensive reference on program evaluation with examples from the health and social science fields. 265 pages.

Fitzpatrick JL, Sanders JR, Worthen BR. *Program Evaluation. Alternative Approaches and Practical Guidelines,* 3rd ed. Boston: Pearson Education, Inc. Allyn & Bacon; 2004.

Comprehensive text on evaluation methods and systematic, detailed approach to design, implementation, and reporting of an evaluation. Excellent use of a longitudinal evaluation problem throughout the text. 555 pages.

Green LW, Lewis FM. *Measurement and Evaluation in Health Education and Health Promotion.* Palo Alto, Calif.: Mayfield Publications; 1986.
Clearly written, comprehensive text with examples from community health and patient education programs with easy applicability to medical education programs. Both quantitative and qualitative methods are included. 411 pages.

Herman JL, ed. *Program Evaluation Kit*, 2nd ed. Newbury Park, Calif.: Sage Publications; 1987.
A user-friendly series of nine handbooks written by various authors, particularly useful for medical educators who are new to the field of evaluation. The subjects include an evaluator's handbook (evaluation framework, kinds of evaluation) and eight "how-to" books on the following: how to focus an evaluation, how to design an evaluation, how to use qualitative methods in evaluation, how to assess program implementation, how to measure attitudes, how to measure performance and use tests, how to analyze data, and how to communicate findings. Nine books ranging from 92 to 176 pages in length.

Whitman NA, Cockayne TW. *Evaluating Medical School Courses: A User Centered Handbook.* Salt Lake City, Utah: University of Utah, School of Medicine; 1984.
Brief handbook to help plan and implement the evaluation of medical school courses, with an emphasis on making the evaluation pertinent for the various evaluation users. The book also introduces the concept of metaevaluation (evaluating your evaluations). 35 pages.

Windsor R, Clark N, Boyd NR, Goodman RM. *Evaluation of Health Promotion, Health Education, and Disease Prevention Programs*. New York: McGraw Hill; 2004.
   Written for health professionals who are responsible for planning, implementing, and evaluating health education or health promotion programs, with direct applicability to medical education. Especially useful are the chapters on process evaluations and cost evaluation. 292 pages.

Measurement

Case SM, Swanson DB. *Constructing Written Test Questions for the Basic and Clinical Sciences,* 3rd ed. (revised). Philadelphia: National Board of Medical Examiners; 2002.
   Written for medical school educators who need to construct and interpret flawlessly written test questions. Frequent examples. Available at www.nbme.org/publications/index.html. Accessed March 5, 2009. 180 pages.

Dillman DA. *Mail and Internet Surveys: The Tailored Design Method,* 2nd ed. Hoboken, N.J.: John Wiley & Sons; 2000.
   Book on how to write questions for, design, and administer surveys. 464 pages.

Downing SM, Haladyna TM. *Handbook of Test Development.* Mahwah, N.J.: Lawrence Erlbaum Associates; 2006.
   Definitive and current handbook on the 12 steps of test development and comprehensive review of issues around testing. 778 pages.

Fink A, ed. *The Survey Kit* (Vols. 1–9). Thousand Oaks, Calif.: Sage Publications; 2002.
   Nine user-friendly, practical handbooks about various aspects of surveys both for the novice and for those who are more experienced but want a refresher reference. The first book is an overview of the survey method. The other handbooks are "how-to" books on asking survey questions; conducting self-administered and mail surveys; conducting interviews by telephone, in person, and by mail; designing surveys; sampling for surveys; measuring reliability and validity; analyzing survey data; and reporting on surveys. Nine books, ranging from 73 to 223 pages in length.

Gronlund NE. *Assessment of Student Achievement,* 8th ed. Boston: Pearson Education; 2006.
   Basic text with review of assessment methods, validity and reliability in planning, preparing and using achievement tests, performance assessments, portfolio assessment, grading reporting, and interpretation of scores. 232 pages.

Miller DC. *Handbook of Research Design and Social Measurement,* 6th ed. Thousand Oaks, Calif.: Sage Publications; 2002.
   The most useful part of this textbook is Part 7 (209 pages), selected sociometric scales and indexes to measure social variables. Scales in the following areas are discussed: social status; group structure and dynamics; social indicators; measures of organizational structure; community; social participation; leadership in the work organization; morale and job satisfaction; scales of attitudes, values, and norms; personality measurements; and others. 786 pages.

Shannon S, Norman G, eds. *Evaluation Methods: A Resource Handbook* 3rd ed. Hamilton, Ont.: Programme for Educational Research and Development, McMaster University; 1996.
   A practical, well-written handbook on evaluation methods for assessing the performance of medical students. Reliability and validity issues are discussed for each evaluation method, including summary reports and ratings; oral examinations; written tests; performance tests; self- and peer assessments; assessment of problem-solving, psychomotor, communication, and critical apprais-al skills; and evaluation of bioethics and professional behavior. 120 pages. Available at www.fhs.mcmaster.ca/perd/publications/pub_evalmethods.htm. Accessed March 5, 2009.

Evaluation Designs

Campbell DT, Stanley JC. *Experimental and Quasi-Experimental Designs for Research*. Chicago: Rand McNally; 1963.
   Succinct, classic text on research/evaluation designs for educational programs. 84 pages.

Cook TD, Campbell DT. *Quasi-Experimentation: Design and Analysis Issues for Field Settings.* Chicago: Rand McNally; 1979.
    Also a classic but in-depth text and follow-up to Campbell and Stanley's book. Thorough discussions of causal inference and types of validity. 405 pages.

Fraenkel JR, Wallen NE. *How to Design and Evaluate Research in Education,* 6th ed. New York: McGraw-Hill; 2006.
    Comprehensive and straightforward review of educational research methods with step-by-step analysis of research and real case studies; interactive CD with quizzes available. Includes basic concepts in statistics. 620 pages.

Qualitative Evaluation

Crabtree B, Miller W, eds. *Doing Qualitative Research*, 2nd ed. Thousand Oaks, Calif.: Sage Publications; 1999.
    Readable book focusing on qualitative research in primary care with many examples. Chapter 1 puts qualitative studies into a taxonomy of research approaches and defines terms. Data collection and analysis strategies are discussed, including audio- and videotape analysis. 406 pages.

Denzin NK, Lincoln YS. *Handbook of Qualitative Research,* 3rd ed. Thousand Oaks, Calif.: Sage Publications; 2005.
    Comprehensive text, useful as a reference to look up particular topics. 1210 pages.

Miles M, Huberman AM. *Qualitative Data Analysis: An Expanded Sourcebook*, 2nd ed. Thousand Oaks, Calif.: Sage Publications; 1994.
    Practical text/useful resource on qualitative data analysis. Chapter 10 focuses on drawing and verifying conclusions, as well as issues of reliability and validity. 338 pages.

Patton MQ. *Qualitative Research & Evaluation Methods,* 3rd ed. Thousand Oaks, Calif.: Sage Publications; 2002.
    Readable, example-filled text emphasizing strategies for generating useful and credible qualitative information for decision making. The three sections of the book cover conceptual issues in the use of qualitative methods; qualitative designs and data collection; and analysis, interpretation, and reporting of such studies. 598 pages.

Richards L, Morse JM. *Read Me First for a User's Guide to Qualitative Methods,* 2nd ed. Thousand Oaks, Calif.: Sage Publications; 2007.
    Readable, introductory book to qualitative research methods. 288 pages.

Statistics

Kanji G. *100 Statistical Tests,* 3rd ed. Thousand Oaks, Calif.: Sage Publications; 2006.
    A handy reference for the applied statistician and everyday user of statistics. An elementary knowledge of statistics is sufficient to allow the reader to follow the formulae given and carry out the tests. All 100 tests are cross-referenced to several headings. Examples are also included. 242 pages.

Norman GR, Streiner D. *PDQ Statistics*. Hamilton, Ont.: B.C. Decker ; 2003.
    This short, well-written book covers types of variables, descriptive statistics, parametric and non-parametric statistics, multivariate methods, and research designs. The authors assume that the reader has had some introductory exposure to statistics. The intent of the book is to help the reader understand the various approaches to analysis when reading/critiquing the results section of research articles. Useful also for planning an analysis in order to avoid misuse and misinterpretation of statistical tests. 218 pages.

Norman GR, Streiner DL. *Biostatistics: The Bare Essentials,* 2nd ed. Lewiston, N.Y.: B.C. Decker; 2000.
    This book conveys the traditional content for a statistics book in an irreverent and humorous tone, packaged for the "do-it-yourselfer." The main sections of the book include the nature of data and

statistics, analysis of variance, regression and correlation, and nonparametric statistics. Three features of the book are helpful: the computer notes at the end of each chapter, which help the reader with the three most common statistical programs; highlighted important points in the text; and sample size calculations with each chapter. 324 pages.

Shott S. *Statistics for Health Professionals*. Philadelphia: W.B. Saunders Co.; 1990.
The author states that after studying this text and working the problems, the reader should be able to select appropriate statistics for most data sets, interpret results, evaluate analyses reported in the literature, and interpret SPSS and SPS output for the common statistical procedures. 418 pages.

Siegel S, Castellan N. *Nonparametric Statistics for the Behavioral Sciences,* 2nd ed. New York: McGraw-Hill; 1988.
Usable text for understanding concepts or as a reference. The information is organized by the characteristics of the data samples (single sample, paired samples, independent samples, measures of association, etc.). It includes examples that illustrate the application of tests to research problems. 399 pages.

SPECIFIC REFERENCES

1. Fitzpatrick JL, Sanders JR, Worthen BR. Evaluation's basic purpose, uses, and conceptual distinctions, Chapter 1. In: Fitzpatrick JL, Sanders JR, Worthen BR. *Program Evaluation: Alternative Approaches and Practical Guidelines*, 3rd ed. Boston: Pearson Education, Allyn & Bacon; 2004. Pp. 4–5.
2. Atasoylu AA, Wright SM, Beasley BW, Cofrancesco J, Macpherson DS, Partridge T, Thomas PA, Bass EB. Promotion criteria for clinician-educators. *J Gen Intern Med.* 2003;18:711–16.
3. Beasley BW, Wright SM, Cofrancesco J Jr., Babbott SF, Thomas PA, Bass EB. Promotion criteria for clinician-educators in the United States and Canada. A survey of promotion committee chairpersons. *JAMA.* 1997;278:723–28.
4. Fleming VM, Schindler N, Martin GJ, DaRosa DA. Separate and equitable promotion tracks for clinician-educators. *JAMA.* 2005;294:1101–4.
5. Hafler JP, Lovejoy FH Jr. Scholarly activities recorded in the portfolios of teacher-clinician faculty. *Acad Med.* 2000;75:649–52.
6. Simpson D, Hafler J, Brown D, Wilkerson L. Documentation systems for educators seeking academic promotion in U.S. medical schools. *Acad Med.* 2004;79:783–90.
7. Green LW, Lewis FM. Formative evaluation and measures of quality, Chapter 2. In: *Measurement and Evaluation on Health Education and Health Promotion*. Palo Alto, Calif.: Mayfield Publications; 1986. Pp. 27–53.
8. Green LW, Lewis FM. *Measurement and Evaluation in Health Education and Health Promotion*. Palo Alto, Calif.: Mayfield Publications; 1986. Pp. 120–21, 366.
9. Shannon S, Norman G, eds. *Evaluation Methods: A Resource Handbook*. Hamilton, Ont.: Program for Educational Development, McMaster University; 1995. Pp. 4–8.
10. Fitzpatrick JL, Sanders JR, Worthen BR. *Program Evaluation. Alternative Approaches and Practical Guidelines*, 3rd ed. Boston: Pearson Publications; 2004. Pp. 400–406.
11. Hafferty FW, Franks R. The hidden curriculum, ethics teaching, and the structure of medical education. *Acad Med.* 1994;69(11):861–71.
12. Hundert EM, Hafferty F, Christakis D. Characteristics of the informal curriculum and trainees' ethical choices. *Acad Med.* 1996;71(6):624–33.
13. Fitzpatrick JL, Sanders JR, Worthen BR. *Program Evaluation. Alternative Approaches and Practical Guidelines,* 3rd ed. Boston: Pearson Publications; 2004. Pp. 212–16.
14. Fitzpatrick JL, Sanders JR, Worthen BR. Identifying and selecting the evaluation questions and criteria, Chapter 12. In: Fitzpatrick JL, Sanders JR, Worthen BR. *Program Evaluation.*

Alternative Approaches and Practical Guidelines, 3rd ed. Boston: Pearson Publications; 2004. Pp. 232–59.

15. Fink A. Evaluation questions and standards of effectiveness, Chapter 2. In: Fink A. *Evaluation Fundamentals: Insights into the Outcomes, Effectiveness, and Quality of Health Programs,* 2nd ed. Thousand Oaks, Calif.: Sage Publications; 2005. Pp. 41–68.

16. Joint Committee on Standards for Educational Evaluation. The program evaluation standards. Available at www.wmich.edu/evalctr/jc/. Accessed March 5, 2009.

17. Coles CR, Grant JG. Curriculum evaluation in medical health care education. *Medical Education.* 1985;19(5):405–22.

18. Green LW, Lewis FM. Selecting and implementing designs for evaluation, Chapter 9. In: *Measurement and Evaluation in Health Education and Health Promotion.* Palo Alto, Calif.: Mayfield Publishing; 1986. Pp. 196–222.

19. Campbell DT, Stanley JC. *Experimental and Quasi-Experimental Designs for Research.* Chicago: Rand McNally; 1963.

20. Fink A. Designing program evaluations, Chapter 3. In: Fink A. *Evaluation Fundamentals: Insights into the Outcomes, Effectiveness, and Quality of Health Programs,* 2nd ed. Thousand Oaks, Calif.: Sage Publications; 2005. Pp. 71–98.

21. Fitz-Gibbon CT, Morris LL. *How to Design a Program Evaluation* (Book 3). In: Herman JL, ed. *Program Evaluation Kit.* Newbury Park, Calif.: Sage Publications; 1987. Pp. 25–127.

22. Cook TD, Campbell DT. *Quasi-Experimentation: Design and Analysis Issues for Field Settings.* Boston: Houghton Mifflin; 1979. Pp. 50–80, 95–146, 341–71.

23. Fitzpatrick JL, Sanders JR, Worthen BR. Collecting evaluative information: design, sampling, and cost choices, Chapter 14. In: Fitzpatrick JL, Sanders JR, Worthen BR. *Program Evaluation. Alternative Approaches and Practical Guidelines,* 3rd ed. Boston: Pearson Education, Allyn & Bacon; 2004. Pp. 303–74.

24. Fraenkel JR, Wallen NE. Internal validity, Chapter 9, and Experimental research, Chapter 13. In: Fraenkel JR, Wallen NE. *How to Design and Evaluate Research in Education,* 6th ed. New York: McGraw-Hill; 2006. Pp. 168–86, 265–304.

25. Windsor R, Clark N, Boyd NR, Goodman RM. Formative and impact evaluations, Chapter 6. In: Windsor R, Clark N, Boyd NR, Goodman RM. *Evaluation of Health Promotion, Health Education, and Disease Prevention Programs.* New York: McGraw Hill; 2004. Pp. 215–63.

26. Shannon S, Norman G, eds. *Evaluation Methods: A Resource Handbook.* Hamilton, Ont.: Programme for Educational Research and Development, McMaster University; 1996. Pp. 25–118.

27. Morris LL, Fitz-Gibbon CT, Lindheim E. Determining how well a test fits the program. In: *How to Measure Performance and Use Tests* (Book 7). In: *Program Evaluation Kit.* Newbury Park, Calif.: Sage Publications; 1987. Pp. 45–67.

28. Lorig K, Stewart A, Ritter P, Gonzalez V, Laurent D, Lynch, J. *Outcome Measures for Health Education and Other Health Care Interventions.* Thousand Oaks, Calif.: Sage Publications; 1996. Pp. 34–89.

29. McDowell I. *Measuring Health: A Guide to Rating Scales and Questionnaires,* 3rd ed. New York: Oxford University Press; 2006.

30. Kassebaum DG. The measurement of outcomes in the assessment of educational program effectiveness. *Acad Med.* 1990;65:293–96.

31. Belfield C, Thomas H, Bullock A, Eynon R, Wall D. Measuring effectiveness for best evidence medical education: a discussion. *Med Teach.* 2001;23:164–70.

32. Miller DC. Assessing social variables: scales and indexes, Part 7, In: Miller DC. *Handbook of Research Design and Social Measurement,* 6th ed. Thousand Oaks, Calif.: Sage Publications; 2002. Pp. 453–660.

33. *Measurement of Nursing Outcomes,* 2nd ed. Waltz CF, Jenkins LS, eds. Volume 1: *Measuring Nursing Performance in Practice, Education, and Research.* 2001. Strickland OL, DiIorio C,

eds. Volume 2: *Client Outcomes and Quality of Care.* 2003. Strickland OL, Dilorio C, eds. Volume 3: *Self Care and Coping.* 2003. New York: Springer Publishing Co.

34. Henerson ME, Morris LL, Fitz-Gibbon CT. *How to Measure Attitudes* (Book 6). In: Fink A, ed. *Program Evaluation Kit.* Newbury Park, Calif.: Sage Publications; 1987. Pp. 39–56, 178–81.

35. Windsor R, Clark N, Boyd NR, Goodman RM. *Evaluation of Health Promotion, Health Education, and Disease Prevention Programs.* New York: McGraw Hill; 2004. Pp. 85–106.

36. Fink A. Collecting information: the right data sources, Chapter 5, and Evaluation measures, Chapter 6. In: Fink A. *Evaluation Fundamentals: Insights into the Outcomes, Effectiveness, and Quality of Health Programs,* 2nd ed. Thousand Oaks, Calif.: Sage Publications; 2005. Pp. 117–162.

37. Afrin LB, Arana GW, Medio FJ, Ybarra AF, Clarke HS Jr. Improving oversight of the graduate medical education enterprise: one institution's strategies and tools. *Acad Med.* 2006;81:419–25.

38. Downing SM. Validity: on the meaningful interpretation of data. *Med Educ.* 2003;37:830–37.

39. Downing SM. Reliability: On the reproducibility of assessment data. *Med Educ.* 2004;38:1006–12.

40. Cook DA, Beckman TJ. Current concepts in validity and reliability for psychometric instruments: theory and application. *Am J of Med.* 2006;119:166.e7–166.e16.

41. Siegel S, Castellan N. *Nonparametric Statistics.* 2nd ed. New York: McGraw-Hill; 1988. Pp. 284–91, 310–11.

42. Crossley J, Davies H, Humphris G, Jolly B. Generalisability: A key to unlock professional assessment. *Med Educ.* 2002;36:972–78.

43. Hatcher L, Stepanski EJ. *A Step-by-Step Approach to Using the SAS System for Univariate and Multivariate Statistics.* Cary, North Carolina: SAS Institute; 1994. Pp. 505–16.

44. Norman GR, Streiner DL. *Biostatistics: The Bare Essentials,* 2nd ed. Lewiston, N.Y.: B.C. Decker; 2000. Pp. 163–77.

45. Stillman P, Swanson D, Regan MB, et al. Assessment of clinical skills of residents utilizing standardized patients: a follow-up study and recommendations for application. *Ann Intern Med.* 1991;114:393–401.

46. Williams RG, Klamen DA, McGaghie WC. Cognitive, social and environmental sources of bias in clinical performance ratings. *Teach Learn Med.* 2003 Fall;15(4):270–92.

47. Downing SM and Haladyna T. Validity threats: overcoming interference with proposed interpretations with assessment data. *Med Educ.* 2004;38:327–33.

48. Mays N, Pope, C. Qualitative research in health care: assessing quality in qualitative research. *BMJ.* 2000:320:50–52.

49. Barbour RS. Checklists for improving rigour in qualitative research: a case of the tail wagging the dog. *BMJ.* 2001;322:1115–17.

50. Giacomini MK, Cook DJ, for the Evidence-based Medicine Working Group. Users' guides to the medical literature, XXIII. Qualitative research in health care: A. Are the results of the study valid? *JAMA.* 2000;284:357–62.

51. Giacomini MK, Cook DJ, for the Evidence-based Medicine Working Group. Users' guides to the medical literature. XXIII. Qualitative research in health care: B. What are the results and how do they help me care for my patients? *JAMA.* 2000;284:478–82.

52. Henry GT, Mark MM. Beyond use: understanding evaluation's influence on attitudes and actions. *American Journal of Evaluation.* 2003;24:293–314.

53. Shott S. *Statistics for Health Professionals.* Philadelphia: W.B. Saunders; 1990. Pp. 347–49.

54. Dimick JB, Diener-West M, Lipsett PA. Negative results of randomized clinical trials published in the surgical literature: equivalency or error? *Arch Surg.* 2001;136:796–800.

55. Fink A. Sampling, Chapter 4. In: Fink A. *Evaluation Fundamentals: Insights into the Outcomes, Effectiveness, and Quality of Health Programs,* 2nd ed. Thousand Oaks, Calif.: Sage Publications; 2005. Pp. 98–115.

56. Fraenkel JR, Wallen NE. Data analysis. Part 3. In: Fraenkel JR, Wallen NE. *How to Design and Evaluate Research in Education,* 6th ed. New York: McGraw-Hill; 2006. Pp. 187–263.
57. Fink A. Analyzing evaluation data, Chapter 8. In: Fink A. *Evaluation Fundamentals: Insights into the Outcomes, Effectiveness, and Quality of Health Programs,* 2nd ed. Thousand Oaks, Calif.: Sage Publications; 2005. Pp. 187–217.
58. Windish DM, Diener-West M. A clinician-educator's roadmap to choosing and interpreting statistical tests. *J Gen Intern Med.* 2006;21:656–60.
59. Baghi H, Noorbaloochi S, Moore JB. Statistical and nonstatistical significance: implications for health care researchers. *Qual Manag Health Care.* 2007;16:104–12.
60. Cohen J. *Statistical Power Analysis for the Behavioral Sciences.* Hillsdale, N.J.: Lawrence Erlbaum Associates; 1988.
61. Morris LL, Fitz-Gibbon CT, Freeman ME. *How to Communicate Evaluation Findings* (Book 9). In: *Program Evaluation Kit.* Newbury Park, Calif.: Sage Publications; 1987. Pp. 9–89.
62. Barman A. Critiques on the objective structured clinical examination. *Ann Acad Med Singapore.* 2005;34(8):478–82.
63. Newble D. Techniques for measuring clinical competence: objective structured clinical examinations. *Med Educ.* 2004;38(2):199–203.
64. Sultana CJ. The objective structured assessment of technical skills and the ACGME competencies. *Obstet Gynecol Clin North Am.* 2006;33(2):259–65.
65. Goff B, Mandel L, Lentz G, Vanblaricom A, Oelschlager AM, Lee D, Galakatos A, Davies M, Nielsen P. Assessment of resident surgical skills: is testing feasible? *Am J Obstet Gynecol.* 2005;192(4):1331–40.
66. Ault G, Reznick R, MacRae H, Leadbetter W, DaRosa D, Joehl R, Peters J, Regehr G. Exporting a technical skills evaluation technology to other sites. *Am J Surg.* 2001;182(3):254–56.

CHAPTER EIGHT

Curriculum Maintenance
and Enhancement

. . . keeping the curriculum vibrant

David E. Kern, M.D., M.P.H., and Patricia A. Thomas, M.D.

THE DYNAMIC NATURE OF CURRICULA

A curriculum that is static gradually declines and dies. A successful curriculum is continually developing. It must respond to evaluation results and feedback, to changes in the knowledge base and the material requiring mastery, to changes in resources (including faculty), to changes in its targeted learners, and to changes in institutional and societal values and needs. A successful curriculum requires *understanding, sustenance,* and *management of change* to maintain its strengths and to promote further improvement. *Innovations*, *networking* with colleagues at other institutions, and *scholarly activity* can also strengthen a curriculum.

UNDERSTANDING ONE'S CURRICULUM

To appropriately nurture a curriculum and manage change, one must understand the curriculum and appreciate its complexity. This includes not only the written curriculum but also its learners, its faculty, its support staff, the processes by which it is administered and evaluated, and the setting in which it takes place. Table 8.1 lists the various areas related to a curriculum that are in need of assessment. Table 8.2 lists some methods of assessing how a curriculum is functioning. *Program evaluation* (discussed in Chapter 7) provides objective and representative subjective feedback on some of these areas. Methods that promote *informal information exchange*, such as internal and external reviews, observation of curricular components, and individual or group meetings with learners, faculty, and support staff, can enrich one's understanding of a curriculum. They can also build relationships that help to maintain and further develop a curriculum.

EXAMPLE: *Community-Based Practice Experience.* The General Internal Medicine Residency Program at an academic medical center has developed a community-based clinical experience for residents in order to expose residents to efficiently operating, real-world primary care practices and to foster learning from a broader range of patient problems than is encountered in the hospital-based medical clinic. Teams of three PGY–2 and PGY–3 residents, one faculty leader, and three or four core clinical preceptors constitute firms at each of four separate community-based practices (CBPs). Residents are assigned every third month to an ambulatory block rotation that includes three sessions per week at their CBP. Representative feedback on the CBP experience is received monthly via a computer-based evaluation system, as well as yearly from more comprehensive questionnaires completed by firm residents and faculty. Practice reports are generated periodically that provide information on the number of different patients seen, number of patients seen per hour scheduled, fee-for-service revenue generated, billing profiles, and referral patterns. Record keeping and preventive care audits are conducted yearly on all CBP providers. Informal feedback on how the CBP experience is functioning is gained at monthly conferences, during which firm residents share experiences with one another and the residency program director. Minutes from quarterly meetings of residents with their faculty advisors, quarterly meetings of residents with program directors, and frequent informal meetings with residents and faculty provide additional information on the quality of these experiences. Finally, strengths, weaknesses, and future directions for the CBP experience are brainstormed every year in a special half-day CBP Retreat, to which all residents, preceptors, firm leaders, clinic administrators, and selected clinic support staff are invited to share their experiences and perspectives. Through these various and complementary mechanisms, the program director develops a good understanding of the CBP experience.

EXAMPLE: *UME Curriculum.* A major revision of the four-year undergraduate medical education (UME) M.D. curriculum at Johns Hopkins was implemented in 1992 with these major themes: integration of basic science content and clinical experience, reduction of lectures and increase of small group case-based teaching, early experience with community-based practicing physicians, strengthening and coordination of social science content into a longitudinal course (the *Physician and Society [PAS] Course*), and increased ambulatory experience in each of the required clerkships (1). Oversight of the curriculum was coordinated by the Educational Policy Committee (EPC) chaired by the Vice Dean for Education. Subcommittees of the EPC included a Year 1 Course Directors committee, a Year 2 committee, and the Clinical Clerkship Directors committee. Each course/clerkship collected student feedback and performance data, which were reviewed by the course director and the appropriate

Table 8.1.   Areas for Assessment and Potential Change

The Written or Intended Curriculum

Goals and objectives	Are they understood and accepted by all involved in the curriculum? Are they realistic? Can some be deleted? Should some be altered? Do others need to be added? Are there new accreditation standards? Are the objectives measurable?
Content	Is the amount just right, too little, or too much? Does the content still match the objectives? Can some content be deleted? Should other content be updated or added?
Curricular materials	Are they being read and used? How useful are the various components perceived to be? Can some be deleted? Should others be altered? Should new materials be added?
Methods	Are they well executed by faculty and well received by learners? Have they been sufficient to achieve curricular objectives? Are additional methods needed to prevent decay of learning? Do any of the methods address the new or important competencies of practice-based learning and improvement, systems-based practice/ teamwork, or professionalism (see Chapter 5)? Should they?
Congruence	Does the curriculum on paper match the curriculum in reality? If not, is that a problem? Does one or the other need to be changed?

The Environment/Setting of the Curriculum

Funding	How is the curriculum funded? Have funding needs changed with the addition of new expectations, additional learners, and/or new technologies?
Space	Is there sufficient space to support the various activities of the curriculum? For clinical curricula, is there sufficient space for learners to see patients, to consult references, and/or to meet with preceptors? Do the residents' clinical practices have the space to support the performance of learned skills and procedures?
Equipment and supplies	Are there sufficient equipment and supplies to support the curriculum while in progress, as well as to support and reinforce learning after completion of the curriculum? For example: Is there audiovisual equipment to support learning of interviewing skills? Are there sufficient, easily accessible references/electronic resources to support clinical practice experiences? Do the residents' clinical practices have the equipment to support the performance of learned skills and procedures?

Table 8.1. *(continued)*

Clinical experience	Is there sufficient concentrated clinical experience to support learning during the course of the curriculum? Is there sufficient clinical experience to reinforce learning after completion of the main curriculum? If there is insufficient patient volume or case mix, do alternative clinical experiences need to be found or do alternative approaches need to be developed, such as a simulated patient program? Are curricular objectives and general programmatic goals (e.g., efficiency, cost-effectiveness, customer service, record keeping, communication between referring and consulting practitioners, and provision of needed services) supported by clinical practice operations? Do support staff members support the curriculum?
Learning climate	Is the climate cooperative or competitive? Are learners encouraged to communicate or hide what they do not know? Is the curriculum sufficiently learner-centered and directed? Is it sufficiently teacher-centered and directed? Are learners encouraged and supported in identifying and pursuing their own learning needs and goals related to the curriculum?
Associated settings	Is learning from the curriculum supported and reinforced in the learners' prior, concomitant, and subsequent settings? If not, is there an opportunity to influence those settings?
Administration of the Curriculum	
Scheduling	Are schedules understandable, accurate, realistic, and helpful? Are they put out far enough in advance? Are they adhered to? How are scheduling changes managed?
Preparation and distribution of curricular materials	Is this being accomplished in a timely and consistent manner?
Collection, collation, and distribution of evaluation information	Is this being accomplished in a consistent and timely manner? If there are several different evaluation forms, can they be consolidated into one form or administered at one time, to decrease respondent fatigue?
Communication	Are changes in and important information about the curriculum being communicated to the appropriate individuals in a user-friendly, understandable, and timely manner?
Evaluation	
Congruence	Is what is being evaluated consistent with the goals, objectives, content, and methods of the curriculum? Does the evaluation reflect the main priorities of the curriculum?
Response rate	Is it sufficient to be representative of learners, faculty, or others involved in or affected by the curriculum?
Accuracy	Is the information reliable and valid?
Usefulness	Does the evaluation provide timely, easily understandable, and useful information to learners, faculty, curriculum coordinators, and relevant others? Is it being used? How?

Table 8.1. *(continued)*

Faculty	
Reliability/accessibility	How reliable are the faculty members in performing their curricular responsibilities? Are they devoting more or less time to the curriculum than expected? How accessible are faculty members in responding to learner questions and individual learner needs? Do faculty members schedule free time for discussion before or after sessions?
Teaching/facilitation skills	How skillful are faculty members at assessing the learners' needs, imparting information, asking questions, providing feedback, promoting practice-based learning and improvement, stimulating self-directed leaning, and creating a learning environment that is open, honest, exciting, and fun?
Nature of the learner-faculty relationship	Is the relationship more authoritative or collaborative? Is it more teacher-centered or learner-centered? For clinical precepting, does the learner see patients on his/her own? Does the learner observe the faculty member seeing patients or in other roles? Are learners exposed to faculty members' professional life outside of the curriculum (e.g., clinical practice, research, community work)? Do learners get to know faculty members as people, and how they balance professional, family, and personal life? Do faculty members serve as good role models?
Satisfaction	Do faculty members feel adequately recognized and rewarded for their teaching? Do they feel that their role is an important one? Are they enthusiastic? How satisfied are faculty members with clinical practice, teaching, and their professional lives in general?
Involvement	To what extent are faculty members involved in the curriculum? Do faculty members complete evaluation forms in a timely manner? Do faculty members attend scheduled meetings? Do faculty members provide useful suggestions for improving the curriculum?
Learners	
Achievement of curriculum objectives	Have cognitive, affective, psychomotor, process, and outcome objectives been achieved? Are learners responsible in meeting their obligations to the curriculum?
Satisfaction	How satisfied are learners with various aspects of the curriculum?
Involvement	To what extent are learners involved in the curriculum? Do they complete evaluation forms in a timely manner? Do they attend scheduled activities and meetings? Do they provide useful suggestions for improving the curriculum?
Application	Do learners apply their learning in other settings and contexts? Do they teach what they have learned to others?

Table 8.2.   Methods of Assessing How a Curriculum Is Functioning

See Program Evaluation (Chapter 7)
Learner/faculty/staff/patient questionnaires
Objective measures of skills and performance
Focus groups of learners, faculty, staff, patients
Other systematically collected data
Regular/periodic meetings with learners, faculty, staff
Special retreats and strategic planning sessions
Site visits
Informal observation of curricular components, learners, faculty, staff
Informal discussions with learners, faculty, staff

committee and presented in rotation to the EPC. The EPC reviewed student scores on the USMLE (U.S. Medical Licensing Examination) Step I and Step II examinations, AAMC (Association of American Medical Colleges) Graduation Questionnaire results, and residency placement. Institutional self-study before the Liaison Committee on Medical Education (LCME) accreditation surveys occurred in 1996 and 2005 and prompted collection of additional data, including residency program directors' surveys, faculty roster results, and alumni surveys.

Electronic curriculum management systems are being used increasingly to provide coordinated information for understanding and managing both subject-focused curricula and complex educational programs, such as an entire medical school curriculum (2).

THE MANAGEMENT OF CHANGE

Overview and Level of Decision Making

Most curricula require midcourse, end-of-cycle, and/or end-of-year changes. Changes may be prompted by informal feedback; evaluation results; accreditation standards; the evolving needs of learners, faculty, institutions, or society; or changes in available resources. *Before expending resources* to make curricular changes, however, it is often wise to *establish that the need for change 1) is sufficiently important, 2) affects a significant number of people, and 3) will persist if it is not addressed.*

It is also helpful to consider *at what level needs should be addressed and changes made*. Minor operational changes that are necessary for the smooth functioning of a curriculum are most efficiently made at the level of the curriculum coordinator or core group responsible for managing the curriculum. More complicated needs that require in-depth analysis and thoughtful planning for change may best be assigned to a carefully selected task group. Other needs may best be discussed and addressed in meetings of learners, faculty, and/or staff. Before implementing major curricular changes, it is often wise to ensure broad, representative support. It can also be helpful to pilot major or complex changes before implementing them fully.

EXAMPLE: *Community-Based Practice Experience.* The firm system described above was implemented in July 1994. Previously, General Internal Medicine (GIM) residents had been assigned to a 4–6 week CBP block rotation at the beginning of their PGY–2 year. Thereafter, residents spent from 0 sessions per month to 1 session per week at their CBP, depending on their hospital rotation. Residents enjoyed their CBP block rotation but had for years complained of the competing demands they felt between inpatient rotations and their CBP experience subsequent to the block rotation. CBP faculty complained of frequent scheduling changes and loss of a resident's identity with a practice subsequent to the ambulatory block month. At a meeting of GIM residents and faculty in November 1993, the firm system described above was brainstormed and discussed. At this and subsequent meetings, the idea received strong support from CBP faculty and GIM residents, who were willing to give up some elective time to accomplish the change. Approval for the change was obtained from the department chair/overall program director. Implementation details were worked out by the GIM residency program director in meetings with the residents, CBP faculty, and chief resident who was responsible for resident scheduling.

EXAMPLE: *UME Curriculum.* Over a decade, a number of changes in the four-year curriculum occurred. With further development and access to the Internet, lectures were videotaped and made available to students through the student intranet, prompting a reevaluation of how formal lecture time should be used in the curriculum. Increasing demands on faculty time left many courses struggling to find expert small group facilitators; course directors responded by introducing more structure to basic science small groups, and the institution developed a small group teaching skills workshop for new small group facilitators. Students requested more learner-centeredness in the *PAS* course, and "selectives" were introduced in years 1 and 2, for content such as "End-of-Life Care" and "Patient Safety." The institution adopted a course-management system (Blackboard) to deliver content more efficiently, which required faculty and staff development. New standards adopted by the LCME included cultural awareness and self-directed learning, which needed to be addressed within the curriculum structure. As ACGME (Accreditation Council for Graduate Medical Education) standards affected resident duty hours, several clerkships adjusted clerkship expectations, with fewer on-call requirements. The USMLE introduced a high-stakes Clinical Skills examination (Step IICS), which prompted increased use of standardized patient methodology for assessment in the clinical years. With the exception of the new Ambulatory Medicine clerkship, directors for each of the clerkships rotated to new faculty within the decade. These substantive changes, which involved several different stakeholders, were discussed at the EPC level and implemented at the course/clerkship director or institutional level, as appropriate.

Accreditation Standards

An important driver of change in medical education curricula are the organizations charged with accreditation at each level of the continuum. In the United States, the national accrediting bodies are the LCME for undergraduate medical education (3), the ACGME for graduate (residency) education (4), and the ACCME (Accreditation Council for Continuing Medical Education) for continuing medical education (5). Curriculum developers should stay abreast of *changing* accreditation standards that will affect their curricula because there is little option but to address these standards explicitly. It is also useful to look at expectations beyond the immediate timeline of the curriculum. For instance, a medical school curriculum must address the LCME standards, but it should also be aware of the ACGME Common Program Requirements. The adoption of the six core competencies in the ACGME Outcomes Project has altered many undergraduate programs' approach to teaching and assessment (see Chapter 5). Attending to these generic competencies in undergraduate, graduate, and postgraduate/continuing medical education curricula can improve coordination throughout the medical education continuum and permit reinforcement and increasing sophistication of learning at each level.

Environmental Changes

Changes in the environment in which a curriculum takes place can *create new opportunities* for the curriculum, *reinforce* the learning that has occurred, and *support* its *application* by learners or create challenges for curriculum coordinators. For example, practice development activities often affect clinical curricula. New institutional or extrainstitutional resources might be used to benefit a curriculum.

> **EXAMPLE:** *Development of Clinical Settings.* A curriculum on gynecology and women's health for internal medicine residents that includes excellent lectures and small group discussions might be hampered by the lack of sufficient clinical training experiences. The development of a women's health program by an associated institution that concentrates on the provision of preventive services for women could improve student and resident training in birth control counseling and management, breast and cervical cancer screening, and osteoporosis prevention, all foci of the curriculum. The development of medical record systems, computerized information systems, and well-trained support staff in the residents' primary care practices to promote and monitor the provision of preventive care services could support the application in real practice of what the residents learn in the curriculum. An incentive system for the faculty in the same practices that rewards the provision of preventive services could create faculty support for the above changes and promote the development of role models for residents and students.

> **EXAMPLE:** *Development of Clinical Settings.* The development of active faculty and staff quality improvement teams as part of a hospitalist service creates opportunities for student, resident, and fellow training in systems-based practice and teamwork.

> **EXAMPLE:** *New Resources.* The provision of databases that track residents' clinical experiences creates the opportunity for assessment of and reflection on their experiences, as well as interventions when appropriate.

> **EXAMPLE:** *UME Curriculum, Organizational Change Opportunity.* Several divisions of the university funded an office to coordinate volunteer opportunities for students in the Schools of Nursing, Medicine, and Public Health. This facilitated the inclusion of service learning as selectives within PAS.

> **EXAMPLE:** *UME Curriculum, Faculty Resources.* In 2005, the School of Medicine funded a College system, in which master clinicians assume teaching of Year 2 *Clinical Skills* and advising over 4 years. The creation and development of this faculty learning community enhanced the quality and consistency of teaching in the *Clinical Skills* course, which had been previously dependent on volunteer faculty.

> **EXAMPLE:** *UME Curriculum, Practice Resources.* In 2007 the community-based practices used in the Ambulatory Medicine clerkship adopted a sophisticated electronic medical record (Logician). Although concerns were raised regarding whether this would be a hindrance to student learning in the sites, a decision was made to provide 2 hours of training for incoming students. Students have easily adapted to the software and developed additional skills of using the software for practice quality and improvement, enhancing their systems-based knowledge.

> **EXAMPLE:** *Community-Based Practice Experience, Organizational Change Challenge.* In 2000, the leadership of the community-based practices and faculty associated with this curriculum transferred out of the Division of General Internal Medicine to an institution-wide organization involving many nonteaching practices. Productivity expectations and the salary structure for the community-based faculty changed. CBP faculty benefits no longer included

the coverage of tuition for continuing medical education (CME) courses. At the same time, the faculty development program, which had trained preceptors in the community-based practices without charge (see example below under Faculty Development), had begun charging tuition through the School of Medicine CME office. Concerns about the loss of clinical productivity while teaching or attending faculty development sessions and the tuition barrier posed challenges to the maintenance of a dedicated, well-trained cadre of clinical preceptors for this core component of the residency. Division and curricular leaders met with leaders of the new expanded CBP organization, so that the teaching function of the involved practices was preserved without loss of clinical productivity for the faculty, and accommodations were made on both sides so that selected new faculty could participate in the faculty development program. Yearly retreats involving the CBP leaders, CBP preceptors, practice administrators, residents, and curricular leaders were initiated to address ongoing challenges, promote the sharing of solutions across practices, and maintain enthusiasm and commitment.

Early adoption of resources must sometimes be tempered with a need to understand the context of the entire curriculum and to strategize for best use.

EXAMPLE: *UME Curriculum, Electronic Student Portfolios.* In 2007, the advising faculty planned to introduce an electronic portfolio for students to organize evaluations and reflective writing and communicate with advisors. The EPC noted that this was the fourth secured electronic system that would be required in the curriculum and recommended that coordination and programming be further developed to simplify student access and maximize its use.

Faculty Development

One of the most important resources for any curriculum is its faculty. As discussed in Chapter 7, a curriculum may benefit from faculty development efforts specifically targeted toward the needs of the curriculum. Institution-wide, regional, or national faculty development programs (see Appendix B) that train faculty in specific content areas, or time management, teaching, curriculum development, management, or research skills, may also benefit a curriculum.

EXAMPLE: *Community-Based Practice Experience.* Almost all of the part-time faculty who serve as ambulatory care preceptors for residents and medical students in the community-based practices associated with the Johns Hopkins Bayview Medical Center have participated in the Teaching Skills portion of the Johns Hopkins Faculty Development Program for Clinician-Educators (6–8). This program provides training in adult learning principles, time management, feedback, precepting, small group teaching, communication, lecturing, and management skills. Some have taken the Longitudinal Program in Curriculum Development and developed curricula for the residency program (9–11) (see also Primary Care Gynecology for Internal Medicine Residents, Appendix A).

EXAMPLE: *UME Curriculum.* Introduction of each technology enhancement required attention to faculty development. The creation of a resource for animated physiology lectures that students view online required a new approach to use of the formal curriculum time and development of teaching plans for this time. Moving from small group teaching to team-based learning required faculty development in facilitating teams, as well as in developing Readiness Tests and Application exercises. The availability of the Simulation Center required faculty development in understanding the uses of simulation, writing simulation cases, and skills in debriefing simulation exercises.

SUSTAINING THE CURRICULUM TEAM

The curriculum team includes not only the faculty but also the support staff and learners, all of whom are critical to a curriculum's success. It is, therefore, important to attend to processes that motivate, develop, and support the team. These processes include orientation, communication, involvement, faculty development and team activities, recognition, and celebration (Table 8.3).

EXAMPLE: *Community-Based Practice Experience.* The above examples demonstrate how a system of informal, formal, and social meetings can increase the involvement of faculty and residents in program assessment and change.

Previously, medical directors and site administrators had been involved in a strategic planning process that identified primary care education as one of the missions of the CBPs. The commitment to education continued when the administration of the CBPs moved from the Division of General Internal Medicine to a different entity within Johns Hopkins Medical Institutions (see example above).

During retreats, CBP faculty, practice administrators, residents, and program leaders identify challenges and new goals, brainstorm new approaches, and sustain their commitment to the CBP resident practice experience.

Clinic preceptors reduce the number of appointments on their clinic schedules on the days that they precept, which allows them to directly supervise and bill for residents while providing focused feedback and teaching. Overall, the scheduling for preceptor and resident is productivity neutral.

Each year, the CBP residents recognize one of the CBP faculty via a special Community-Based Teaching Award.

Community-based preceptors are given faculty appointments and some benefits, such as free access to some of the medical school's CME courses and to the university's library and computer network.

Periodic meetings with CBP office staff orient them to the goals of the clinical practice curriculum, invite feedback on and suggestions for improving the curriculum, and develop in them a sense of involvement and commitment to the curriculum.

EXAMPLE: *UME Curriculum.* An infrastructure of several curriculum teams maintains the UME program. This structure begins with course directors, their faculty, and administrative staff, who report to Year committees and ultimately to the EPC. Coordination of these teams allows coordination and consistency as changes are introduced and policies made, such as grading and absence policies, introduction of new technology, and awareness of innovation in related courses.

THE LIFE OF A CURRICULUM

A curriculum that does not keep pace with the needs of its learners, its faculty, its institution, its resources, patients, and society does a disservice to its constituents and is likely to deteriorate or die prematurely. One that does keep pace is likely to continually change and improve. After a few years, it may differ markedly from its initial form. As health problems and societal needs evolve, even a well-conceived curriculum that has been carefully maintained and developed may appropriately be downscaled or come to an end.

Table 8.3. Methods of Motivating, Developing, and Supporting a Curriculum Team

Method	Mechanisms
Orientation and Communication	
▪ Goals and objectives	▪ Syllabi/handouts
▪ Guidelines/standards	▪ Meetings
▪ Evaluation results	▪ Memos/e-mails
▪ Program changes	▪ Newsletters
▪ Rationale for above	▪ Web site
▪ Learner, faculty, staff, patient experiences	
Involvement of Faculty, Learners, Staff	▪ Questionnaires/interviews
▪ Goal and objective setting	▪ Informal one-on-one meetings
▪ Guideline development	▪ Group meetings
▪ Curricular changes	▪ Task group membership
▪ Determining evaluation and feedback needs	▪ Strategic planning
Team Activities	▪ Team teaching/co-teaching
	▪ Faculty development activities
	▪ Retreats
	▪ Task groups to analyze/assess needs
	▪ Strategic planning groups
Recognition and Celebration	▪ Private communication
	▪ Public recognition
	▪ Rewards
	▪ Parties and other social gatherings

EXAMPLE: *Managed Care Curriculum.* In the 1990s, capitated (HMO) insurance was on the ascendancy in the United States, and the majority of the CBP patients were covered under HMO insurance. A managed care curriculum was introduced into the GIM residency program. Subsequently, the prevalence of HMO-insured patients dropped in the United States and the CBPs. The course was renamed the Medical Practice and Health Systems Curriculum. The curriculum content evolved from one with emphasis on capitated care to one that emphasizes systems-based practice, including quality improvement theory and practice, patient safety, U.S. health insurance systems, health systems finance and use, medical informatics, practice management, and teamwork.

EXAMPLE: *UME Curriculum, Resource Changes.* In the Year 1 "Molecules and Cells" course, virtual microscopy replaced slide sets and microscopes, and students had online access to the full array of slides through the Internet. This increased the efficiency of learning histology and allowed introduction of more interactive laboratories and student teaching of content.

EXAMPLE: *UME Curriculum, Societal Needs.* As initially implemented in 1992, the purpose of the "Physician and Society" course was to "teach students that medicine does not exist in a social vacuum." Objectives were written in ethics, history of medicine, cultural anthropology, sociology, disease prevention, global health, drama, and the visual arts (1). Reflecting changes in the health care environment (12) and educational needs (13) for modern physicians, the course was renamed in 2006 as the "Patient, Physician and Society" (PPS) course and reorganized to address six major domains: Professionalism, Personal (self-care and awareness), Behavioral Medicine, Social (cultural awareness and health care disparities), Public Health, and Organizational Medicine (health policy, medicolegal, and health care financing).

EXAMPLE: *UME Curriculum, Major Revision of Basic Science Teaching*. A burgeoning of knowledge in the biomedical sciences, heralded by the Human Genome Project, continued to challenge the curriculum leadership to reformulate the content of the four-year curriculum, to prepare physicians for twenty-first century medicine. As course directors attempted updates in the curriculum, it became more difficult to justify the original organization of the biomedical content into a year of "normal" (e.g., human anatomy, physiology, metabolism) and a year of "abnormal" (e.g., pathophysiology, pathology). A decision was made to reorganize the approach to teaching the science of medicine from societal and genetic perspectives, emphasizing individual variability affected by genetics, social factors, and environmental factors. In 2004 a task force was convened to design this new approach. The ultimate design began with a grounding in the tools of modern science, termed "Scientific Foundations," followed by a "Genes to Society" course, which reviewed each system through a hierarchical perspective from molecular biology to population health. This was an additional degree of integration beyond the 1992 revision and required recruitment of all important stakeholders to this effort. Basic science faculty were enthused by the approach because it modeled translational research. Additional time for basic science teaching was built into the clinical biennium as well to bring students with appreciation of clinical medicine back to the study of basic science.

NETWORKING, INNOVATION, AND SCHOLARLY ACTIVITY

A curriculum can be strengthened not only by improvements in the existing curriculum per se, environmental changes, new resources, faculty development, and processes that support the curricular team but also by networking, ongoing innovation, and associated scholarship.

Networking

Faculty responsible for a curriculum at one institution can benefit from and be invigorated by *communication with colleagues at other institutions* (14). Conceptual clarity and understanding of one's own curriculum are usually enhanced as one prepares it for publication or presentation. New ideas and approaches may come from the comments of those who review one's manuscript, or from the interchange that occurs when one presents one's own work to colleagues and hears about or experiences colleagues' work. Multi-institutional efforts can produce scholarly products (see below), such as annotated bibliographies (15), articles (16–17), texts (18–20), and curricula (21–22) that improve on or transcend the capabilities of faculty at a single institution. The opportunity for such interchange and collaboration can be provided at professional meetings and through professional organizations.

EXAMPLE: *Interest Group at a Professional Organization*. There are usually one to a few internal medicine faculty responsible for teaching medical consultation on surgical, obstetric, and psychiatric patients at any single institution. The Medical Consultation Interest Group of the Society of General Internal Medicine has provided the opportunity for such faculty to meet yearly, discuss issues electronically, update medical knowledge, share curricula and teaching approaches, and engage in collaborative writing and research (23).

EXAMPLE: *Professional Organization.* The American Academy on Communication in Health-care (24) sponsors courses, meetings, and interest groups for teachers of interviewing skills and the psychosocial domain of medical practice that provide opportunities for faculty development, the sharing of curricula and teaching approaches, collaborative work relevant to curricula, and collaborative research.

Innovation and Scholarly Activity

Scholarly inquiry can enrich a curriculum by increasing the breadth and depth of knowledge and understanding of its faculty, by creating a sense of excitement among faculty and learners, and by providing the opportunity for learners to engage in scholarly projects. Scholarly activities may include original research or critical reviews in the subject matter of the curriculum or in the methods of teaching and learning that subject matter. Such scholarship can result in not only publications for curriculum developers but also other forms of dissemination (see Chapter 9). Scholarship can arise from means other than the original development, implementation, and evaluation of a curriculum. Once developed, curricula provide ongoing opportunities for innovation that can form the basis of scholarship. The need for innovation is often heralded by learner and faculty assessments, as well as opportunities to use new educational methods. Support for innovation can come from networking and the habits of scholarly inquiry.

EXAMPLE: *Mentored Scholarly Activity by Learners.* A curriculum in informatics and evidence-based medicine requires that each PGY–1 resident complete and present a critical review of a preventive, diagnostic, or treatment modality of her/his choice at the end of the one-month rotation. This project creates the opportunity for residents and their faculty mentors to apply the critical thinking, clinical decision making, literature search, and computer slide preparation skills that are emphasized in the curriculum.

EXAMPLE: *UME Curriculum, Reflective Writing Seminar.* GIM faculty and fellows joined a professor from the Writing Seminars program on the university campus to teach medical students in a popular reflective writing "selective" for the above-described PPS curriculum. The selective helped students communicate meaningful interactions with patients in a skillful manner that promoted self-awareness, reflection, and empathy. During the first year, one medical student had her paper accepted by a prominent medical journal (25), and the curriculum developers submitted a paper on the curriculum for publication and presented their work at three professional meetings.

EXAMPLE: *Scholarly Activity by Faculty.* Faculty involved in a curriculum development project on domestic violence became interested in its prevalence and clinical characteristics among female primary care patients. They assembled a team to conduct a study (26–28) that took place in the community-based practices described in previous examples. They received support from an institutional research grant and from the administration of the practices. The faculty expertise and new knowledge that resulted from this study have enriched the domestic violence curriculum, which became integrated into the gynecology/women's health curriculum.

CONCLUSION

Attending to processes that maintain and enhance a curriculum helps the curriculum remain relevant and vibrant. These processes help a curriculum to evolve in a direction of continuous improvement.

QUESTIONS

For the curriculum you are coordinating, planning, or would like to be planning, please answer or think about the following questions:

1. As curriculum coordinator, what methods will you use (Table 8.2) to *understand* the curriculum in its complexity (Table 8.1)?

2. How will you implement *minor changes? Major changes?*

3. Will evolving *accreditation standards* affect your curriculum?

4. Could *environmental or resource changes* provide opportunities for your curriculum? Can you stimulate positive changes, or build on new opportunities? Do environmental or resource changes present new challenges? How should you respond?

5. Is *faculty development* required or desirable?

6. What methods (Table 8.3) will you use to maintain the *motivation and involvement* of your faculty and your support staff?

7. How could you *network* to strengthen the curriculum, as well as your own knowledge, abilities, and productivity?

8. Are there *related scholarly activities* that you could encourage, support, or engage in that would strengthen your curriculum, help others engaged in similar work, and/or improve your faculty's/your own promotion portfolio?

GENERAL REFERENCES

Bland CJ, Schmitz, CC, Stritter FT, Henry RC, Aluise JJ. *Successful Faculty in Academic Medicine: Essential Skills and How to Acquire Them*. New York: Springer Publishing; 1990.
This book comprehensively addresses faculty skills that are essential for success in academic medicine and how these skills should be learned. The authors describe a model faculty development curriculum focusing on the five domains of education, administration, research, written communication, and professional academic skills. An excellent resource for faculty development. 315 pages.

DeAngelis C, ed. *The Johns Hopkins University School of Medicine Curriculum for the Twenty-first Century.* Baltimore: Johns Hopkins University Press; 1999.
This monograph describes in detail the history of the JHUSOM curriculum and changes leading to a major revision in 1992, with detailed descriptions of new courses and plans for evaluation. 248 pages.

Dyer WG, Dyer WG Jr., Dyer JH. *Team Building: Proven Strategies for Improving Team Performance,* 4th ed. San Francisco: John Wiley & Sons; 2007.
Practical, easy-to-read book, now in its 4th edition, written by three business professors, a father and his two sons. Useful for leaders and members of committees, task forces, and other task-oriented teams, for anyone engaged in collaboration. 240 pages.

King JA, Morris LY, Fitz-Gibbon CT. *How to Assess Program Implementation*. Newbury Park, Calif.: Sage Publications; 1987.
Maintenance and continual improvement of a program involves evaluation. The focus of this book is on planning and executing an evaluation of how well a program has been implemented. The

appendix contains over 300 questions for an implementation evaluation of all aspects of a program, which in turn can be used for initial program planning or subsequent program modification. 143 pages.

Scholtes PR. *The Team Handbook for Educators: How to Use Teams to Improve Quality*. Madison, Wisc.: Joiner Associates; 1994.
An easy-to-use manual on how to assemble and run teams. Focus is on quality improvement, but generally applicable. 304 pages.

Whitman N. Managing faculty development. In: Whitman N, Weiss E, Bishop FM, eds. *Executive Skills for Medical Faculty*. Salt Lake City, Utah: University of Utah School of Medicine; 1989. Pp. 99–106.
Managing faculty development to improve teaching skills is discussed as a needed executive function. Five strategies are offered to promote education as a product of the medical school: rewards, assistance, feedback, connoisseurship (developing a taste for good teaching), and creativity. 8 pages.

SPECIFIC REFERENCES

1. DeAngelis C, ed. *The Johns Hopkins University School of Medicine Curriculum for the Twenty-first Century.* Baltimore: Johns Hopkins University Press; 1999.
2. Watson EG, Moloney PJ, Toohey SM, Hughes CS, Mobbs SL, Leeper JB, McNeil HP. Development of eMed: a comprehensive, modular curriculum-management system. *Acad Med.* 2007;82:351–60.
3. Liaison Committee for Medical Education. *Functions and Structure of a Medical School: Standards for Accreditation of Educational Programs Leading to the M.D. Degree* (revised 2008). Available at www.lcme.org. Accessed March 11, 2009.
4. Accreditation Council for Graduate Medical Education. *Common Program Requirements.* Available at www.acgme.org. Go to Review Committees or Program Directors and Coordinators, then Common Program Requirements. Accessed March 11, 2009.
5. Accreditation Council for Continuing Medical Education. "Accreditation Requirements: ACCME Essential Areas and Their Elements". Available at www.accme.org. Accessed March 11, 2009.
6. Cole KA, Barker LR, Kolodner K, Williamson P, Wright SM, Kern DE. Faculty development in teaching skills: an intensive longitudinal model. *Acad Med.* 2004;79(5):469–80.
7. Knight AM, Cole KA, Kern DE, Barker LR, Koldner K, Wright SM. Long-term follow-up of a longitudinal faculty development program in teaching skills. *J Gen Intern Med.* 2005;20(8): 721–25.
8. Knight AM, Carrese JA, Wright SM. Qualitative assessment of the long-term impact of a faculty development programme in teaching skills. *Med Educ.* 2007;41:592–600.
9. Windish DM, Aysegul Gozu A, Bass EB, Thomas PA, Sisson SD, Howard DM, Kern DE. A ten-month program in curriculum development for medical educators: 16 years of experience. *J Gen Intern Med.* 2007;22:655–61.
10. Gozu A, Windish DM, Knight AM, Thomas PA, Kolodner K, Bass EB, Sisson SD, Kern DE. Long-term outcomes of a ten-month program in curriculum development: a controlled study. *Med Educ.* 2008;42:684–92.
11. Houston TK, Connors RL, Cutler N, Nidiry MA. A primary care musculoskeletal clinic for residents: success and sustainability. *J Gen Intern Med.* 2004;19:524–29.
12. Institute of Medicine. *Improving Medical Education: Enhancing the Behavioral and Social Science Content of Medical School Curricula.* Washington, D.C.: National Academies Press; 2004.

13. AAMC Institute for Improving Medical Education. *Educating Doctors to Provide High Quality Medical Care: A Vision for Medical Education in the United States*. Washington, D.C.: AAMC; 2004.
14. Woods SE, Reid A, Arndt JE, Curtis P, Stritter FT. Collegial networking and faculty vitality. *Fam Med.* 1997;29(1):45–49.
15. Rao NR, Kramer M, Saunders R, Twemlow SW, Lomax JW, Dewan MJ, Myers MF, Goldberg J, Cassimir G, Kring B, Alami O. An annotated bibliography of professional literature on international medical graduates. *Acad Psychiatry.* 2007;31(1):68–83.
16. Williamson PR, Smith R, Kern DE, Lipkin M Jr., Barker LR, Hoppe RB, Florek J. The medical interview and psychosocial aspects of medicine: block curricula for residents. *J Gen Intern Med.* 1992;7:235–42.
17. Holmboe ES, Bown JL, Green M, Gregg J, DiFrancesco L, Reynolds E, Alguire P, Battinelli D, Lucey C, Duffy D. Reforming internal medicine residency training: a report from the Society of General Internal Medicine's Task Force for Residency Reform. *J Gen Intern Med.* 2005;20:1165–72.
18. Lipkin ML Jr., Putnam SM, Lazare A, eds. *The Medical Interview: Clinical Care, Education, and Research.* New York: Springer-Verlag; 1995.
19. ACP Governors' Class of 1996. *Learning from Practitioners: Office-Based Teaching of Internal Medicine Residents.* Philadelphia: American College of Physicians; 1995.
20. Deutsch SL, Noble J, eds. *Community-Based Teaching: A Guide to Developing Education Programs for Medical Students and Residents in the Practitioner's Office.* Philadelphia: American College of Physicians; 1997.
21. *CDIM/SGIM Core Medicine Clerkship Guide*, 3rd ed., 2006. Available at Alliance for Academic Internal Medicine (AAIM) Web site, www.im.org/, then go to AAIM Alliance Sites, CDIM. Accessed March 11, 2009.
22. *Graduate Education in Internal Medicine, A Resource Guide to Curriculum Development: The Report of the Federated Council for Internal Medicine Task Force on the Internal Medicine Residency Curriculum*, 2nd ed, 2002. Available at www.acponline.org/education_recertification/education/training/fcim/. Accessed March 11, 2009.
23. Society of General Internal Medicine. Available at www.sgim.org. Go to About Us, then Interest Groups. Accessed March 11, 2009.
24. American Academy on Communication in Healthcare. Available at www.aachonline.org. Accessed March 11, 2009.
25. Shapiro AE. An uneasy understanding. *Ann Intern Med.* 2007 Dec 4;147(11):811–12.
26. McCauley J, Kern DE, Kolodner K, Dill L, Schroeder AF, DeChant HK, Ryden J, Bass EB, Derogatis LR. The "battering syndrome": prevalence and clinical characteristics of domestic violence in primary care internal medicine practices. *Ann Intern Med.* 1995;123:737–46.
27. McCauley J, Kern DE, Kolodner K, Dill L, Schroeder AF, DeChant HK, Ryden J, Derogatis LR, Bass EB. Clinical characteristics of adult female primary care patients with a history of childhood abuse: unhealed wounds. *JAMA.* 1997;277:1362–68.
28. McCauley J, Kern DE, Kolodner K, Bass EB. Relationship of low severity violence to women's health. *J Gen Intern Med.* 1998;13:687–91.

CHAPTER NINE

Dissemination

. . . making it count twice

David E. Kern, M.D., M.P.H., and Eric B. Bass, M.D., M.P.H.

DEFINITION

Dissemination refers to efforts to promote consideration or use of a curriculum or related products (e.g., needs assessment or evaluation results) by others. It also refers to the delivery of the curriculum or segments of the curriculum to new groups of learners.

WHY BOTHER?

The dissemination of a curriculum or related work can be important for several reasons. Dissemination can do the following:

- *Help address a health care problem:* As indicated in Chapter 2, the ultimate purpose of a curriculum in medical education is to address a problem that affects the health of the public or a given population (1, 2). To maximize the positive impact of a curriculum, it is necessary to share the curriculum or related work with others who are dealing with the same problem.
- *Stimulate change:* Innovative curricular work can create excitement and stimulate change in educational programs and medical institutions (3).
- *Provide feedback to curriculum developers:* By disseminating curriculum-related work, curriculum developers can obtain valuable feedback from others who may have unique perspectives. This external feedback can promote further development of one's curriculum and curriculum-related work (see Chapter 8).
- *Increase collaboration:* Dissemination efforts may lead to increased exchange of ideas between people within an institution or in different institutions who are interested in the same issues. Such interchange may lead to active collaboration. The resulting teamwork is likely to lead to development of an even better curriculum or to other products that would not have been developed by individuals working separately.
- *Prevent redundant work:* Others may be struggling with the same issues that require curriculum development and evaluation. By disseminating a curriculum, curriculum developers can minimize the extent to which different people expend time and energy repeating work that has been done elsewhere. Instead, they can devote their time and energy building on what has already been accomplished.

    EXAMPLE: *Prevention of Redundancy.* Internal medicine residency programs all must provide training in ambulatory medicine. When a Web-based curriculum in ambulatory care medicine was developed for internal medicine residency programs, more than 80 residency programs subscribed to it. By subscribing to the curriculum, residency program directors were able to build on an existing resource without each one having to create the same core set of learning materials. In addition, the income from subscriptions has permitted the curriculum developers to regularly update the curriculum's topic-based modules, thereby continuing to save time for all users of the curriculum (4, 5).

- *Help curriculum developers achieve recognition and academic advancement:* Medical school faculty may devote a substantial amount of time to the development of curricula but have difficulties achieving academic advancement if this portion of their overall work is not recognized as representing significant scholarship. Properly performed, curriculum development is a recognized form of scholarship (6–8). Promotion committees and department chairs report that they value clinician-educators' accomplishments in curriculum development (9–11). Educational portfolios detailing these accomplishments are increasingly being used to support applications for promotion (12–14). One important criterion for judging the significance of scholarly work is the degree to which the work has been disseminated and has had an impact at a local, regional, national, or international level.

EXAMPLE: *Benefits of Dissemination.* Faculty developed innovative curricula for internal medicine residents and primary care practitioners on interviewing skills and the psychosocial domain of medical practice starting in 1979. Dissemination of this and related curricula occurred in workshops and in published articles (15–17). This dissemination was of value to faculty at other institutions who were independently working on ways to enhance clinical training in this area. It generated feedback and promoted interactions and discussions that led to improvements in the original curriculum. It also led to collaborative work that resulted in additional publications (18–21). As a result of the successful dissemination of this curriculum-related work, the curriculum developers gained national recognition for their work. The medical school's promotion and tenure committee cited this recognition as an important achievement when the scholarly activities of responsible faculty members were reviewed. The curriculum developers were approved for promotion.

Are dissemination efforts worth the time and effort required? In many cases, the answer is yes, even for individuals who do not need academic advancement. If the curriculum developer performed an appropriate problem identification and general needs assessment, as discussed in Chapter 2, the curriculum will likely address an important problem that has not been adequately addressed previously. If this is the case, the curriculum is likely to be of value to others. The challenge is to decide how the curriculum should be disseminated and how much time and effort the curriculum developer can realistically devote to dissemination efforts. The final decision involves a trade-off between the degree of dissemination desired and the amount of time that the curriculum developer can afford to spend on dissemination.

PLANNING FOR DISSEMINATION

Curriculum developers who wish to disseminate work related to their curriculum should start planning for dissemination when they start planning their curriculum (i.e., *before* implementation) (22). To ensure a product worthy of dissemination, curriculum developers will find it helpful to follow rigorously the principles of curriculum development described in this book, particularly with respect to those steps related to the part of their work they wish to disseminate. They may also find it useful to think in advance of the characteristics of an innovation that contribute to its diffusion or dissemination. It is important to develop a coherent strategy for dissemination that clarifies the purposes of one's dissemination efforts (see above), addresses ethical and legal issues related to the protection of subjects and intellectual property, identifies what is to be disseminated, delineates the target audience, and determines venues for dissemination. A realistic assessment of the time and resources available for dissemination is necessary to ensure that the dissemination strategy is feasible. These topics are discussed in the following sections of this chapter.

DIFFUSION OF INNOVATIONS

If the curriculum developer wants to disseminate all or parts of an actual curriculum, it is worthwhile to review what is known about the diffusion of innovations. Factors identified by Rogers (23) that promote the likelihood and rapidity of adoption of an innovation include the following:

- *Relative advantage*—the degree to which an innovation is perceived as superior to existing practice.
- *Compatibility*—the degree to which an innovation is perceived by the adopter as similar to previous experience, beliefs, and values.
- *Simplicity*—the degree to which a new idea is perceived as relatively easy to understand and implement.
- *Trialability*—the degree to which an innovation can be divided into steps and tried out by the adopter.
- *Observability*—the degree to which the innovation can be seen and appreciated by others.

Additional factors include impact on existing social relations, modifiability, reversibility, time investment, risk/uncertainty, and commitment (24).

> **EXAMPLE:** *Diffusion of Problem-Based Learning.* Problem-based learning (PBL) is an approach to education that presents problems to small groups of students and engages them in analysis of the problems, elaboration of prior knowledge, acquisition of new knowledge, application of the knowledge to problem solving, and collaboration. A faculty facilitator is usually involved. Since its introduction at McMaster University in the 1970s, the use of PBL has spread internationally. While evidence of its efficacy is mixed, it appears to have several advantages and satisfies all of the above conditions promoting diffusion (25).

According to the conceptual model described by Rogers (23), individuals pass through *several stages* when deciding whether to adopt an innovative idea. These stages include 1) acquisition of *knowledge* about an innovation, 2) *persuasion* that the innovation is worth considering, 3) a *decision* to adopt the innovation, 4) *implementation* of the innovation, and 5) *confirmation* that the innovation is worth continuing.

One of the main implications of the diffusion theory and research is that efforts to disseminate an innovative curriculum should involve more than just communication of knowledge about the curriculum. The dissemination strategy should include efforts to *persuade* individuals of the need to consider the curriculum innovation. Efforts at persuasion are best directed at individuals who are most likely to make decisions about implementation of a curriculum or who are most likely to influence other individuals' attitudes or behavior regarding implementation of a curricular innovation. The dissemination strategy also should include efforts to identify barriers (26) to curricular transfer and to *support* those individuals who decide to implement the curriculum. Such efforts usually require direct interpersonal communication, through professional meetings, telephone conversations, or electronic mail. In some cases, a site visit may be necessary to achieve optimal communication. Regardless of the mode of communication, it usually is best to identify a specific individual in a targeted institution who will lead the effort to transfer an innovative curriculum to that institution.

Ideally, a collaborative relationship will develop between the original curriculum developer and the adopting group. A *collaborative approach is ideal* because most curricula require modifications when transferred to other settings. Moreover, the establishment of an ongoing collaborative relationship generally strengthens the curriculum for all users and stimulates further innovation and products.

PROTECTION OF SUBJECTS

If publication of curriculum-related work is anticipated, the work is likely to be considered educational research. While federal regulations governing research in the United States categorize many educational research projects as exempt from the regulations if the research involves the study of normal educational practices or records information about learners in such a way that they cannot be identified, institutional review boards (IRBs) often differ in their interpretation of what is exempt. It is wise for curriculum developers to check in advance with their IRBs. IRBs will be concerned about whether learners, faculty, patients, or others could incur harm as a result of participation. Issues such as informed consent, confidentiality, and the use of incentives to encourage participation in a curriculum may need to be considered (27). Failure to consult one's IRB before implementation of the curriculum can have adverse consequences for the curriculum developer who later tries to publish research about the curriculum (28). (See Chapter 6, Implementation, Scholarship, and Chapter 7, Evaluation and Feedback, Address Ethical Concerns, for additional details.)

INTELLECTUAL PROPERTY AND COPYRIGHT ISSUES

When considering dissemination of curriculum-related work, curriculum developers need to address intellectual property issues, with respect to both copyrighted content in the curriculum and protecting their own intellectual property. A curriculum that is used locally for one's own learners generally falls under the exceptions contained in the Copyright Act, often referred to as fair use privilege provided by Section 107 of U.S. copyright law (Title 17 of the U.S. Code) (29). "Fair use" provides for use of material without the author's permission if it is being used for teaching, scholarship, or research, and it generally implies no commercial use of the material. With the ease of online dissemination that has occurred recently, the law is being interpreted more narrowly by universities. Once work, such as a syllabus, a presentation, or a multimedia site with images, is disseminated, it may no longer fall under fair use guidelines. Careful attention to the proper use of copyrighted materials may require additional citations and/or written permissions from publishers for use of graphs and images. If the curriculum developer is a member of a university, the curriculum developer should be familiar with the university's copyright policy and seek expertise before disseminating the work.

Most universities have multiple resources to assist faculty in understanding these issues. Additional resources include the Association of Research Libraries (30), the American Libraries Association Office of Intellectual Freedom (31), and the "Crash Course in Copyright," maintained by the University of Texas (32).

Curriculum developers may wish to protect their disseminated products from unlawful use, alteration, or dissemination beyond their control. One approach is to license the material, and most universities have expertise to assist with this process as well. Yale University maintains a Web site with resources for licensing digital information (33).

WHAT SHOULD BE DISSEMINATED?

One of the first decisions to make when developing plans for disseminating curriculum work is to *determine whether the entire curriculum, parts of the curriculum, or curriculum-related work should be disseminated.* The curriculum developer can refer to the problem identification and general needs assessment to determine the extent of the need for the curriculum and to determine whether the curriculum truly represents a new contribution to the field. The results of the evaluation of a curriculum will also help determine whether any aspect of the curriculum is worth disseminating.

In some cases, dissemination efforts will focus on promoting adoption of a *complete curriculum* or *curriculum guide* by other sites. Often this requires some allowance for modifications to meet the unique needs of the learners at these sites.

> **EXAMPLE:** *Complete Curriculum.* The Healer's Art is a 15-hour, quarter-long elective that has been taught annually at the University of California, San Francisco, since 1993 and has been disseminated to 60 medical schools. The course's educational strategy is based on a discovery model that uses reflection on recollections and experiences related to session themes, and it draws on approaches and theories from fields such as humanistic psychology, formational theory, and cognitive and Jungian psychology. The course addresses professionalism, meaning, and the human dimensions of medical practice. Faculty development workshops, guidebooks, and curricular materials prepare faculty to plan and implement the course at their institutions (34–36).

> **EXAMPLE:** *Curriculum Guide.* Members of the Society of General Internal Medicine and the Clerkship Directors in Internal Medicine, under a contract from the federal Health Resources and Services Administration (HRSA), designed a curriculum guide for improving existing core clerkships in internal medicine. The guide described the need for the curriculum, specific learner objectives, proposed educational strategies, and methods of evaluation. This guide was published by HRSA and distributed to internal medicine clerkship directors in all U.S. medical schools (37). The work also was disseminated through presentations at meetings of the American Association of Medical Colleges, the Clerkship Directors in Internal Medicine, and the Society of Internal Medicine. A follow-up survey demonstrated that clerkship directors in 80 of the 125 medical schools in the United States had used the guide (38). The objectives were subsequently updated (39).

In other cases, it is appropriate to limit dissemination efforts to *specific products of the curriculum development process* that are likely to be of value to others. We provide examples below of products of the curriculum development process that have been disseminated through publication in peer-reviewed journals, although curricular work can also be disseminated through presentations, workshops, and courses delivered at other institutions and at professional meetings, as well as through books (see Healer's Art example above and Gynecology and Curriculum Development examples in Appendix A).

The problem identification and general needs assessment (Step 1) may yield new insights about a problem that warrant dissemination. This may occur when a comprehensive review of the literature on a topic has been performed, or when a systematic survey on the extent of a problem has been conducted.

> **EXAMPLE:** *Step 1, Systematic Review.* A systematic review of teamwork training interventions in medical student and resident education addressed a topical issue, revealed that existing curricula employed some sound educational methods, and found that those that included more teamwork principles achieved greater efficacy (40).

EXAMPLE: *Step 1, Systematic Survey.* A national survey of faculty development in depart-ments of medicine in U.S. teaching hospitals revealed that a minority of them offered faculty development in educational skills. For those that did, the study reported on the methods used and content addressed and identified areas of need (41).

The targeted needs assessment (Step 2) may yield unique insights about the need for a curriculum that merit dissemination because the targeted learners are reasonably representative of other potential learners. When this occurs, the methods employed in the needs assessment will need to be carefully described so that other groups can determine whether the results of the needs assessment are valid and applicable to them.

EXAMPLE: *Step 2.* A survey of targeted learners in internal medicine, neurology, and family practice residency programs at three teaching hospitals found that residents rated most principles of professionalism highly important to medical practice but difficult to incorporate into daily practice. Duty hour requirements created special challenges (42).

In some cases, the formulation of learning objectives for a topic (Step 3) may, by itself, represent an important contribution to a field, thereby calling for some degree of dissemination.

EXAMPLE: *Step 3.* A team of educators used a systematic, evidence-based consensus-building process to establish agreement about educational competencies and learning ob-jectives in disaster preparedness for hospital-based health care workers (43).

In other cases, it may be worthwhile to focus the dissemination efforts on specific educational methods (Step 4) and/or on implementation strategies (Step 5).

EXAMPLE: *Step 4.* Faculty at the University of Kentucky worked with community partners to develop a novel training program written in lay terms on the protection of human subjects for community workers involved in community-based research. The program was novel enough to merit publication even though it had not yet undergone rigorous evaluation (44).

EXAMPLE: *Steps 4 and 5.* The Harvard Medical School–Cambridge integrated clerkship was piloted in 2004-05 with eight volunteer medical students. The objective of the innovation was to restructure clinical education to address the inadequacies of hospital-based experiences as effective learning opportunities for chronic care, continuity of care, and humanism. A dedicated group of faculty from the medical school collaborated with clinicians to design this unique approach to the clinical year. A variety of obstacles needed to be overcome, including fiscal, cultural, political, and operational ones (45). Following successful results for the pilot, the curriculum was expanded to include all clinical teaching sites and all students at Harvard Medical School.

Most often, however, the results of the evaluation of a curriculum (Step 6) are the focus of dissemination efforts because people are more likely to adopt an innovative approach, or abandon a traditional approach, when there is evidence regarding the efficacy, or lack of efficacy, of the approach.

EXAMPLE: *Step 6.* Curriculum developers demonstrated in a randomized controlled trial that trained residents participating in a 13 hour, 6 month teaching skills curriculum performed better than untrained residents on a 3.5 hour, eight-station structured teaching examination, rated by 50 medical students. The students used a unique structured assessment form for each station. All forms were based on a validated instrument for rating clinical teachers (46).

EXAMPLE: *Step 6.* Curriculum developers used self-reporting of skills, activities, and impact in pre-post and long-term follow-up survey studies of participants versus a comparison group, as well as the cataloging of curricular products of participants, to assess the efficacy of a longitudinal faculty program in curriculum development (47, 48).

WHO IS THE TARGET AUDIENCE?

Dissemination efforts may be targeted at individuals within one's institution, individuals at other institutions, or individuals who are not affiliated with any particular institution. The ideal target audience for dissemination of a curriculum depends on the nature of the curriculum-related work being disseminated.

EXAMPLE: *Determination of Target Audience.* The ideal audience for disseminating a curriculum for medical students on delivering primary care to a culturally diverse, inner-city, indigent population might be the faculty and deans of medical schools located in major cities. In contrast, a curriculum on ethical issues in genetic testing may be worth disseminating more widely because the targeted learners include health care providers in practice as well as those in training.

HOW SHOULD CURRICULUM WORK BE DISSEMINATED?

Once the purpose and content of the dissemination and the target audience have been defined and available resources identified, the curriculum developer must choose the most appropriate modes of dissemination (see Table 9.1 and text below). Ideally, the curriculum developer will use a variety of dissemination modes to maximize impact.

Presentations

Usually, the first mode of dissemination involves *written or oral* presentations to key people *within the setting where the curriculum was developed*. These presentations may be targeted at potential learners or at faculty who will need to be involved in the curriculum. The presentations may also be directed at leaders who can provide important support or resources for the curriculum.

Sometimes it may be appropriate to disseminate curriculum-related work, such as a timely needs assessment, before implementation of the curriculum at the curriculum developer's own institution. Once a curriculum has been established within the setting of its origin, dissemination to *other sites* is appropriate. An efficient way to disseminate curriculum-related work to other sites is to present it at regional, national, or international *meetings of professional societies*. A workshop or minicourse is an appropriate format for presenting the content or methods of a curriculum. A presentation that follows a research abstract format is appropriate for presenting results of a needs assessment or a curriculum evaluation. Guidelines have been published for research presentations (49). As illustrated in Table 9.2, information from the six-step curriculum development cycle can fit nicely into the format for an abstract presentation.

Multi-institutional Interest Groups

In some cases, presentation of curriculum work may occur within multi-institutional interest group meetings of professional societies. Once an interest group is created,

Table 9.1.   Modes of Disseminating Curriculum Work

- Presentations of abstracts, workshops, or courses to individuals and groups within specific institutions
- Presentations of abstracts, workshops, or courses at regional, national, and international professional meetings
- Creation of a multi-institutional interest group
- Use of electronic communication systems
    Submission of curricular materials to a Web-based educational clearinghouse
    Preparation and distribution of instructional audiovisual recordings
    Creation and distribution of instructional interactive software
- Publication of an article in a professional journal
- Publication of a manual, book, or book chapter
- Preparation of a press release

back-and-forth dissemination among members of the group may occur in a number of ways, such as in-person meetings, telephone contact, or electronic mail.

EXAMPLE: *Multi-institutional Interest Group.* The American Society for Bioethics and Humanities (ASBH) created a task force to address the ACGME General Competencies, particularly with regard to required educational goals for professionalism and ethics. The task force collected and disseminated information about residency programs with syllabi in professionalism, patient care, interpersonal and communication skills, and systems-based practice. The task force presented its findings at a national ASBH meeting, and a model curriculum was developed. An interest group on residency education was also formed, and interest group members can present their curricular innovations at the interest group meeting. A peer-reviewed syllabus exchange project is also available for use by ASBH members.

Electronic Communication Systems

The emergence of computer-based communication systems, such as the Internet, provides a tremendous opportunity for curriculum developers to share curriculum materials with anyone having access to a computer. *Written curricular materials*, *instructional visual and sound recordings*, *interactive instructional software*, and *measurement instruments used in needs assessment and/or curriculum evaluation* can be shared widely using computer-based systems, as well as by hard copy, digital versatile disk (DVD), compact disk (CD), or audio- or videotape. Interpersonal educational methods used for achieving affective and psychomotor objectives are less amenable to such transfer, although there are exceptions.

EXAMPLE: *Web-based Curriculum on Communication Skills.* The American Academy on Communication in Healthcare and Drexel University College of Medicine cosponsor a curriculum on communication skills that includes the demonstration of key skills in 40 different learning modules. The curriculum involves video encounters with standardized patients and provides text commentary on the interviews, key principles, evidence-based recommendations, and skills checklists (50).

Educational clearinghouses, such as MedEdPORTAL, which publishes peer-reviewed curricular materials (51), are now mostly electronic and provide the opportunity to disseminate one's work widely. Information about the existence of an educational clearinghouse for a particular clinical domain generally can be obtained from the

Table 9.2.   Format for a Curriculum Development Abstract Presentation or Manuscript

I. Introduction
    A. Rationale
        1. Problem identification
        2. General needs assessment
        3. Targeted needs assessment
    B. Purpose
        1. Goals of curriculum
        2. Goals of evaluation: evaluation questions

II. Materials and Methods
    A. Setting
    B. Subjects/power analysis if any
    C. Educational intervention
        1. Relevant specific measurable objectives
        2. Relevant educational strategies
        3. Resources: faculty, other personnel, equipment/facilities, costs*
        4. Implementation strategy*
        5. Display or offer of educational materials*
    D. Evaluation methods
        1. Evaluation design
        2. Evaluation instruments
            a. Reliability measures if any
            b. Validity measures if any
            c. Display (or offer) of evaluation instruments
        3. Data collection methods
        4. Data analysis methods

III.   Results
    A. Data: including tables, figures, graphs, etc.
    B. Statistical analysis

IV.   Conclusions and Discussion
    A. Summary and discussion of findings
    B. Contribution to existing body of knowledge, comparison to work of others*
    C. Strengths and limitations of work
    D. Conclusions/implications
    E. Future directions*

* These items are usually omitted from presentations.

professional societies that have a vested interest in educational activities in that domain. (See Appendix B for additional clearinghouse information.)

> **EXAMPLE:** *Web-based Clearinghouse for Palliative Care.* The End of Life/Palliative Education Resource Center (EPERC) is an educational resource site for health professional educators involved in palliative care education that includes resource material such as course syllabi and guides; cases; standardized patient materials; slide presentations; CD-ROMs; articles; books; links to other Web sites; and concise, practical, peer-reviewed, evidence-based sum-

maries on key topics (Fast Facts). Its complete database of peer-reviewed educational materials is now based at the American Academy of Hospice and Palliative Medicine, to which materials can be submitted (52, 53).

Publication

One of the most traditional, but still underused, modes of disseminating medical education work is publication in a paper or electronic *medical journal or textbook*. When a curriculum developer seeks to disseminate a comprehensive curriculum, it may be wise to consider preparation of a book or manual. On the other hand, the format for original research articles can be used to present results of a needs assessment or a curriculum evaluation (Table 9.2). The format for review articles or meta-analyses can be used to present results of a problem identification and general needs assessment. An editorial or special article format sometimes can be used for other types of work, such as discussion of the most appropriate learning objectives or methods for a needed curriculum.

Many journals will consider articles derived from curriculum work. Curriculum developers who wish to publish work related to their curriculum should prepare their manuscript using principles of good scientific writing (22). Their manuscript will have an increased chance of being accepted by a journal if the results of the curriculum work are relevant to the majority of the readers of that journal and if that journal has a track record of publishing medical education articles (Table 9.3). Manuscripts should follow the Instructions for Authors provided by the journal to which they are submitted and, for instructions not specified, by the Uniform Requirements for Manuscripts Submitted to Biomedical Journals published by the International Committee of Medical Journal Editors (ICMJE) (54). Curriculum evaluations will most likely be accepted for publication by peer-reviewed journals if they satisfy common standards of methodological rigor (55–57). Table 9.4 displays criteria that may be considered by reviewers of an original article on a curriculum. Seldom do even published curricular articles satisfy all of these criteria. Nevertheless, the criteria can serve as a guide to curriculum developers interested in publishing their work. Methodological criteria for controlled trials (58), systematic review articles and meta-analyses (57, 59, 60), and reports of nonrandomized educational, behavioral, and public health interventions (61) have been published elsewhere.

Media Coverage

Curriculum developers should consider whether their work would have sufficient interest to the lay public to consider issuing a press release. If so, they should contact the public affairs office in their institution to request assistance in preparing a press release. Sometimes a press release will lead to requests for interviews or publication of articles in lay publications, either of which will bring attention to the curricular work.

WHAT RESOURCES ARE REQUIRED?

To ensure a successful dissemination effort, it is important for the curriculum developer to identify the resources that are required. While the dissemination of curricular work can result in significant benefits to both curriculum developers and others, it is

Table 9.3.   Peer-reviewed Journals and Sites That Are Likely to Publish Curriculum-related Work

Medical education journals and sites

    Academic Medicine (www.academicmedicine.org)[†]

    Advances in Health Sciences Education (www.springer.com/education/journal/10459)[‡]

    Advances in Physiology Education (http://advan.physiology.org)[‡]

    American Journal of Pharmaceutical Education (www.ajpe.org)[†]

    BMC Medical Education (www.biomedcentral.com/bmcmededuc/)[§]

    Education for Health (www.educationforhealth.net)[§]

    Education for Primary Care (www.radcliffe-oxford.com/journals/J02_Education_for
       _Primary_Care/)[§]

    Journal of Cancer Education (www.informaworld.com/smpp/title~db=all~content=g793703
       083~tab=summary)[∥]

    Journal of Continuing Education in the Health Professions (www.jcehp.com)[†]

    Journal of Dental Education (www.jdentaled.org)[†]

    Journal of Nursing Education (www.journalofnursingeducation.com)[†]

    Journal of Veterinary Medical Education (www.jvmeonline.org)[†]

    MedEdPORTAL (www.aamc.org/mededportal/)[§]

    Medical Education (www.mededuc.com)[†]

    Medical Education Online (www.med-ed-online.org)[§]

    Medical Teacher (www.medicalteacher.org)[†]

    Nurse Education Today (www.nurseeducationtoday.com)[†]

    Patient Education and Counseling (www.elsevier.com/wps/find/journaldescription.cws
       _home/505955/description)[∥]

    Teaching and Learning in Medicine (www.siumed.edu/tlm/)[†]

General medical journals

    Academic Emergency Medicine (www.wiley.com/bw/journal.asp?ref=1069-6563)[†]

    Academic Pediatrics, formerly *Ambulatory Pediatrics* (www.ambulatorypediatrics.org)[‡]

    Family Medicine (www.stfm.org/fmhub/fmhub.html)[†]

    Journal of General Internal Medicine (www.springer.com/medicine/internal/journal/11606)[†]

    Journal of the American Geriatric Society (www.wiley.com/bw/journal.asp?ref=0002-8614)[†]

    Journal of Hospital Medicine (www3.interscience.wiley.com/journal/111081937/home)[¶]

    Journal of Palliative Medicine (www.liebertpub.com/publication.aspx?pub_id=41)[∥]

    Journal of Professional Nursing (www.aacn.nche.edu/publications/jpn.htm)[†]

    Pediatrics (http://pediatrics.aappublications.org/)[‡]

    Progress in Community Health Partnerships (www.press.jhu.edu/journals/progress_in
       _community_health_partnerships/)[§]

Specialty journals

    American Journal of Obstetrics and Gynecology (http://journals.elsevierhealth.com/
       periodicals/ymob)[‡]

    American Journal of Surgery (http://americanjournalofsurgery.com/)[†]

    Academic Radiology (www.academicradiology.org)[†]

    Academic Psychiatry (http://ap.psychiatryonline.org/misc/ifora.dtl)[†]

    Clinical Anatomy (http://www3.interscience.wiley.com/journal/37476/home)[∥]

    Journal of the American College of Surgeons (www.journalacs.org)[**]

Table 9.3.   *(continued)*

Journal of Surgical Research (www.journalofsurgicalresearch.com)‖
Journal of Urology (www.jurology.com)‖

Note: In addition to considering the journals listed above, curriculum developers are advised to read the Instructions for Authors of the journals in their specialty area and to review past issues of those journals to see what types of curriculum-related work, if any, they have published. All Web sites accessed July 11, 2009.

† ≥50 curriculum-related publications January 2003 to July 2008 or ≥20 January 2006 to July 2008, ISI Web of Science search.

‡ ≥30 curriculum-related publications January 2003 to July 2008 or ≥15 January 2006 to July 2008, ISI Web of Science search.

§ Not included in ISI Web of Knowledge databases.

‖ ≥20 curriculum-related publications January 2003 to July 2008 or ≥10 January 2006 to July 2008, ISI Web of Science search.

¶ Eight curriculum-related publications January 2006 to July 2008, ISI Web of Science search.

** 16 curriculum-related publications January 2003 to July 2008, nine January 2006 to July 2008, ISI Web of Science search.

also necessary for the curriculum developer to ensure that the use of limited resources is appropriately balanced among competing needs.

Time and Effort

Disseminating curricular work almost always requires considerable time and effort of the *individual or individuals responsible*. Unless one is experienced in disseminating curricular work, it is wise to multiply one's initial estimates of time and effort by a factor of 2–4, which is likely to be closer to reality than the original estimate. Submissions of already developed curricular products to an educational clearinghouse or Web site require the least time and effort. More time and effort are required for presentations of abstracts, workshops, and courses. Still more time is required for the creation of instructional interactive software and audiovisual recordings. Publications generally require the most time and effort.

Personnel

In addition to the curriculum developer, other personnel may be helpful or necessary for the dissemination effort. The creation of instructional audiovisual recordings or computer software may require the involvement of *individuals with appropriate technical expertise*. Individuals with research and/or statistical expertise can help make needs assessments and evaluation research publishable. Collaborative approaches with *colleagues* permit the sharing of workload, can help group members maintain interest and momentum, and can provide the type of creative, critical, and supportive interactions that result in a better product than would have been achieved by a single individual. The identification of a *mentor* can be helpful to individuals with little experience in disseminating curricular work.

Table 9.4.   Criteria That May Be Considered in the Review of an Original Article on a Curriculum or Curriculum-related Work

Rationale
- Is there a well-reasoned and documented need for the curriculum or curriculum-related work? (Problem Identification and General Needs Assessment)

Setting
- Is the setting clearly described?
- Is the setting sufficiently representative to make the article of interest to readers? (External validity)

Subjects
- Are the learners clearly described? (Specific profession and specialty within profession; educational level [e.g., third-year medical students, PGY–2 residents, or practitioners]; needs assessment of targeted learners; sociodemographic information)
- Are the learners sufficiently representative to make the article of interest to readers? (External validity)

Educational Intervention
- Are the relevant objectives clearly expressed?
- Are the objectives meaningful and congruent with the rationale, intervention, and evaluation?
- Are the educational content and methods described in sufficient detail to be replicated? (If written description is incomplete, are educational materials offered in an appendix or elsewhere?)
- Are the required resources adequately described (e.g., faculty, faculty development, equipment)?

Evaluation Methods
- Are the methods described in sufficient detail so that the evaluation is replicable?
- Is the evaluation question clear? Are independent and dependent variables clearly defined?
- Are the dependent variables meaningful and congruent with the rationale and objectives for the curriculum? (For example, is performance/behavior measured instead of competence/skill, or skill instead of knowledge, when those are the desired or most meaningful effects?) Are the measurements objective (preferred) or subjective? Where in the hierarchy of outcomes are the dependent variables (patient/health care outcomes > behavior/performance > skills/competence > knowledge or attitudes > satisfaction or perceptions)?
- Is the evaluation design clear and sufficiently strong to answer the evaluation question? Could the evaluation question and design have been more ambitious?
    Is the design single or multi-institutional? (latter enhances external validity)
    Has randomization and/or a control group been used?
    Are long-term as well as short-term effects measured?
- Has a power analysis been conducted to determine the likelihood that the evaluation would detect an effect of the desired magnitude?
- Are raters blinded to the status of learners?
- Are the measurement instruments described or displayed in sufficient detail? (If incompletely described or displayed, are they offered or referenced?)
- Do the measurement instruments possess content validity (see Chapter 7)? Are they congruent with the evaluation question?

Table 9.4. *(continued)*

- Have inter- and intra-rater reliability and internal consistency validity been assessed? (See Chapter 7.)
- Are there other forms of validity evidence for the measurement instruments (e.g., relationship to other variables evidence, such as concurrent and predictive validity)? (Desirable, but frequently not achieved in curricular publications; see Chapter 7.)
- Are the reliability and validity sufficient to ensure the accuracy of the measurement instruments? Have the measurement instruments been used elsewhere? Have they attained a level of general acceptance? (Rarely are the last two criteria satisfied.)
- Are the statistical methods (parametric vs. nonparametric) appropriate for the type of data collected (nominal, ordinal, numerical; normally distributed vs. skewed; very small vs. larger sample size)? Are the specific statistical tests appropriate to answer the evaluation question? Have potentially confounding independent variables been controlled for by random allocation or the appropriate statistical methods?
- Are the evaluation methods, as a whole, sufficiently rigorous to ensure the internal validity of the evaluation and to promote the external validity of the evaluation?

Results
- Is the response rate adequate?
- Have educational significance/effect size been assessed? (See Chapter 7.)
- Are the results of sufficient interest to be worthy of publication? (The paper's Introduction and Discussion can help address this question.)

Conclusions
- Are the conclusions justified based on the methodology of the study or report?
- Are the strengths and limitations of the methodology acknowledged?
- Has the contribution of the work to the literature been accurately described?

Equipment and Facilities

Equipment needs for dissemination are generally minimal and usually consist of equipment that is already accessible to health professional faculty, such as audiovisual equipment or a personal computer. Occasionally, software programs may need to be purchased. *Facilities or space* for presentations are usually provided by the recipients. Occasionally a studio may be required for the development of audiovisual recordings.

Funds

Faculty may need to have time protected from other responsibilities in order to accomplish a dissemination effort. Technical consultants may require support. Funds may also be required for the purchase of necessary new *equipment* or the rental of *facilities*. Sometimes a faculty member's institution is able to provide such funding. Sometimes external sources can provide such funding (see also Chapter 6 and Appendix B). Well-funded curricula are often of higher quality than those that are poorly funded, and they typically fare better when it comes to publishing work related to the curricula (55, 56).

HOW CAN DISSEMINATION AND IMPACT BE MEASURED?

To determine whether dissemination efforts have the desired impact on target audiences, curriculum developers should make an effort to measure the effectiveness of dissemination. Quantitative and qualitative measurements can be helpful in assessing the degree of dissemination and impact of one's work.

For *journal articles*, journal impact factor and sometimes immediacy factor and cited half-life are used as measures of the influence of the journal in which one's work is published. Such information is available at Thomson Reuters's ISI (Institute for Scientific Information) Web of Knowledge (62). An alternative measure, the SCR-SCImago Journal Rank (SJR), attributes different weights to citations depending on the prestige of the citing journal without including self-citations (63). Curriculum developers may want to consider journal impact factors or SJRs in deciding to which journals to submit their manuscript. Perhaps a more important measure of dissemination is the number of times one's work has been cited in other journal articles. Both types of information can be provided by a *citation index*, such as the ISI (Institute for Scientific Information) Web of Knowledge (64) or Scopus (65).

Both the ISI Web of Knowledge and Scopus can also provide a measure, called an *h-index*, for authors who have had a number of publications in a field. The *h*-index reflects both the number of publications an author has had and the number of citations per publication. The index was developed to improve on simpler measures such as the total number of citations or publications (66). The *h*-index works properly only for comparing academicians working in the same field, such as education. Desirable *h*-indices vary widely among different fields, such as medical student education, biochemistry, and clinical cardiology research.

For *curricular materials*, one can *keep track of the number of times they have been requested by others*. This is easiest for Web-based material, where one can build in a tracking mechanism for access and completion. MedEdPORTAL, for example, provides authors with usage reports that provide a list of users that have viewed the full abstract of their posted materials (51). The report contains the name, institution, country, e-mail address, and date the resource was last accessed. There is an understanding that authors may contact users to determine if and how they used the resource.

For other forms of dissemination, impact can be measured in a variety of ways. For *books*, one can keep track of *sales*, *book reviews*, and *communications* regarding one's book. For *workshops* and *presentations*, one can keep track of the *number* and *locations* of those that are peer reviewed and requested. Another measure of dissemination is *media coverage* of one's work, which can be assessed by running an Internet search for any news coverage of the work.

Most of the above provide quantitative information about the dissemination of one's work. A curriculum developer can elect to collect additional information, including qualitative information, about how their ideas and curricular materials have been used, as well as the impact they have had, through either *informal communications* or *systematic assessment strategies*. For example, one can build evaluation strategies into the use of a disseminated electronic curriculum.

EXAMPLE: *Systematic Evaluation Strategy to Assess Dissemination.* A Web-based curriculum in ambulatory care medicine was developed for internal medicine residency programs, and over 80 residency programs have subscribed to it. Information on use of modules and resident performance is routinely collected. Periodic surveys of the program directors or curriculum administrators at each site assess how the curriculum is used (4, 5). The curriculum is also structured to generate reports related to each module (67–70).

CONCLUSION

The dissemination of a new or improved curriculum can be valuable to the curriculum developer and curriculum, as well as to others. To be effective in disseminating a curriculum or products of a curriculum development process, the curriculum developer must develop a coherent strategy that determines what is worth disseminating, employs appropriate modes of dissemination, and makes the best use of available time and resources. When dissemination efforts are done well, measurement of degree and impact of the dissemination can be very rewarding.

QUESTIONS

For a curriculum that you are coordinating, planning, or would like to be planning, please answer or think about the following questions:

1. What are the *reasons* why you might want to disseminate part or all of your work?

2. *Which* steps in your curriculum development process would you expect to lead to a discrete *product* worth disseminating to other individuals and groups?

3. *Describe a dissemination strategy* (target audiences, modes of dissemination) that would fulfill your reasons for wanting to disseminate part or all of your work. Usually this requires more than one mode of dissemination (see Table 9.1).

4. *Estimate the resources, in terms of time and effort, personnel, equipment/facilities, and costs,* that would be required to implement your dissemination strategy. Is the strategy feasible? Would you need to identify mentors, consultants, or colleagues to help you develop or execute the dissemination strategy? Multiply your estimate of needed time and effort by a factor of 2–4 (which is likely to be closer to reality). Would your plans for dissemination need to be altered or abandoned?

5. What would be a *simple strategy for measuring the degree/impact of your dissemination efforts*? Consider your goals for dissemination and the importance of documenting the degree and impact of your dissemination.

6. Imagine the *pleasures and rewards* of a successful dissemination effort. Could you afford to abandon your goals for dissemination?

GENERAL REFERENCES

Bauman LJ, Stein REK, Ireys HT. Reinventing fidelity: the transfer of social technology among settings. *Am J of Community Psychology.* 1991;19:619–39.

Thoughtful discussion of barriers to program diffusion and guidance as to how to implement a program in different sites with different personnel and client populations.

Garson A, Gutgesell HP, Pinsky WW, McNamara DG. The 10-minute talk: organization, slides, writing and delivery. *Am Heart J.* 1986;111(1):193–203.
 Practical instruction on giving 10 minute oral presentations before a professional audience.

Kern DE, Branch WT, Green ML, Bass EB, et al. Making it count twice: how to get curricular work published. Available at www.sgim.org/userfiles/file/AMHandouts/AM05/handouts/WG06.pdf. Accessed March 11, 2009.
 Practical tips from the editors of the first medical education issue of the Journal of General Internal Medicine on planning curricular work so that it is likely to be publishable, on preparing curriculum-related manuscripts for publication, and on submitting manuscripts to journals and responding to editors' letters. 24 pages.

Oldenburg B, Parcel GS. Diffusion of innovations, Chapter 14. In: Glanz K, Rimer BK, Lewis FM, eds. *Health Behavior and Health Education,* 3rd ed. San Francisco: Jossey-Bass; 2002. Pp. 312–34.
 This chapter discusses various aspects of diffusion theory and their practical application in the development and implementation of broad-based health behavior change interventions.

Rogers EM. *Diffusion of Innovations,* 5th ed. New York: Free Press; 2003.
 Classic text that presents a useful framework for understanding how new ideas are communicated to members of a social system. 551 pages.

Westberg J, Jason H. *Fostering Learning in Small Groups: A Practical Guide.* New York: Springer Publishing Co.; 2004.
 Practical book, drawing on years of experience, on practical strategies for planning and facilitating small groups. Can be applied to giving workshops. 288 pages.

Westberg J, Jason H. *Making Presentations: Guidebook for Health Professions Teachers.* Boulder, Colo.: Center for Instructional Support, Johnson Printing; 1991.
 User-friendly resource for health professionals on all aspects of preparing and giving presentations, stage fright, audiovisuals, and strategies to enhance presentations. 89 pages.

SPECIFIC REFERENCES

1. Golden AS. A model for curriculum development linking curriculum with health needs. In: Golden AS, Carlson DG, Hogan JL, eds. *The Art of Teaching Primary Care.* Springer Series on Medical Education, Vol. 3. New York: Springer Publishing Co.; 1982. Pp. 9–25.
2. Ludmerer KM. *Time to Heal: American Medical Education from the Turn of the Century to the Era of Managed Care.* Oxford: Oxford University Press; 1999.
3. Sharf BF, Freeman J, Benson J, Rogers J. Organizational rascals in medical education: mid-level innovation through faculty development. *Teaching and Learning in Medicine.* 1989;1:215–20.
4. Sisson SD, Hughes MT, Levine D, Brancati FL. Effect of an Internet-based curriculum on post-graduate education. A multicenter intervention. *J Gen Intern Med.* 2004 May;19(5 Pt 2):505–9.
5. Sisson SD, Rastegar DA, Rice TN, Hughes MT. Multicenter implementation of a shared graduate medical education resource. *Arch Intern Med.* 2007;167:2476–80.
6. Glassick CE, Huber MR, Maeroff GI. *Scholarship Assessed: Evaluation of the Professoriate.* San Francisco: Jossey-Bass; 1997.
7. Glassick CE. Boyer's expanded definitions of scholarship, the standards for assessing scholarship, and the elusiveness of the scholarship of teaching. *Acad Med.* 2000;75:877–880.
8. Simpson D, Fincher RM, Hafler JP, Irby DM, Richards BF, Rosenfeld GC, Viggiano TR. *Advancing Educators and Education: Defining the Components and Evidence of Educational*

Scholarship. Washington, D.C.: Association of American Medical Colleges; 2007. P. 9. Available at www.aamc.org/. Go to "Publications, Browse by Title." Accessed March 11, 2009.

9. Lubitz RM. Guidelines for the promotion of clinician-teachers. *J Gen Intern Med.* 1997;12(Suppl 1):S71–78.

10. Atasoylu AA, Wright SM, Beasley BW, et al. Promotion criteria for clinician-educators. *J Gen Intern Med.* 2003;18:711–16.

11. Beasley BW, Wright SM, Cofrancesco J Jr., Babbott SF, Thomas PA, Bass EB. Promotion criteria for clinician-educators in the United States and Canada. A survey of promotion committee chairpersons. *JAMA.* 1997;278:723–28.

12. Fleming VM, Schindler N, Martin GJ, DaRosa DA. Separate and equitable promotion tracks for clinician-educators. *JAMA.* 2005;294:1101–4.

13. Hafler JP, Lovejoy FH Jr. Scholarly activities recorded in the portfolios of teacher-clinician faculty. *Acad Med.* 2000;75:649–52.

14. Simpson D, Hafler J, Brown D, Wilkerson L. Documentation systems for educators seeking academic promotion in U.S. medical schools. *Acad Med.* 2004;79:783–90.

15. Kern DE, Grayson M, Barker LR, Roca RP, Cole KA, Roter D, Golden AS. Residency training in interviewing skills and the psychosocial domain of medical practice. *J Gen Intern Med.* 1989;4:421–31.

16. Roter DL, Cole KA, Kern DE, Barker LR, Grayson MA. An evaluation of residency training in interviewing skills and the psychosocial domain of medical practice. *J Gen Intern Med.* 1990;5:347–54.

17. Roter DL, Hall JA, Kern DE, Barker LR, Cole KA, Roca RP. Improving physicians' interviewing skills and reducing patients' emotional distress: a randomized clinical trial. *Arch Intern Med.* 1995;155:1877–84.

18. Williamson PW, Smith R, Kern DE, Lipkin ML Jr., Barker LR, Hoppe R, Florek J. The medical interview and psychosocial aspects of medicine: residency block curricula. *J Gen Intern Med.* 1992;7:235–42.

19. Branch WT Jr., Kern DE, Gracey K, Haidet P, Weissmann P, Mitchell G, Inui T, Novak TL. Teaching the human dimensions of care in clinical settings. *JAMA.* 2001;286:1067–74.

20. Kern DE, Branch WT Jr., Jackson JL, Brady DW, Feldman MD, Levinson W, Lipkin M Jr. Teaching the psychosocial aspects of care in the clinical setting: practical recommendations. *Acad Med.* 2005;80(1):8–20.

21. Gracey CF, Haidet P, Branch WT, Weissmann P, Kern DE, Mitchell G, Frankel R, Inui T. Precepting humanism: strategies for fostering the human dimensions of care in ambulatory settings. *Acad Med.* 2005;80(1):21–28.

22. Kern DE, Branch WT, Green ML. Making it count twice: how to get curricular work published. Available at www.sgim.org/userfiles/file/AMHandouts/AM05/handouts/WG06.pdf. Accessed March 11, 2009.

23. Rogers EM. *Diffusion of Innovations,* 5th ed. New York: Free Press; 2003. Pp. 219–66.

24. Oldenburg B, Parcel GS. Diffusion of innovations, Chapter 14. In: Glanz K, Rimer BK, Lewis FM, eds. *Health Behavior and Health Education,* 3rd ed. San Francisco: Jossey-Bass; 2002. Pp. 312–34.

25. Sanson-Fisher RW, Lynagh MC. Problem-based learning: a dissemination success story? *Med J Aust.* 2005;183(5):258–60.

26. Bauman LJ, Stein REK, Ireys HT. Reinventing fidelity: the transfer of social technology among settings. *Am J of Community Psychology.* 1991;19:631–35.

27. Roberts LW, Geppert C, Connor R, Nguyen K, Warner TD. An invitation for medical educators to focus on ethical and policy issues in research and scholarly practice. *Acad Med.* 2001;76(9):876–85.

28. Tomkowiak JM, Gunderson AJ. To IRB or not to IRB? *Acad Med.* 2004 Jul;79(7):628–32.

29. Copyright Act of 1976, Pub. L. No. 94–553, 90 Stat. 2541 (for the general revision of copyright law, title 17 of the United States Code, and for other purposes), October 19, 1976.

30. Association of Research Libraries. Copyright and Intellectual Property Policies. Available at www.arl.org/pp/ppcopyright/. Accessed March 11, 2009.
31. American Libraries Association Office of Intellectual Freedom. Available at www.ala.org/. Go to Issues and Advocacy, Copyright. Accessed March 11, 2009.
32. Crash Course in Copyright, maintained by the University of Texas. Available at www.utsys tem.edu/ogc/intellectualproperty/cprtindx.htm. Accessed March 11, 2009.
33. Yale University Library. Council on Library and Information Resources. Liblicense: licensing digital information: a resource for librarians. Available at www.library.yale.edu/~llicense/index.shtml. Accessed, March 11, 2009.
34. Raman RN, O'Donnell JDF, Rabow MW. The Healer's Art: education in meaning and service. *J Cancer Educ.* 2008;23(1):65–67.
35. Institute for the Study of Health and Illness at Commonweal. The Healer's Art. Available at www.commonweal.org/ishi/programs/healers_art.html. Accessed March 11, 2009.
36. Rabow MW, Srubel J, Remen RN. Authentic community as an educational strategy for advancing professionalism: a national evaluation of the Healer's Art curriculum. *J Gen Intern Med.* 2007;22(10):1422–28.
37. Goroll AH, Morrison G, Bass EB, Fortin AH, Mumford L. *Core Medicine Clerkship Guide.* Washington, D.C.: Health Resources and Services Administration; 1995.
38. Jablonover RS, Blackman DJ, Bass EB, Morrison G, Goroll AH. Evaluation of a national curriculum reform effort for the medicine core clerkship. *J Gen Intern Med.* 2000;15:484–91.
39. CDIM/SGIM Core Medicine Clerkship Curriculum Guide Version 3.0 Update Taskforce. *Core Medicine Clerkship Version 3.0.* Clerkship Directors in Internal Medicine/Society of General Internal Medicine Curriculum. 2006. Available at Alliance for Academic Internal Medicine (AAIM) Web site, www.im.org/, then go to AAIM Alliance Sites, CDIM. Accessed March 11, 2009.
40. Chakraborti C, Boonyasai RT, Wright SM, Kern DE. A systematic review of teamwork training interventions in medical student and resident education: a systematic review. *J Gen Intern Med.* 2008;23(6):846–53.
41. Clark JM, Houston TK, Kolodner K, Branch WT Jr., Levine R, Kern DE. Teaching the teachers: a national survey of faculty development in departments of medicine of U.S. teaching hospitals. *J Gen Intern Med.* 2004;19:205–14.
42. Ratanawongsa N, Bolen S, Howell EE, Kern DE, Sisson SD, Larriviere D. Residents' perceptions of professionalism in training and practice: barriers, promoters, and duty hour requirements. *J Gen Intern Med.* 2006;21(7):758–63.
43. Hsu EB, Thomas TL, Bass EB, Whyne D, Kelen GD, Green GB. Healthcare worker competencies for disaster training. BMC *Med Educ.* 2006;6:19.
44. Hatcher J, Schoenberg NE. Human subjects protection training for community workers: an example from Faith Moves Mountains. *Progress in Community Health Partnerships.* 2007;1:257–65.
45. Ogur B, Hirsh D, Krupat E, Bor D. The Harvard Medical School–Cambridge integrated clerkship: an innovative model of clinical education. *Acad Med.* 2007;82(4):397–404.
46. Morrison EH, Rucker L, Boker JR, et al. The effect of a 13-hour curriculum to improve residents' teaching skills: a randomized trial. *Ann Intern Med.* 2004;141:257–63.
47. Windish DM, Gozu A, Bass EB, Thomas PA, Sisson SD, Howard DM, Kern DE. A ten-month program in curriculum development for medical educators: 16 years of experience. *J Gen Intern Med.* 2007;22:655–61.
48. Gozu A, Windish DM, Knight AM, Thomas PA, Kolodner K, Bass EB, Sisson SD, Kern DE. Long-term follow-up of a ten-month program in curriculum development: a cohort study. *Med Educ.* 2008;42:684–92.
49. Garson A, Gutgesell HP, Pinsky WW, McNamara DG. The 10-minute talk: organization, slides, writing and delivery. *Am Heart J.* 1986;111(1):193–203.
50. doc.com. Available at www.aachonline.org/. Accessed March 11, 2009.
51. MedEdPORTAL. Available at www.aamc.org/mededportal. Accessed March 11, 2009.

52. End of Life/Palliative Education Resource Center. Available at www.eperc.mcw.edu. Accesssed March 11, 2009.
53. American Academy of Hospice and Palliative Medicine. End of Life/Palliative Care Educational Resources. Available at www.aahpm.org/resources/. Accessed March 11, 2009.
54. International Committee of Medical Journal Editors (ICMJE). Uniform Requirements for Manuscripts Submitted to Biomedical Journals: Writing and Editing for Biomedical Publication Updated October 2007. Available at www.icmje.org. Accessed March 11, 2009.
55. Reed DA, Cook DA, Beckman TJ, Levine RB, Kern DE, Wright SM. Association between funding and quality of published medical education research. *JAMA*. 2007;298:1002–9.
56. Reed DA, Beckman TJ, Wright SM, Levine RB, Kern DE, Cook DA. Predictive validity evidence for medical education research study quality instrument scores: quality of submissions to *JGIM*'s medical education supplement. *J Gen Intern Med*. 2008;23(7):903–7.
57. Reed D, Price EG, Windish DM, Wright SM, Gozu A, Hsu EB, Beach MC, Kern DE, Bass EB. Challenges in systematic reviews of educational intervention studies. *Ann Intern Med*. 2005;142:1080–89.
58. Consolidated Standards of Reporting Trials (CONSORT) statement, guidelines, and checklist. Available at www.consort-statement.org/. Accessed March 11, 2009.
59. Stroup DF, Berlin JA, Morton SC, Olkin I, Williamson GD, Rennie D, Moher D, Becker BJ, Sipe TA, Thacker SB. Meta-analysis of observational studies in epidemiology: a proposal for reporting. Meta-analysis of Observational Studies in Epidemiology (MOOSE) group. *JAMA*. 2000;283:2008–12.
60. Moher D, Cook DJ, Eastwood S, Olkin I, Rennie D, Stroup DF. Improving the quality of reports of meta-analyses of randomised controlled trials: the QUOROM statement. Quality of Reporting of Meta-analyses. *Lancet*. 1999;354:1896–1900. Also available at www.consort-statement.org/index.aspx?o=1065. Accessed March 11, 2009.
61. Des Jarlais DC, Lyles C, Crepaz N, TREND Group. Improving the reporting quality of nonrandomized evaluations of behavioral and public health interventions: the TREND statement. *Am J Public Health*. 2004;94:361–66.
62. ISI Web of Knowledge. Available at www.isiwebofknowledge.com. Go to ISI Web of Knowledge, then Select a Database, then Journal Citation Reports. Accessed March 11, 2009.
63. SCImago. 2007. SJR—SCImago Journal and Country Rank. Available at www.scimagojr.com. Accessed March 11, 2009.
64. ISI Web of Knowledge. A citation index that is part of the Web of Science sponsored by Thomson Reuters. Available at www.isiwebofknowledge.com. Go to ISI Web of Knowledge, then Web of Science, enter information, click Search, then click Create Citation Report. Accessed March 11, 2009.
65. Scopus. A citation index sponsored by Elsevier. Available at www.scopus.com/scopus/home.url. Information on Scopus available at www.info.scopus.com. Accessed March 11, 2009.
66. Hirsch JE. An index to quantify an individual's scientific research output. *Proc Natl Acad Sci USA*. 2005;102:16569–72.
67. Cosgrove SE, Perl TM, Song X, Sisson SD. Ability of physicians to diagnose and manage illness due to category A bioterrorism agents. *Arch Intern Med*. 2005;165:2002–6.
68. Sisson SD, Rice TN, Hughes MT. Physician knowledge of national cholesterol guidelines before and after an interactive curriculum. *Am J Cardiol*. 2007;99:1234–35.
69. Ashar BH, Rice TN, Sisson SD. Physicians' understanding of the regulation of dietary supplements. *Arch Intern Med*. 2007 May 14;167(9):966–69.
70. Dy SM, Hughes M, Weiss C, Sisson S. Evaluation of a Web-based palliative care pain management module for housestaff. *J Pain Symptom Manage*. 2008 Apr 25. [Epub ahead of print]

Example Curricula

This appendix provides three examples of curricula that have progressed through all six steps of curriculum development. The reader may want to review one or more of these examples to see how the various steps of the curriculum development process can relate to one another and be integrated into a whole.

The curricula were chosen to demonstrate differences in learner level and longevity. One focuses on medical students (Chronic Disease and Disability), one on residents (Primary Care Gynecology), and one on faculty (Longitudinal Program in Curriculum Development). The Chronic Disease and Disability curriculum was developed as part of the Longitudinal Program in Curriculum Development in 2005–6, was introduced as an elective rotation in 2006–7, and will become a required rotation in the new Johns Hopkins medical school curriculum to be implemented in 2009–10. The Primary Care Gynecology curriculum was initially developed as part of the Longitudinal Program in Curriculum Development in 1993–94, implemented in 1994–95, and further developed by a second project in Longitudinal Program in Curriculum Development in 2004–5. The Longitudinal Program in Curriculum Development was implemented in 1987–88 as part of a faculty development grant and has been in operation since. The latter two examples have progressed to the stage of dissemination.

CHRONIC DISEASE AND DISABILITY FOR MEDICAL STUDENTS

R. Samuel Mayer, M.D., Amit A. Shah, M.D., Barbara J. de Lateur, M.D., M.S., and Patricia A. Thomas, M.D.

This curriculum was developed in 2005–6 as part of the Curriculum Development Workshop of the Johns Hopkins University (JHU) Faculty Development Program. The development team included Drs. R. Samuel Mayer and Barbara de Lateur, of the Department of Physical Medicine and Rehabilitation (PM&R) of JHU, and Dr. Amit Shah, a geriatrics fellow at the time and now a faculty member at University of Texas Southwestern Medical School. In the process of a major curriculum reform, the medical school curriculum committee recognized the paucity of training that medical students receive in chronic illnesses and disabling conditions. The curriculum committee approved a required *advanced* four-week clerkship in the senior year.

Step 1: Problem Identification and General Needs Assessment

The authors used literature searches and an Internet search for ideal curricula in preparing this step. Other helpful online data included the Association of American Medical College (AAMC) Graduation Questionnaire and CurrMIT curriculum management software (see Chapter 2 and www.aamc.org/meded/curric/start.htm, accessed March 12, 2009).

Problem Identification	In the United States, 125 million people have chronic illnesses, which account for more than three-quarters of all health care expenses (1–3). Nearly 50 million individuals over the age of 5 have at least one disability, and that excludes institutionalized patients (4). About one-half of these people have a severe disability limiting a significant life activity (5).
Current Approach	Patients with chronic illness and disability perceive their physicians as poorly prepared to deal with the issues most pertinent to their quality of life (3, 6). Furthermore, there is growing evidence of safety concerns among patients with chronic illness as they transition through a fragmented health care system (7, 8).
	Medical student/resident training is driven by the emphasis on acute hospital/inpatient medicine. Greater than 75% of the time of most students and residents is spent in these acute settings, thus greatly limiting exposure to those issues that are not addressed in the inpatient setting. Because of this structure, physicians in training may attach less value to the care of chronic illness.
	Graduating medical students recognize inadequacies in their training for providing the future care of the chronically ill and disabled. The 2005 AAMC Medical School Graduation Questionnaire (GQ) is revealing (9). In it 28% of students said their training in patient follow-up was inadequate, 30% said time spent learn-

ing about long-term health care was inadequate, 45% said more time should be devoted to instruction in pain management, 45% felt that they needed more knowledge about health care systems, and 33% noted that they were insufficiently trained in the utilization of community health resources. These students matriculated into medical school with both positive and negative attitudes about individuals with disability and chronic illness (10–12). They generally have an idealistic outlook toward serving these patients but somewhat low expectations for what individuals with disability can achieve. Unfortunately, as time goes on in their medical training, students develop increasingly negative attitudes about caring for the chronically ill (12).

The inadequacies of the current training system that are sensed by graduating medical students are confirmed by practicing physicians. Darer et al. (13) surveyed 1236 practicing physicians (half primary care, half specialists) in the United States in 2000–2001; more than half of respondents reported inadequate training in each of 10 chronic care competencies. These competencies were end-of-life care, coordination of home and community care services, management of geriatric syndromes, psychosocial aspects of chronic illness, assessment of caregiver needs, chronic pain management, nutrition, interdisciplinary teamwork, and assessing developmental milestones in disabled children. Negative attitudes that form during earlier training were also confirmed by this survey. With the exception of family practitioners, only a minority (range by specialty group, 34%–46%) of the physicians said their medical school and residency training left them feeling positive about taking care of patients with chronic illnesses.

These data strongly support the need for curriculum reform in medical schools nationwide. Current teaching in medical schools tends to be fragmented. A survey of CurrMIT, the AAMC online repository of medical school curricula, shows that knowledge about chronic illness and disability is primarily attained through disparate lectures in the epidemiology, pathophysiology, and pharmacology of specific diseases during the preclinical years. During clinical rotations, much of the bedside teaching centers on disease-specific management rather than a holistic view of the bio-psychosocial needs of the patient. Elective courses in geriatrics and rehabilitation are offered at some medical schools, but a small minority make them a requirement for all students. Physical diagnosis courses teach rudimentary skills in social history and almost never touch on functional evaluation.

Several authors have written about chronic illness care competencies that ought to be covered in medical training (14–18). A recent survey of course directors demonstrates that, although there is agreement about certain competencies that all medical students

should have, there is considerable variation in the implementation and addressing of these competencies (18). Furthermore,
a search of the literature reveals no "best practices guidelines"
or published curricula for teaching students approaches to the
care of the chronically ill and disabled. Few medical schools offer
courses in chronic illness, disability, PM&R, and geriatrics, which
often address chronic illness and disability. One of the best developed and closest to a "model curriculum" is a long-standing
course offered by the University of Washington. Students learn
aspects of rehabilitation, geriatrics, and palliative medicine during
a four-week rotation. Complete course details are available online
at http://courses.washington.edu/conj690/ (accessed March 12,
2009).

Ideal Approach   An ideal curriculum would help learners develop knowledge,
skills, and attitudes to effectively care for patients with chronic
illness and disability. Major areas of knowledge would include
epidemiology of disability and chronic illness, falls, incontinence,
dementia and cognitive deficits, mood disorders, chronic pain,
polypharmacy, and childhood development. Key skills are teamwork, patient communication, rehabilitation prescriptions, functional evaluation, anticipatory management, transition among
levels of care, and utilization of resources for optimizing indepen-
dence. Negative attitudes, such as viewing chronic illness as "in-
curable, life altering and terminal," (11) can be improved through
innovative teaching techniques such as patient presentations on
stereotypes, team meetings and home visits, and simulated experiences such as a day in a wheelchair, which help students
to develop empathy and a sense of empowerment. A survey of
course directors reveals some consensus about which of these
topics are felt to be most important for medical students (18).
Noting that the growing prevalence of chronic illness has implications for nearly all physicians regardless of specialty, the survey
concluded that the overall focus needs to be on quality-of-life
issues for individuals with disability and chronic illness. The ideal
format for this type of a curriculum would include both clinical
experiences and didactics about key points and would be longitudinal and integrated with other courses and experiences.

Step 2: Needs Assessment of Targeted Learners

For this step, the authors used school-specific data from the AAMC Graduation
Questionnaire and developed the first-ever survey of Johns Hopkins University School
of Medicine (JHUSOM) alumni, 5–10 years after graduation.

Targeted Learners   We identified our targeted learners for this curriculum as medical
students at the JHUSOM in their clinical years (third/fourth year).
We chose this group for several reasons. Medical school (rather

than later in residency training) provides an opportunity for all future physicians to be exposed to Chronic Disease and Disability (CDD) issues, irrespective of their ultimate choice of medical specialty or career direction. We believe strongly that the knowledge, skills, and attitudes for managing people with chronic disease and disability are applicable to all physicians. Many Johns Hopkins medical students go into academic medicine, and thus we have an opportunity to train the teachers of tomorrow. Many also ultimately attain leadership roles in medicine and thus will have tremendous impact on the future direction of health care. Early career exposure will give students the tools necessary to address the care of complex and chronically ill patients and thus may mitigate the negative attitudes that often develop during the course of training.

Targeted Environment	JHUSOM students have intense exposure to acute tertiary care settings in nearly all of their clinical rotations. Their faculty role models often defer the concerns of chronic illness to the primary care providers and fail to give explicit teaching or importance to the skills of CDD. Given the nature of CDD, a longitudinal experience would be most ideal, but it would be difficult to coordinate and integrate into the curriculum. A self-contained rotation is easier to administer and may be more goal directed.
Needs Assessment	Currently CDD topics are not covered in any one place in the curriculum. Informal interviews of current Hopkins medical students revealed a feeling of "just being expected to pick it up." Medical students often felt overwhelmed by complex and chronically ill patients. JHUSOM-specific data about CDD topic areas were extracted from the Pham et al. study of course directors (18). In the core rotations of pediatrics, ambulatory care, and internal medicine, there is a clear lack of attention paid to a number of key issues in chronic disease and disability, despite the fact that the course directors felt that these were important to include in the medical school curriculum. These issues included cognitive impairment, incontinence, falls prevention, pain, polypharmacy, nutrition, functional limitations, rehabilitation prescription, caregiver needs, and end-of-life care. Currently, intense exposure in CDD topics occurs only in electives (i.e., in geriatrics and PM&R). Only a relatively few JHUSOM students (approximately 15 per year) currently take these electives.
Survey of JHUSOM Alumni	We surveyed alumni of JHUSOM who had graduated 5–10 years earlier. Our survey addressed the following questions: How do former JHUSOM students feel about the training they received in CDD topics? What is the JHUSOM student's preferred modality to

learn CDD topics? What will be the best way to supplement clinical experiences? What topics are most critical to cover, considering their importance to practice and the paucity of coverage in the current curriculum? We chose this group because we felt that they were recent enough graduates to reflect the current curriculum, yet experienced enough to know the needs of the "real-world" practitioner. We used an e-mail-based questionnaire that was sent to 279 alumni. A total of 135 people answered the introductory questions, and 122 (44%) completed the full survey. The alumni survey was analyzed by dividing responses into adequate (4 or 5 on a 5-point Likert scale) or inadequate (1–3) training and important (4–5) or unimportant (1–3) subject matter.

Fifty-one percent of respondents felt that medical school inadequately trained them to care for chronically ill and disabled patients, and 64% felt that the time in the curriculum devoted to issues of chronic disease and disability was inadequate. Specific topics that stood out as large discrepancies between training adequacy and importance to practice were teamwork with allied health professionals, polypharmacy, chronic pain, access to care, psychosocial aspects of chronic disease, communication with chronically ill or disabled patients, nutrition, and functional evaluation.

The open-ended responses received were also enlightening. We received 277 written comments to our questionnaire. Prominent themes that emerged included the following:

1. Experiences at JHUSOM that best taught them about CDD issues (114 responses): there were numerous responses about the pediatric chronic care hospital experience being useful. Learning during medicine and psychiatry clerkships was mentioned frequently. Experiences with the geriatrics department were also mentioned frequently. Home visits (in either geriatrics or pediatric HIV patients) were also mentioned frequently. Here is an example:

> As a medical student on the pediatric basic clerkship we were required to pay a home visit with the social worker to the home of one of the pediatric patients on the service with a chronic medical problem. In my case we went to see a young girl with congenital HIV who had been admitted during our clerkship with PCP pneumonia. She was being raised by her uncle and his partner. Listening to how these two dedicated gentlemen organized their lives around the life of their young charge, her medicines and appointments, and still strived to let her play and be like other kids was really the best experience in medical school that I had on the "tip of the iceberg" phenomenon of what living with a chronic illness means and how difficult what may be "prescribed" in the hospital is in terms of translating it to a patient's real life setting in the most

dedicated circumstances. Who ever designed that component of the pediatric clerkship really did all the medical students a great service. That experience has stayed with me when many other didactic experiences have faded away.

2. There were 86 responses giving advice about what CDD areas should be developed in the curriculum. Chronic pain training was listed several times, as were teaching of communication skills, multidisciplinary teamwork, and addressing quality-of-life issues. One person's response was representative:

> That physicians need to be comprehensive and detail-oriented about all the possible needs of patients, and to always try to put themselves in the patient's position, or to think about how they would want the patient treated if it were his or her own family member. To take the time with patients and to listen—as patients really notice and get frustrated/dislike physicians who don't seem to care. Especially in the Internal Medicine field, to realize how important continuity of care is for patients with chronic and complex diseases. To understand that it's normal for people to be depressed, often, or at times, about having a disability or chronic medical illness, and that you've gotta talk to patients about it. How to manage multiple medical illnesses in a patient so that they can try to lead a normal life and be as productive as they would have been without all of the medical problems. That medical insurance is complex, expensive, and really frustrating for everybody, rich and poor.

3. Open-ended questions about teaching methods (77 responses) revealed that most thought that direct patient care with increased exposure was the most important. Interdisciplinary exposure, home visits, and increased outpatient exposure were also listed. Here is one example response:

> At the bedside, in a clinic. Teaching it in a classroom gives too skewed a view which can be depressing and pessimistic as well as unrealistic. Students need to see an infant with cerebral palsy to not only see how it affects that infant's life but the family's life as well, and not only in an adverse manner but also in the ways it demonstrates the triumph of life and family love over a medical disability. That is, not only is living with disability (or raising an infant with a disability) life-changing and sometimes tragic, it can also be an amazing demonstration of what is truly important in life and how, despite medical tragedies, infants and families still live good lives with love.

School-specific AAMC Graduation Questionnaire Data

We reviewed the 2005 AAMC survey of exiting medical students. This is conducted at each accredited medical school annually. In the 2005 AAMC survey of exiting medical students, 73.0% of JHU students felt that their training was inadequate in nutrition (compared to 51.1% of all schools' graduates), 40.5% in geriatrics (compared to 24.4%), 51.4% in pain management (compared to 44.7%), 29.7% in continuity of care (compared to 19.8%), and 45.9% in palliative care (compared to 22.9%).

Step 3: Goals and Objectives

Building on the information obtained in Step 2, and cognizant of the resources available to them, the authors wrote specific learning objectives for the curriculum. These are presented in Table A.1, which emphasizes the attention given to congruence among objectives, educational strategies, and learner evaluation.

Goals	The overarching goal for the curriculum is that all graduating students of the Johns Hopkins University School of Medicine will possess the knowledge, skills, and attitudes to provide compassionate and high-quality care for individuals with chronic diseases and disabilities.
Objectives	Objectives are divided into cognitive, psychomotor, and affective domains. We have tied each objective to the educational strategy (Step 4) and the evaluation technique (Step 6). (See Table A.1.) We carefully worded each objective so that it would be measurable, achievable, and meaningful to the learners. We felt that the affective objectives (attitudes) were paramount to the overall success of the clerkship; these were also the most difficult to write and to evaluate.

Step 4: Educational Strategies

This clerkship was planned as a month-long, mandatory advanced clinical clerkship for senior medical students. Some students may take the rotation during their third year as their schedules allow. Prerequisites are successful completion of the first and second years. The clerkship will focus on issues of chronic disease and disability in a variety of clinical settings and will have concurrent didactic work, discussion groups, and simulation exercises to achieve its objectives.

Clinical Experience	Students will select two of four primary clinical sites for their rotation, each for two-week blocks. Each clinical site serves a different population in terms of age, diagnoses, and social situations, so that students can tailor the rotation to their interests. These sites will serve as a "home base" for the students, but there will be a common centralized didactic program and overlap among the sites for outpatient and community experiences. Each site will accommodate two to four students at a time. Sites will be assigned by order of student preference, but a lottery may be necessary if a particular site is oversubscribed.

Table A.1.   Objectives, Educational Strategies, and Evaluation

Objective	Educational Strategy	Evaluation
Knowledge		
State the prevalence and understand the impact of chronic disease and disabilities	Internet module	Internet module quiz
Define principles of interdisciplinary team management	Clinical exposure, reflection, discussion group	Participation passport, reflection journal entry
Discuss the evaluation and management of patients with chronic pain	Internet module, clinical exposure, discussion group	Internet module quiz
Delineate nutritional issues in patients with chronic diseases and disabilities	Internet module, clinical exposure	Internet module quiz
Identify polypharmacy issues in chronically ill patients	Internet module, discussion group	Internet module quiz
Describe management of urinary bladder, bowel, and sexual dysfunction in patients with disabilities	Internet module, clinical exposure	Internet module quiz
Identify limitations and resources in health care finances for the chronically ill and disabled patient	Internet module, discussion group	Internet module quiz
Skills		
Demonstrate effective, empathic, and culturally sensitive communication	Discussion groups, clinical exposures, patient simulations	360 degree observation
Demonstrate approaches to affect behavioral changes in health promotion for persons with chronic illness	Discussion groups, clinical exposures, role-playing	Faculty observation
Perform a detailed functional evaluation, including delineation of impairments, activity limitations, and participation restrictions	Internet module with video demonstrating an ideal evaluation; structured templates, clinical exposures	Faculty observation of student functional evaluation on a patient, and participation passport
Prescribe routine rehabilitation services and durable medical equipment	Structured templates, clinical exposure	Participation passport
Write progress notes, sign-offs and discharge summaries that optimize continuity of care	Structured templates, clinical exposure	Faculty observation

Table A.1. *(continued)*

Objective	Educational Strategy	Evaluation
Attitudes		
Describe the impact of chronic illness and disability on individuals, families, and society	Group discussion, reflection, simulation exercises	Reflection journal entry, participation passport
Participate in interdisciplinary goal setting with patients and families	Clinical exposure	360 degree observation, participation in team meetings as documented by passport
Demonstrate empathic attitudes toward individuals with disability and chronic illness	Group discussion, clinical exposure, reflection, simulation exercises	ATDP*/UCLA Geriatrics Attitudes Scale, 360 degree observation

* Attitudes Towards Disabled Persons.

	All sites will include experiences on an inpatient rehabilitation unit, visits to a subacute or chronic care facility, outpatient clinics that emphasize care of disabled and chronically ill patients, and home visits. Inpatient acute care will be de-emphasized. Students will participate in interdisciplinary team meetings and patient/family conferences.
Internet Modules	Knowledge-based objectives will be primarily addressed in self-study Internet modules posted on Blackboard. The modules will take approximately 20–30 minutes to complete, and students will be required to complete one or two modules weekly. The modules will include interactive pre- and postquizzes. Instructors will be available for e-mail questions, and there will be a *Frequently Asked Questions* (FAQs) bulletin board.
	Topics will include epidemiology and socioeconomic impact of chronic disease and disability; interdisciplinary team concepts; pain management; polypharmacy; nutrition; and bladder, bowel, and sexual dysfunction.
Discussion Groups	Discussion groups will meet 3–4 hours weekly at a central location for all 10 students on the clerkship. They will be led by faculty members, fellows, senior residents, or allied health professionals, as well as actual patients in some of the groups. There will be problem-based learning and interactive role-playing incorporated into the sessions. Topics for discussion will include attitudes toward people with chronic disease and disability, team communication skills, socioeconomic issues, functional evaluation, polypharmacy, and pain management.

Simulation Exercises One of the main goals of this clerkship is to improve attitudes that students have toward the disabled and chronically ill. We hope to increase empathy through simulation exercises that will be highly interactive and engaging. Students will experience some of what it is like to have a disability or chronic disease. They will be required to participate in at least two simulation activities. These may include time in a wheelchair as a "paraplegic" individual; time as a hemiparetic, aphasic, or hemianopsic stroke survivor (simulated with knee immobilizer, hand splint, or goggles); time as a visually impaired individual (specialized goggles); and a day as an individual with several chronic diseases who takes multiple medications (done with placebo candies and a restricted diet). Students will maintain a journal and then join in a discussion group to follow that week.

Step 5: Implementation

The clerkship will be offered 12 months a year, and as it is mandatory, 120 students will rotate through annually. This amounts to 10 students per month.

Resources   Implementation of this clerkship will require substantial personnel resources, as well as some space and equipment needs. As it is currently only being piloted as an elective, much of the implementation is only in the planning stage at the time of this publication.

Personnel:

Faculty: Leadership is crucial for success of this new program. It will involve multiple clinical sites and faculty from two different departments: Physical Medicine and Rehabilitation and the Division of Geriatrics. This will run most smoothly with two course codirectors, one from each department. The course codirectors will be responsible for course development and maintenance, oversight of all didactic content, clinical operations, and coordination. They will need to identify appropriate faculty and clinical facilities. They will have oversight of the evaluation process for students, faculty, and the overall program. They will need to observe the overall clinical experience and the learning environment. They will make frequent site visits and hold periodic feedback sessions. They will lead at least one discussion group each per month. Support was awarded for 0.25 FTE for each codirector.

Due to the interdisciplinary and patient-focused nature of this clerkship, we think that an advisory council will promote the interest of all stakeholders. We would like this committee to be composed of patient advocates, faculty, therapists, nurses, and student representatives. The council will meet quarterly to review program evaluations and do strategic planning.

Faculty will provide the backbone of teaching for the clerkship. We need to assure adequate training for them. We have arranged faculty retreats on educational topics, and we also include educational topics in grand rounds. We have identified core faculty to lead small group discussions. Because these will recur every month of the year, we need a rotating schedule for faculty participation in these groups. The group leaders are not only physicians but also, as appropriate, psychologists, social workers, therapists, and nurses. We also utilize geriatric fellows and senior PM&R residents for some of the discussion groups.

Support Staff: Support staff are critical to the smooth operation of this program. A 1.0 FTE administrative assistant will serve as the clerkship coordinator. This coordinator will facilitate student scheduling and site assignment with the registrar and faculty scheduling with the course codirectors. S/he will monitor and collate student and faculty evaluations. S/he will maintain Blackboard. S/he will also assist in preparation of lecture materials, scientific papers, and presentations.

Facilities and Equipment: Our facility space needs and equipment needs will be less costly. We will need a 20 person conference room one-half day per week for the small group discussions. We will need to borrow wheelchairs and splints for our patient simulations. We have already purchased low vision simulation goggles.

Online Learning: We will need to develop Internet modules that will be delivered with the institutional content management software (Blackboard); most of this cost is faculty time. Based on previous experience with Internet learning modules, 20 hours per topic will be needed for development.

Support	*Internal Support:* Internal funding support will come from the dean's office, the Department of PM&R, and the Division of Geriatrics. *External Support:* Interest from private foundations has been identified, and the authors are currently applying for private foundation support.
Barriers	*Curricular Time:* Securing time in the curriculum, especially during the clinical years, when students were most anxious for flexibility, was a major barrier to the introduction of a new clinical curriculum. Dr. Patricia Thomas, associate dean of curriculum, was actively involved in the curriculum reform process and mentored the development of the curriculum through the workshop year, and she actively supported its inclusion in the new curricu-

lum. The clerkship codirectors facilitated the issue of flexibility by accepting students with minimal clerkship experience into the advanced clerkship.

Faculty Resources and Recruitment: The School of Medicine (SOM) was fortunate that the faculty of two departments were enthused to have more opportunity to teach medical students. Nevertheless, it was critical that support be given to those with major teaching and administrative commitments such as this curriculum would require. A line item for codirectors and the clerkship coordinator was included in the dean's budget for the new curriculum (see Resources above).

Student Support: While students involved in the curriculum reform process have been relatively quiet about the new requirement, the first year of implementation will be critical to understanding student reaction to the new rotation.

Introduction	The rotation has been made available as an elective before full implementation of the new clinical curriculum, which will take place in spring of 2010. Feedback from volunteers during the elective will be used to improve the curriculum before its full implementation.

Step 6: Evaluation and Feedback

Evaluation itself is a powerful teaching methodology and drives the curriculum. We have designed tools to evaluate both the students (learners) and the program.

Users	Users of the evaluation include students, participating faculty, codirectors of the rotation, and the medical school curriculum committee.
Uses	The individual student assessments will contribute to the School of Medicine e-portfolio system of student evaluation, to document competency in several institutional objectives, such as medical knowledge, patient care, understanding the social context of medicine, and knowledge of systems-based care. The course codirectors and faculty will review program evaluations to improve the effectiveness of the rotation in achieving objectives. Course codirectors will also use evaluation to recruit faculty and to disseminate the curriculum beyond the institution. The medical school curriculum committee will rely on course evaluations and student outcomes to document accreditation standards and to justify resources of faculty time, student time, and monetary support for the rotation.
Resources	Collection of student performance assessment will be built into the online modules and the activities of the clerkship in most instances. Collation of results will be done by the clerkship coordina-

Table A.2. Participation Passport

	Date(s) Completed	Signature of Faculty
Required Activity		
Team meetings at two locations		
Family conference		
Home visit		
Functional H&P		
Observe: PT session		
Observe: OT session		
Observe: Speech (SLP) session		
Simulation exercise: Disability		
Simulation exercise: Chronic illness		
Prescription for rehab therapies or DME		
Optional for Honors Grade		
Reflection journal		Submit journal to course director
Community reintegration center visit		
Day hospital visit		
Nursing home visit		

tor. Because this clerkship will run 12 months a year, it is anticipated that a 1.0 FTE coordinator will be needed to support the implementation, including the evaluation activities of the clerkship.

Evaluation Questions	Are the objectives of the clerkship being met? Are the attitudes of learners toward individuals with disability different for those who have completed the rotation as compared to their peers who have not? What are the strengths and weaknesses of the rotation? How could it be improved?
Evaluation Design	Pre- and posttest design (O_1.....X....O_2) will be used for Internet knowledge quizzes. Attitudinal surveys will use a posttest design with a cohort comparison. Cohort comparisons of the AAMC GQ

regarding adequacy of exposure to chronic illness, etc., will be examined. The remainder of learner and program evaluations will be posttest design only.

Evaluation Methods and Instruments	*Learner Evaluations:*

Participation Passport (see Table A.2): Much of this course is experiential in nature, and so the participation passport will help to ensure that students know which experiences they are expected to have during the month and evaluate the completion of these experiences. The second purpose of the passport is to help to communicate to the teacher (attending physicians, therapists, etc.) why the student is there and what they are expected to teach the student on that particular day. Orientation to the goals of the session using the passport will facilitate ongoing learner feedback from the attending faculty or therapist. This communication is particularly important given that students will be at multiple clinical sites and will have multiple teachers, which will vary from month to month and day to day.

Internet Quizzes: We plan pre- and postquizzes with each Internet module (5–10 short modules per month). This is the most efficient way to evaluate students for knowledge-based objectives and also can be used to help focus the learner on key points that should have been learned from the module or lecture. The aggregate data can also be used to measure the effectiveness of each module.

Reflection Journals: Reflection journals can be a powerful tool to guide learners' introspection with respect to the experiences they are having during the clerkship, and to potentially effect attitudinal changes by making the learner aware of their own biases and assumptions about the chronically ill patient. Focused journaling will help enrich the discussion groups because the learner will have already thought through the discussion topics. This writing will also provide qualitative feedback about the course.

360 Degree Evaluations: Students will be evauated by not only attending physicians but also other team members and possibly patients. The 360 degree evaluations teach the student about the importance of working well with all team members and focus on communication skills.

Program Evaluation:

End of Rotation: Standardized course evaluation forms will be used for formative and summative program evaluation. Summative student evaluations will be through the existing online evaluation system and linked to the educational objectives.

Feedback Session: At the last didactic session each month, we will ask for verbal feedback regarding aspects of clerkship that could be improved.

Compilation of Participation: The participation passports will be reviewed in aggregate to assure that students are able to attend and complete all elements.

Passports: This should meet LCME requirements for quantitative assessment of student procedures and experiences.

Attitudinal Surveys: The Attitudes Towards Disabled Persons (ATDP) (19, 20) and UCLA Geriatric Attitudes Scale (21) will be administered to a control group of students who have not taken the course and then administered on completion of the clerkship.

Alumni Survey: We will repeat the alumni survey (described in Step 2) for those graduating after implementation of the required clerkship.

Ethical Concerns	*Confidentiality in Surveys, Reflection, and Journaling:* The following questions have arisen during curriculum development and will be addressed by the codirectors: Will attitudinal surveys use unique identifiers or de-identified codes? Who will have access to survey results? How should students be assured of anonymity? Should student reflective writing and journals be made public, e.g., form the basis of discussion groups and be available for review by instructors? Should permission be obtained from students before this writing is shared?
	Simulation Exercises: There is potential for harm to students in the simulation exercises (falls, accidents, emotional stress). Should consent be obtained from individual students for participation in the simulation?
	Resource Allocation: Because most of the learner evaluations are built into the teaching activities and other coordination of the clerkship, it is not felt that resource allocation will be an issue. Evaluations of the clerkship will be done online in a system that is already institutionalized and will not require additional cost.
Data Collection	The clerkship coordinator will oversee the evaluation system, to ensure that data are being collected, and will be responsible for collating data for the codirectors.
	Learner Evaluations: Internet quizzes and online evaluations will be collected and collated online. Students are responsible for collecting and maintaining the passports, which will be reviewed by the clerkship director at the conclusion of the clerkship. Reflective writing will be done in the student's institutional e-portfolio, which has a function to share or not share elements of the portfolio.

Program Evaluations: The Graduation Questionnaire is completed online and compiled by the AAMC. Alumni surveys will also be done online, working with the SOM's alumni survey. Attitudinal surveys will be done on paper and entered manually into spreadsheets by the clerkship coordinator. Student evaluations of the clerkship will be done online.

Data Analysis	Descriptive statistics will be used to look at mean differences in pre- and posttest assessments of knowledge and attitudinal surveys and to calculate effect size. Selective comments from 360 degree evaluations, review of passports, and small group discussions will be used to write narrative evaluations for each student. There are no plans at present to collate the reflective writing of students, although a qualitative thematic analysis could be undertaken in the future.
Reporting of Results	*Learner Evaluations:* Grades and narrative evaluations are reported to the Registrar and will become part of the individual's student record, as well as the JHUSOM Student Database.

Program Evaluations: De-identified aggregated data will be reported to the JHUSOM Educational Policy and Curriculum Committee, as part of its internal review procedure for each course. It is anticipated that aggregated data will form the basis for future dissemination of the clerkship in publication or workshops, as well as for justifying external funding.

REFERENCES

1. Hoffman C, Rice D, Sung HY. Persons with chronic conditions, their prevalence and costs. *JAMA.* 1996;276:1473–79.
2. Hwang W, Weller W, Ireys H, Anderson G. Out-of-pocket medical spending for care of chronic conditions. *Health Aff (Millwood).* 2001;20:267–78.
3. Institute of Medicine (U.S.). Committee on Quality of Health Care in America. *Crossing the Quality Chasm: A New Health System for the 21st Century.* Washington, D.C.: National Academy Press; 2001.
4. Waldrop J, Stern SM, U.S. Census Bureau. *Disability Status, 2000.* Vol. C2KBR–17. Washington, D.C.: U.S. Dept. of Commerce, Economics and Statistics Administration, U.S. Census Bureau; 2003.
5. Kraus LE, Stoddard S, Gilmartin D, National Institute on Disability and Rehabilitation Research, InfoUse. *Chartbook on Disability in the United States, 1996.* Washington, D.C.: The Institute: For sale by the U.S. G.P.O., Supt. of Docs.; 1996.
6. Campbell C, McGauley G. Doctor-patient relationships in chronic illness: insights from forensic psychiatry. *BMJ.* 2005;330:667–70.
7. Coleman EA, Berenson RA. Lost in transition: challenges and opportunities for improving the quality of transitional care. *Ann Intern Med.* 2004;141:533–36.
8. Coleman EA, Boult C, American Geriatrics Society Health Care Systems Committee. Improving

the quality of transitional care for persons with complex care needs. *J Am Geriatr Soc.* 2003;51:556–57.

9. AAMC. Medical school graduation questionnaire, all schools report. Available at www.aamc .org/data/gq/allschoolsreports/2005.pdf. Accessed March 12, 2009.

10. Fitzpatrick SB, O'Donnell R, Getson P, Sahler OJ, Goldberg R, Greenberg LW. Medical students' experiences with and perceptions of chronic illness prior to medical school. *Med Educ.* 1993;27:355–59.

11. Turner J, Pugh J, Budiani D. "It's always continuing": first-year medical students' perspectives on chronic illness and the care of chronically ill patients. *Acad Med.* 2005;80:183–88.

12. Davis BE, Nelson DB, Sahler OJ, McCurdy FA, Goldberg R, Greenberg LW. Do clerkship experiences affect medical students' attitudes toward chronically ill patients? *Acad Med.* 2001;76:815–20.

13. Darer JD, Hwang W, Pham HH, et al. More training needed in chronic care: a survey of US physicians. *Acad Med.* 2004;79:S41–48.

14. Stephenson A, Collerton J, White P. Teaching medical students about long-term illness. *Acad Med.* 1996;71:549–50.

15. Jerant AF, Levich B, Balsbaugh T, Barton S, Nuovo J. Walk a mile in my shoes: a chronic illness care workshop for first-year students. *Fam Med.* 2005;37:21–26.

16. DeBusk RF, West JA, Miller NH, Taylor CB. Chronic disease management: treating the patient with disease(s) vs. treating disease(s) in the patient. *Arch Intern Med.* 1999;159:2739–42.

17. Cohen AJ. Caring for the chronically ill: a vital subject for medical education. *Acad Med.* 1998;73:1261–66.

18. Pham HH, Simonson L, Elnicki DM, Fried LP, Goroll AH, Bass EB. Training U.S. medical students to care for the chronically ill. *Acad Med.* 2004;79:32–40.

19. Yuker HE, Block JR, Campbell WJ. A scale to measure attitudes toward disabled persons. Albertson, N.Y.: Human Resources Center; 1960. Study No. 5.

20. Tervo RC, Azuma S, Palmer G, Redinius P. Medical students' attitudes toward persons with disability: a comparative study. *Arch Phys Med Rehabil.* 2002;83:1537–42.

21. Reuben DB, Lee M, Davis JW, et al. Development and validation of a geriatrics attitudes scale for primary care residents. *J Am Geriatr Soc.* 1998;46:1425–30.

PRIMARY CARE GYNECOLOGY FOR INTERNAL MEDICINE RESIDENTS

Leah Wolfe, M.D., and Janice Ryden, M.D.

This curriculum was initially developed in 1993–94 as part of the curriculum development arm of the Johns Hopkins Faculty Development Program for Clinician Educators. It was first implemented during the 1994–95 academic year as part of the General Internal Medicine (GIM) Residency Program based at Johns Hopkins Bayview Medical Center (JHBMC) and remains an integral part of that program's curriculum for PGY–2 (Postgraduate Year 2) and PGY–3 residents more than a decade later. Faculty who collaborated in its initial development included three internists (Richard H. Baker, M.D., Jeannie McCauley, M.D., and Janice Ryden, M.D.), one of whom was a medical education fellow at the time, and two gynecologists (Jessica Bienstock, M.D., and Vanessa Cullins, M.D.), one of whom was a gynecology–public health fellow at the time. In 2004–5, a separate focused module on pelvic examination was developed by Dr. Leah Wolfe for all PGY–1 internal medicine residents in the program.

This curriculum was chosen as an example for a number of reasons. First, it covers a general content area that is still in need of enhancement in most internal medicine residency programs. Second, it has involved a multidisciplinary working group that has been essential to the development and maintenance of the curriculum. Third, it is a "real-world" example of a curriculum that has evolved since its inception in response to changing curricular needs and has adapted to embrace changes in leadership and program administrative demands.

Step 1: Problem Identification and General Needs Assessment

This needs assessment has evolved since the initial curriculum development effort, based on experience with the curriculum and an evolving literature. Because the initial literature search in 1993 revealed only a few relevant references, the curriculum developers conducted informal interviews with a number of primary care internists, gynecologists, and internal medicine residents. The results of the interviews and literature search are summarized in the following table.

Problem Identification	Women's health issues are common in medical practice. Sixty percent of internists' patients are women. Breast and cervical cancer screening is an important component of preventive care. Other women's health issues commonly encountered in primary care include menopause, osteoporosis, domestic violence, vaginal infections/sexually transmitted diseases, use of medications during pregnancy, family planning/birth control, premenstrual syndrome, amenorrhea, dysfunctional uterine bleeding, and gynecologic emergencies.
	Many internists have been inadequately trained to meet the women's health needs of their patients (1–4).
	Most gynecologists have not been trained to provide nongynecologic care to female patients.

As a result, many women receive fragmented health care (5, 6).

Women's health care may also be inefficient in that some care is duplicated, routine care often requires visits to two separate physicians, and surgically trained gynecologists may spend much time providing routine/preventive care and less time performing higher level consultations and surgery.

Current Approach	*Society:* There is pressure from some managed care insurers and providers to provide care efficiently and to limit unnecessary referrals. There is increasing public pressure on health care providers to address the health care needs of women (7). *Patients:* Patients may fail to be screened appropriately for early detection of disease. Some patients may identify a gynecologist as their primary care physician and fail to seek other general medical preventive interventions, such as cardiac risk factor modification. Internists' referrals can cause fragmentation of care and additional time burden on patients. Patients may have a preference for a female provider or gynecologist for gynecologic care (8). *Physicians:* Internists report lack of knowledge, skills, and training in this area (2, 3). They frequently refer patients for routine gynecologic care (9), and some may not perceive the provision of routine gynecologic care as their role. *Medical Educators:* Internal medicine residents report lack of adequate training in this area (2, 4). Some residencies have developed women's health curricula and/or provide residents with experience in women's health outpatient clinics.
Ideal Approach	*General Internists* should do the following: ▪ be able to perform breast and pelvic exams and provide women's preventive care with confidence and competence; ▪ be proficient at managing women's health problems that are common in primary care practice, recognizing that whether specific problems are managed by the primary care physician or gynecologist may vary depending on setting (e.g., rural vs. urban) and patient preference; ▪ be proficient at recognizing and initially managing gynecologic emergencies; ▪ refer appropriately to gynecologic specialists, recognizing that the indications for referral may vary depending on setting. *Medical Educators* should provide internal medicine residents with an education that does the following: ▪ addresses biases, attitudes, and beliefs of residents with respect to the role of an internist;

- instructs residents in performance of breast and pelvic exams using simulated models and real patients, with observation and feedback by supervisors;

- ensures that the structure of the residents' continuity practice promotes the provision of routine gynecologic care;

- provides training in the appropriate provision of women's preventive care;

- provides training in the recognition, diagnosis, and management of women's health problems common in primary care practice;

- exposes residents to internists who are knowledgeable in primary care gynecology and women's health, who can serve as teachers and role models.

Step 2: Needs Assessment of Targeted Learners

To assess learning needs of the residents in the JHBMC program, three methods were chosen: 1) questionnaire of all internal medicine residents, 2) chart audit of all internal medicine residents in their hospital-based ambulatory Medical House Staff Practice (MHSP), and 3) informal discussion with selected internal medicine residents and faculty.

Targeted Learners	*PGY–2 and PGY–3 GIM Residents:* Based on demands from GIM residents and the GIM Program Director, the career path of GIM residents, the availability of curricular time, and the results of the targeted needs assessment, it was decided that the curriculum should be integrated into the ambulatory block rotations of all GIM track residents. More than 80% of GIM track residents pursue generalist careers. Most traditional track residents (more than 75%) pursue subspecialty training; they would be able to take the curriculum, if they chose, during elective rotations.
Initial Needs Assessment	*Survey Results (November, 1993; PGY–1, PGY–2, and PGY–3 Residents):* - Number of pelvic exams/Pap smears: mean was 11/4 for all residents and 17/6 for GIM residents, with a range of 0–100/ 0–20; results probably influenced by inexperience of PGY–1 residents and by an "outlier" resident who performed many pelvic exams despite barriers. - Location of pelvic exams: emergency room was the primary site for clinical experience, followed by community-based practices and the hospital-based Medical House Staff Practice (MHSP). - Barriers to providing gynecologic care in MHSP: lack of support from clinic staff, time, and poor facilities were seen as

major barriers by all residents; although residents' perceptions of the importance of learning the pelvic examination may have been a barrier in some instances, in initial surveys most residents (and particularly GIM residents) acknowledged the value of this skill for internists.

- Anticipated future need: GIM residents, on average, predicted that, in the future, they would have to do gynecologic exams "occasionally" to "frequently"; all residents felt that they would have to do them "rarely" to "occasionally."

- Desire for gynecologic curriculum: GIM residents "definitely," and all residents "probably," wanted a gynecology curriculum; GIM residents preferred 2 weeks, all residents 1 week.

- Desired content: topics in order of preference for GIM residents were hormone replacement, abnormal vaginal bleeding, pelvic and Pap exams, contraception, sexually transmitted diseases and vaginitis, gynecologic emergencies, domestic violence, pelvic pain, amenorrhea, recurrent urinary tract infections, medications in pregnancy, endometriosis, breast exam and breast cancer, gynecologic cancers, preconception counseling, premenstrual tension, rape, gynecology in the HIV+ patient, and gynecologic endocrinology. Analysis by all residents was similar, except that all residents rated medications in pregnancy several places higher.

Audit Results:

- 82% of eligible female patients under age 50 in the MHSP had received a Pap smear:

  - 87.5% were done in gynecology clinic

  - only 12.5% were done in MHSP

- Of the 18% of female patients who did not receive a Pap smear, 75% had a cervix and thus might have benefited from screening.

Informal Discussion:

- Gynecology teaching occurs in an inconsistent and haphazard manner in relation to a resident's clinical experience.

- A Gynecology elective was available but viewed as being poorly organized. It was only occasionally taken by residents, predominantly GIM residents.

- Curricular time could be made available during the GIM residents' ambulatory block time.

Steps 1 and 2 confirmed the need for a primary care gynecology curriculum for internists, defined the targeted learners and location for the curriculum, and identified desired and needed content areas.

Step 3: Goals and Objectives

An important aspect of this curriculum was identifying the interface between GIM and obstetrics-gynecology: defining the problems and procedures for which internists should be expected to have competency, as well as guidelines for appropriate referrals. There was a paucity of literature on this interface at the time the curriculum was developed. The developers of this curriculum used the results of problem identification, needs assessments, expert opinion, and their own clinical experiences to identify the goals and objectives for this curriculum. They were tempered by resource constraints, including faculty and curricular time. For example, performance objectives were not included because the curriculum faculty did not have the resources to perform yearly audits. The goals and objectives below are updates to reflect the 2007–8 version of the GIM gynecology curriculum, which has been reorganized to reflect the U.S. ACGME's (Accreditation Council for Graduate Medical Education) six core competencies.

Goals	GIM residents will do the following:
	<ul><li>*Patient Care:* become proficient in obtaining focused history and performing an accurate examination in Gynecology; recognize "can't miss" diagnoses and conditions requiring emergency management in gynecology.</li><li>*Medical Knowledge and Skill Development:* acquire knowledge and skills necessary to recognize and manage common diseases in gynecology that may present to primary care physicians; learn to do simple office procedures in gynecology that are appropriate for primary care practice.</li><li>*Systems-Based Practice:* understand when and how to refer patients with a problem in gynecology; become familiar with support services and community and education resources for patients with gynecology problems.</li><li>*Practice-Based Learning and Improvement:* access and use educational resources, databases, and guidelines for gynecology problems.</li><li>*Interpersonal Communication Skills and Professionalism:* continue development and assessment of these core competencies in the context of the gynecology curriculum.</li></ul>
Objectives	*Cognitive Objectives:* By completion of the gynecology curriculum, residents will demonstrate accurate knowledge of the following: <ul><li>the rationale and current recommendations for cervical cancer screening;</li></ul>

- the appropriate management and referral for abnormal Pap smear results;

- the recognition, diagnosis, and treatment of vulvovaginitis and sexually transmitted diseases;

- the recognition and management of premenstrual syndromes;

- the diagnosis and management of amenorrhea and dysfunctional uterine bleeding;

- counseling and management of symptoms of menopause;

- the benefits and risks of postmenopausal hormone replacement therapy, and how to counsel patients effectively on its use;

- the diagnosis and management of chronic pelvic pain;

- preconception counseling;

- contraception counseling, including the efficacy, risks, and benefits of birth control options, and the appropriate prescribing and management of oral contraceptives;

- the usual presentation, diagnostic approaches, options for treatment, early management, and appropriate referral of patients with common gynecologic malignancies;

- the screening for, resources for, and management of domestic violence;

- resources enabling the appropriate and safe prescribing of medications during pregnancy;

- resources for women's health/gynecology information and guidelines.

Affective Objectives: By completion of the gynecology curriculum, residents will do the following:

- rate proficiency in these areas of women's health as important and relevant for general internal medicine practice.

Psychomotor Objectives: By completion of the gynecology curriculum, residents will be able to do the following:

- perform pelvic examinations accurately and with sensitivity to the comfort of the patient;

- perform Pap smears accurately.

Process Objectives: By the end of their residency, GIM residents will have done the following:

- completed the pelvic examination and gynecology curriculum;

- performed a minimum of six observed pelvic exams using a proficiency checklist;

- seen a case mix of patients in their ambulatory gynecologic, primary care practice, and emergency department experiences that includes >80% of problems included in the curriculum.

Step 4: Educational Strategies

Having specified learning objectives, the authors chose educational strategies that would facilitate the achievement of knowledge objectives through structured didactic sessions and the achievement of associated skills through supervised simulated and real clinical experiences. The attitudinal objective would be met through discussion and through improved comfort in managing gynecologic issues as the residents' experience and competency increased.

Content	Content areas include those listed above under "Objectives" in Step 3, Goals and Objectives.
Methods	*Lectures/Discussions:* For PGY–2 and 3 residents, 1 to 1.5 hour lecture/discussion sessions were developed for each topic area, were divided among faculty, and were incorporated into the residency's noon conference and ambulatory didactic curriculum. This allowed non-GIM residents access to the didactic portion of the curriculum and promoted more efficient use of *faculty* time. Lectures were initially videotaped for use by residents as needed. Later, an online learning module on gynecology for the internist, through the Johns Hopkins Internet Learning Center, replaced some of this. For PGY–1 residents, there is a 3 hour lecture/discussion/demonstration (repeated four times per year) on the pelvic examination. *Syllabus Material:* Concise, practical, clinically relevant handouts were initially prepared for each content area. Some of these were later replaced by a textbook, published by the American College of Physicians, which was coedited by one of the original curriculum development team members (see below). As noted above, online learning modules, created by two of the original curricular team members, replaced some of the original syllabus material. *Standardized Patient:* The pelvic exam curriculum introduced in 2005 for PGY–1 residents includes a 2 to 2.5 hour module, in addition to the 3 hour lecture/discussion/demonstration session mentioned above, during which a standardized patient trained as a genitourinary teaching associate (GTA) provides residents with experience practicing the pelvic exam and feedback on their performance.

Clinical Experience:

- Supervised clinical experience in gynecology setting for three (later expanded to four) sessions per week for 1 month of each resident's training, including emphasis on techniques of pelvic examination and obtaining Pap smears.

- General Internal Medicine clinical experience: community-based practice experience structured to expect and support the efficient provision of primary gynecologic care by internists; support staff in MHSP primed to assist during pelvic exams; eventual completion of new ambulatory building greatly improved facilities and space available for performance of gynecologic exams in the MHSP; starting in 2005, MHSP attending physicians trained to supervise, complete observation checklists, and provide feedback to residents on two observed pelvic exams per year.

Step 5: Implementation

The authors met with the GIM Residency Program Director and determined that the ideal time for the curriculum would be during one of eight of the GIM residents' month-long ambulatory block rotations. Each block rotation currently includes 3 half-days of community-based GIM practice, 1 half-day of MHSP, 1 half-day of visits to a Home-Care panel of patients, 4 half-days of related subspecialty clinical experience (in this case, gynecology), and 1 half-day of small group didactics. During most months of the year, one GIM resident is assigned to the Gynecology clinical rotation, which includes four sessions per week of office-based gynecology over a month-long period. During PGY–1, two 3–4 hour sessions on the pelvic examination, one with a faculty member and one with a GTA, are integrated into an existing communications skills, psychosocial, and physical examination rotation. The concurrent general internal medicine clinical experiences permit residents to apply newly acquired gynecologic competencies in their general internal medicine practices.

Resources   *Personnel: Faculty:*

- Curriculum Development: two internist clinician-educator faculty, one internist medical education fellow, one gynecologist faculty, and one gynecology fellow met for 2–4 hours per week for about 9 months to develop and pilot parts of the curriculum.

- Gynecology Clinical Experience: three to four clinic sessions per week precepted by a gynecology faculty member.

- Lectures/Discussions: 14–16 hours per month plus preparation time, for 4 months every 2 years. Faculty time was subsequently reduced to 8–10 hours per year plus preparation time with the introduction of Web-based interactive learning modules through the Johns Hopkins Internet Learning Center.

- Pelvic Exam Curriculum: In addition to the 4 hours of small group didactic teaching and discussion led by a faculty member 4 times per year, four pelvic exam practice sessions with a plastic model and GTA per year (one per month) were added, at a cost of approximately $1,000 per year.

Personnel: Support Staff: GIM secretary spends 1–4 hours per month constructing schedules, copying syllabus materials, and tallying evaluation results.

Facilities: Conference room for lecture/discussion. Clinic space for gynecologic exams.

Equipment: A plastic pelvic model. Videotape equipment to tape lectures.

Funding: The Faculty Development Program, which included workshops on curriculum development and curriculum mentors, was supported in part by a federal grant. Partial salary support from a federal GIM residency grant was provided to one internist and one gynecologist during the initial development period and to one gynecologist during the first year of implementation. The plastic pelvic model was obtained with grant funds. The GIM division provided the videotaping equipment. Funding for the GTA sessions for the interns is provided by the residency program.

Support	*External Support:* The development and implementation of a primary care gynecology curriculum were supported in part by a federal grant obtained by the GIM Residency Program. Gynecology faculty who precept in the program do so on a volunteer basis. *Internal Support:* The GIM Division Co-Chiefs, the GIM Residency Grant Project Director, and the GIM Residency Director commissioned and strongly supported the curriculum. Internist faculty release time for teaching is supported by the GIM Division. Residents requested and strongly supported the curriculum. It is now fully integrated into the ongoing internal medicine residency program curriculum.
Administration	One internist serves as Curriculum Coordinator. She coordinates the lecture/discussion series, the updating of syllabus material, review of evaluation results, and communication among faculty regarding the curriculum. GIM and Department of Medicine secretaries assist in scheduling, copying syllabus material, and tallying evaluation results. Gynecology secretaries coordinate the scheduling of gynecologic clinic sessions with the GIM secretary and gynecology faculty.
Barriers	*Faculty from outside the Department/Division:* The devotion of faculty time from other departments/divisions was secured in the first years through support from a federal GIM residency training

grant, but subsequently it has been on a volunteer basis. Despite periodic faculty turnover, the coordinators of the curriculum have continued to recruit enthusiastic and committed gynecology faculty to participate.

Change in Clinical Venues over Time: At several junctures, due to loss of funding, faculty, or other support, venues for the clinical component of the curriculum changed. The GIM gynecology clinical curriculum, in its 14th year in 2008, continues to include four sessions per week, three in a general gynecology clinic and now one session per week in a gynecology clinic for HIV-infected women.

Faculty Turnover: The development of a team of internists and gynecologists involved in the development and implementation of the curriculum has permitted the curriculum to manage transient and permanent faculty turnover. The original curriculum coordinator left in 2003, and the leadership role was assumed by an incoming GIM residency director with an interest in women's health. That person took responsibility for organizing the clinical curriculum on an ongoing basis and for updating and modifying the didactic portion of the curriculum to interdigitate more effectively with overall changes in the didactic curriculum for the residency program. Since its implementation, more than eight different gynecology faculty members have participated as preceptors, and three are currently providing the core clinical experiences. Faculty are asked to commit as preceptors for a full academic year, and detailed resident schedules are prepared for that entire academic year several months in advance. This helps to minimize transitions of faculty that can potentially disrupt the residents' learning experience.

Introduction	The curriculum was developed as a *mentored project* in the Johns Hopkins Faculty Development Program for Clinician Educators (FDP) during 1993–94. The curriculum was constructed after a careful needs assessment and the assurance of divisional and resident support. The full curriculum was *piloted* before full implementation *on other team members*. Some lectures/discussions were piloted on *colleagues* in the FDP. The Gynecology clinical experience was piloted on two *interested interns*. The curriculum was *fully implemented on all PGY–2 and PGY–3 GIM residents* during 1994–95 and has remained an integral part of the GIM residency curriculum since that time. The PGY–1 pelvic exam curriculum was developed in 2004–5 and fully implemented in the fall of 2005.

Step 6: Evaluation

Because of limited resources, the evaluation was kept simple. Data collection was integrated into the curriculum schedule. The major goals of the evaluation were to provide formative information that the residents can use to achieve curricular objectives and that the faculty can use to monitor the quality of and improve the curriculum. Time and resources were not allocated to tally pretest data; pretest data were used solely for formative individual evaluation.

Users	Residents, curriculum faculty, GIM residency director, department chair/overall residency program director.
Uses	Formative information to help residents achieve learning objectives; formative information for curriculum coordinator and faculty to guide improvement of curriculum; summative information for GIM residency director on resident performance and program effectiveness/worthiness of continued support.
Resources	Curriculum faculty and secretaries. No additional funding.
Evaluation Questions	What percentage of residents score ≥85% on the knowledge posttest?
	What percentage of residents are able to perform a competent, supervised pelvic exam as determined by their supervisor?
	What are the strengths of the curriculum? What are its weaknesses? How can the curriculum be improved?
Evaluation Designs	O_1-X-O_2: Knowledge test, pelvic exam competency checklist (formative individual).
	$X-O$: Knowledge test (summative program).
	Pelvic exam competency checklist (summative individual and program).
	End of rotation Department of Medicine global evaluation form on each resident, completed by gynecology clinical attending (summative individual).
Evaluation Methods and Instruments	*Gynecology Knowledge Test:* A self-administered multichoice knowledge test covering the most important knowledge objectives of the curriculum was delivered at the start and end of the gynecology rotation for the first several years of the curriculum. By focusing the residents on the key content of the curriculum and providing them with the correct answers after taking the test, it served as a formative evaluation tool for each resident (formative individual evaluation). Tallying the results of the anonymous posttests for all residents permitted faculty to determine how effective their lectures/discussions were in achieving learner cognitive objectives (summative program evaluation). After several years, this instrument was replaced by an online gynecology learning

module available through the Johns Hopkins Internet Learning Center/Curriculum in Internal Medicine. The online module was authored by two of the original collaborators in the Gynecology curriculum and is a case-based learning module that incorporates pre- and posttests for learners' self-assessment.

Pelvic Exam Competency Checklist: Residents were initially given a lecture on the pelvic exam and received a copy of a pelvic exam checklist to be used with the gynecology attending at the outset and close of the rotation to highlight areas of performance strengths and weaknesses (formative individual evaluation). The gynecology attending also used checklist performance to assist in completion of the end-of-rotation global evaluation form (formative and summative individual evaluation). Starting in 2005, a new pelvic exam skills checklist was introduced in the MHSP for use by internal medicine attendings doing direct observation of residents in this setting, and a new focused curriculum on pelvic examination was initiated for all PGY–1 internal medicine house staff (see below).

Standard Department of Medicine Global Evaluation Form: Completed by gynecology faculty member at the end of the clinical experience. It rates residents on several attribute scales (e.g., knowledge, independent learning, gathering of clinical information, oral and written presentation, clinical reasoning ability and judgment, organization and efficiency, rapport with patients and family, integrity, humaneness of patient care, response to constructive criticism) and asks for written comments on resident performance.

End-of-Curriculum Evaluation Form: Elicits residents' ratings of adequacy with which each content area was covered, whether they would recommend the curriculum to others, and written comments on curriculum strengths, weaknesses, and suggestions for improvements.

Ethical Concerns	Patients are made aware of the learner evaluation process and are asked for consent before evaluation pelvic exams. Residents perform pelvic examinations without supervision only after the attending is convinced of their competence. End-of-curriculum evaluation forms are completed by residents anonymously to promote uninhibited ratings and comments and to protect residents against any retaliation for unflattering ratings or comments.
Data Collection	End-of-curriculum knowledge tests were originally administered and collected during the last lecture/discussion session. Later, these were absorbed into a more comprehensive internal medicine curriculum via the Johns Hopkins Internet Learning Center (ILC). End-of-curriculum evaluation forms are collected at the end of each month to permit assessment of both the lecture/discus-

sion/ILC series and the clinical component of training. Global evaluation forms are returned to the residency program director by the gynecology attendings at the end of the clinical component of the rotation.

Data Analysis	End-of-curriculum evaluation forms are tallied by the GIM residency secretary, with written comments transcribed verbatim.
Reporting of Results	Collated yearly results are reviewed and discussed yearly by the curriculum faculty and residency program leadership and shared with program faculty.

Residents' ratings of the curriculum have been consistently high, comparing favorably with parallel evaluations of other segments of the GIM clinical curriculum. For example, in a pooling of data from 1998 to 2001, GIM residents rated the gynecology rotation (on a scale from 1 to 5) 4.55 as a clinical experience, 4.77 for quality of precepting, and 4.82 for impact and usefulness. Ratings were somewhat lower for syllabus (4.00) and logistics (3.77), reflecting in part some of the ongoing challenges of scheduling regular precepting sessions with several busy gynecology faculty.

Over this same period of time (1998–2001), on a 20 question knowledge test administered before and following the rotation, there was a statistically significant difference of 2.85 points between pre- and posttest scores (13.15/20 points pretest, and 16.00/20 posttest, $p=.01$). However, the conditions under which the knowledge tests were administered (nonchaperoned) and the fact that the same instrument was used only several weeks apart limit the validity of these data. The knowledge tests were primarily intended as a formative self-evaluation tool.

Curriculum Maintenance and Enhancement

The major anticipated challenge of this curriculum was to maintain a viable, enthusiastic team of faculty who would periodically update and revise the curriculum to meet evolving need. Despite this challenge and considerable turnover since its inception in the faculty responsible for oversight and delivery, the curriculum has continued to be a vital component of the GIM residents' education, and components have been expanded to non-GIM house staff as well.

Understanding the Curriculum and Managing Change	It is the job of the curriculum coordinator to maintain a good understanding of the curriculum through review of evaluation results, occasional observation of didactic and clinical sessions, and discussion with curriculum faculty, residents, and the GIM residency director (who receives feedback from residents). In this case, coordination of the curriculum was ultimately passed on

from the original curriculum coordinator to an incoming GIM residency director, who assumed responsibility for scheduling, faculty communication, and coordination of the didactic portion of the curriculum in 2003.

Evolution of Educational Resources for the Curriculum: As noted below, several members of the original curriculum development team engaged in "spin-off" projects that led to the development of nationally available learning resources for gynecology in internal medicine. Once available, these resources were ultimately embraced as core reading/didactic material for the ongoing gynecology curriculum at JHBMC.

Development of a Curriculum on Pelvic Examination for PGY–1 House Staff: The GIM residency director who assumed oversight of the gynecology curriculum in 2003 conducted an assessment in 2001 identifying persistent needs for focused instruction in the pelvic examination. In 2001, 43% of GIM and 75% of non-GIM internal medicine house staff still reported that they had performed 10 or fewer pelvic examinations during residency. A total of 33% of GIM house staff and 75% of non-GIM house staff reported that they provided routine gynecologic care to less than 10% of their eligible MHSP patient panel. This led to the development of a separate pelvic examination curriculum for all (not just GIM) internal medicine residents at JHBMC, to begin at the start of the PGY–1 year rather than in PGY–2 or PGY–3 as it had in the initial curriculum. This curriculum, also developed through the curriculum development arm of the Johns Hopkins Faculty Development Program and implemented in the fall of 2005, consists of a 3 hour introductory small group session, followed by a 2 to 2.5 hour intensive training session with a pelvic exam simulated patient-instructor. This curriculum prepares PGY–1 house staff to provide pelvic exams and Pap smears for their continuity patients in the MHSP from the very beginning of their tenure in that practice. A pelvic examination direct observation tool was developed as part of this curriculum and is used by attending faculty in the MHSP to facilitate formative evaluation and feedback on performance of these exams in the clinic. The forms are also forwarded to the residency program director for use in summative evaluation. Residents are encouraged to invite attending faculty for direct observation at every opportunity. Approximately $1,000 per year is provided by the residency program to support the simulated patient-instructor training sessions.

Possible Further Expansion of Curriculum to Non-GIM House Staff: Currently, non-GIM house staff are free to use elective time to gain additional gynecologic clinical experience during their PGY–2 and PGY–3 years and have done so with increasing frequency. The residency program leadership is looking for ways to incorporate a focused gynecology clinical experience into the core curriculum for non-GIM house staff as well.

Sustaining the Curriculum Team/ Related Activities that Strengthen the Curriculum	*Networking/Scholarly Activity:* ▪ The curriculum team *presented portions of the lecture/ discussion curriculum at two national meetings* of the Society of General Internal Medicine (SGIM) and *at a regional continuing medical education course* for practicing primary care clinicians. The team won a junior faculty award for education at one of the SGIM meetings. ▪ The original series of lectures/didactics developed for this curriculum inspired the addition of an annual featured "Women's Health Grand Rounds" at Johns Hopkins Bayview Medical Center, which is ongoing. ▪ The original curriculum coordinator coedited and collaborating faculty members contributed chapters to a book, *Practical Gynecology: A Guide for the Primary Care Physician*, which was initially published in 2002 by the American College of Physicians and is now in its second edition (10). ▪ The curriculum coordinator and another project team member coauthored an Internet-based learning module entitled "Gynecology" for the Johns Hopkins Internet Learning Center/Internal Medicine Curriculum, which is updated on an annual basis and is now used nationally by more than 80 internal medicine residency programs.

Dissemination

Based on their problem identification and general needs assessment (Step 1), the curriculum developers anticipated a broad audience among primary care clinicians for their curriculum. As noted above, national dissemination of components of this curriculum has already occurred through some "spin-off" projects, including a book and an Internet-based learning module.

Target Audience	Practicing primary care practitioners, and internal medicine and other generalist practitioners in training.
Reasons for Dissemination	The major reasons were to help address the health care problem identified in Step 1, to motivate and invigorate the curricular team, and to help the curriculum developers to achieve recognition and academic advancement. A further benefit has been enrichment through interchange and collaboration with colleagues.
Content	The content for dissemination has been the curricular material itself. There is a continued need for practical, evidence-based, well-organized presentations of gynecology and women's health topics that are oriented to primary care clinicians. The initial cur-

ricular evaluation was designed for internal, predominantly for-mative purposes and was not thought to have the scientific rigor that would make it appropriate for dissemination. The literature search for Step 1 was limited, and although an original needs assessment of targeted residents was performed, it was not felt that it was sufficiently representative of residents or practicing internists to warrant dissemination.

Methods	Workshops/Minicourses: see above (Curriculum Maintenance and Enhancement).
	Book: see above (Curriculum Maintenance and Enhancement).
	Internet-based Learning Module: see above (Curriculum Mainte-nance and Enhancement).
Resources	Secretarial support and funds for travel to conferences have been provided by the GIM division.

REFERENCES

1. Martin G, Curry R, Yarnold P. The content of internal medicine residency training and its rele-vance to the practice of medicine: implications for primary care curricula. *J Gen Intern Med.* 1989;4:304–8.
2. Coodley GO, Elliot DL, Goldberg L. Internal medicine training in ambulatory gynecology. *J Gen Intern Med.* 1992;7:636–39.
3. Kern D, Parrino T, Korst D. The lasting value of clinical skills. *JAMA.* 1985;254:70–76.
4. Linn LS, Brook RH, Clark VA, et al. Evaluation of ambulatory care training by graduates of internal medicine residencies. *J Med Educ.* 1986;61:293.
5. Council on Graduate Medical Education. Fifth report: women and medicine. Rockville, Md.: U.S. Department of Health and Human Services; 1995.
6. Clancy CM, Massion CT. American women's health: a patchwork quilt with gaps. *JAMA.* 1992;268:1918–20.
7. Doyal, L. Promoting women's health. *WHO Reg Publ Eur Ser.* 1991;37:283–311.
8. Lurie N, Slater J, McGovern P, et al. Preventive care for women: does the sex of the physician matter? *N Engl J Med.* 1993 Aug 12;329(7):478–82.
9. Kwolek DS, et al. Assessing the need for faculty development in women's health among inter-nal medicine and family practice teaching faculty. *Journal of Women's Health and Gender-Based Medicine.* 1999;8:1195–1201.
10. Ryden J, Blumenthal PD, Charney P, eds. *Practical Gynecology: A Guide for the Primary Care Physician,* 2nd ed. Philadelphia: American College of Physicians Press; 2009.

LONGITUDINAL PROGRAM IN CURRICULUM DEVELOPMENT

David E. Kern, M.D., M.P.H.

This curriculum was developed as part of a faculty development grant proposal to the Bureau of Health Professions, Health Resources and Services Administration, U.S. Public Health Service, in 1986 and implemented as part of the Johns Hopkins Faculty Development Program for Clinician-Educators in 1987–88. Faculty involved in its initial development included David E. Kern, M.D., M.P.H., Donna H. Howard, R.N., Dr.P.H., L. Randol Barker, M.D., Sc.M., Penelope R. Williamson, Sc.D., and Laura Mumford, M.D. Faculty involved in its subsequent development, in addition to Drs. Kern and Howard, have included Eric B. Bass, M.D., Karan A. Cole, Sc.D., Mark T. Hughes, M.D., Stephen D. Sisson, M.D., Patricia A. Thomas, M.D., and Leah Wolfe, M.D.

Step 1: Problem Identification and General Needs Assessment

This needs assessment has evolved since the original application based on faculty needs and an evolving literature.

Problem Identification	• Deficiencies have been demonstrated in the knowledge, skills, and behaviors of practicing physicians and graduating students and residents, as well as in related health care outcomes (1–7).
	• Professional organizations, including the Liaison Committee on Medical Education, the Accreditation Council for Graduate Medical Education (ACGME), and the American Academy of Continuing Medical Education, have called for curricular changes to enhance the ability of physicians to fulfill their societal contract of providing quality medical care (8–17).
	• Medical education requires ongoing curriculum development (CD) to incorporate new knowledge and competencies (18).
Current Approach	• Medical schools and residency programs are required to define learning objectives and methods for their trainees (13–14).
	• Soon they will be expected to demonstrate the attainment of program objectives and trainee competence (17).
	• Despite demands for curricular change, most faculty in academic medical centers have no formal instruction in education or CD (19, 20).
	• Curricula produced are often suboptimal and do not follow curriculum development principles (21, 22).
	• Funding for medical education is limited, yet it results in better research and development (23–26).
	• At the time of the inception of the program, a few faculty development programs existed, but they did not focus on CD.

Ideal Approach	• Curriculum developers should be trained in knowledge and skills to produce high-quality curricula.
	• Generic approaches to CD have been articulated by Taba, Tyler, Yura, and others (27–30).
	• McGaghie et al. and Golden articulated the importance of linking curricula in medical education to health care needs (31, 32).
	• A six-step approach that derives from the above was developed for this curriculum and has been articulated in a standard, widely used book on the subject (22).
	• At the time of this curriculum's inception, other faculty development programs existed, but they tended not to focus on CD or had not published on their programs' results. Since then, a few publications have described faculty training programs that included training in curriculum development (33–37).
	• The methods chosen for our CD program were similar to methods used in research training and other CD programs (33–39): skills training sessions, independent projects, and regular meetings with and feedback from mentors. To help with time management, provide additional support, and stimulate progress, we decided to include periodic deadlines, work-in-progress presentations, and the oral and written presentation of a final project.

Step 2: Targeted Needs Assessment

Targeted Learners	• Initially GIM faculty and fellows from Johns Hopkins Medical Institutions and the geographic region.
	• Subsequently expanded to faculty and fellows from all divisions and departments.
Needs Assessment/ Targeted Learners	• Based on the curriculum developers' knowledge and informal information gathering, no faculty training in CD existed at Johns Hopkins at the time of the program's inception. No survey was done.
	• Later a survey of all medical schools was performed as part of a national project (20).
Needs Assessment/ Targeted Learning Environment	• There were no related curricula available to faculty.
	• There were no funds available to support such a program.
	• There was little demand/awareness of need by institutional leaders.

- However, the department chair and other institutional leaders were pleased by the opportunity for external funding.

- As the program was successfully implemented, it came to be viewed as an important resource for improving educational programs.

- As the approach taught gained wide recognition, such an approach has come to be expected as part of an institution-wide curriculum reform.

Step 3: Goals and Objectives

Goals	The overarching goal of the program is for participants to develop the knowledge, attitudes, and skills required to design, implement, evaluate, and disseminate effective medical curricula.
Objectives	By the end of the program, participants will do the following:

1. They will be proficient in the six steps of curriculum development:

    a. problem identification and general needs assessment

    b. targeted needs assessment

    c. goals and objectives

    d. educational strategies: content and methods

    e. implementation

    f. evaluation and feedback

2. They will have applied their knowledge and skills of these steps by having designed, piloted, and formulated plans for the implementation of a curriculum in medical education relevant to the needs of their own institution and their own professional career(s).

3. They will have developed the skills necessary for presenting their work to the academic community. These skills include 1) verbal presentation of one's work and 2) preparation of a paper describing one's work, for the purposes of obtaining support for funding, sharing information, or publication. With respect to their curriculum, they will have presented their work orally before a professional audience and completed a written paper describing their work.

By one year after completion of the program, participants will have implemented their curriculum.

Step 4: Educational Strategies

The educational strategies were based on the ideal approach as identified in Step 1: Problem Identification and General Needs Assessment. Educational methods were selected to be congruent with the type of educational objectives. Knowledge objectives were addressed through readings and mini-lectures during workshops and reinforced through discussion and application of the knowledge. Psychomotor objectives were taught by having participants develop, present, and write up a real curriculum, supported by ongoing mentoring, discussion, and feedback; participants were supported by having protected time and having the project broken down into component steps with associated deadlines. Affective objectives were addressed by immersing participants in a logical approach to curriculum development supported by the existing educational literature, enabling them to have a successful experience, and exposing them to other successful curricular development examples and projects.

Content	• The six steps of curriculum development.
	• Literature searching skills.
	• Survey design skills.
	• Obtaining institutional review board approval for educational projects.
	• Presenting, writing up, and submitting for publication curriculum-related work.
	• Finding and applying for funding support for curriculum-related work.
Methods	One-half day per week, 10 month longitudinal program that includes the following:
	• Workshops on each of the CD steps and related topics.
	• Readings (handouts, CD text, and selected articles on the above topics).
	• A mentored project, with participants organized into curriculum teams focused on the development of a predetermined curriculum (participants apply and are organized into curricular teams before acceptance to the program). The process includes the following:
	• protected time for independent work
	• deadlines for outlines and written drafts of each CD step
	• meetings with experienced facilitators for 1 hour every 4–6 weeks to discuss progress and receive written feedback on their work
	• end-of-year paper on their curriculum
	• end-of-year presentation before a professional audience

- Work-in-progress sessions where participants present their needs assessment instruments, curricular segments, evaluation instruments, and other aspects of their work to facilitators and other course participants.

Step 5: Implementation

Implementation of a program that resembled an ideal approach was greatly helped by sufficient external funding.

Resources   *Personnel:*

- Two to four faculty experienced in CD, teaching skills, and mentoring facilitate each year, depending on the number of curricular projects (generally two projects per faculty member); invited faculty give selected workshops (e.g., on obtaining IRB approval and disseminating one's work). Salary support is based on activities provided by faculty members: 5% FTE for facilitating and presenting at total group sessions, 1.5% FTE for each curriculum mentored.

- Administrative Assistant for overall Faculty Development Program, which also includes a longitudinal program in teaching skills and a special programs/consulting arm (0.8 FTE, of which about 0.3 FTE is devoted to CD). Provides general administrative, communications, evaluations, scheduling, and secretarial support.

- One Sc.D. faculty member serves as director of the overall Faculty Development Program. She provides overall direction for the various arms of the Johns Hopkins Faculty Development Program and interfaces with the CME office at a leadership level regarding CME requirements and financial issues (5% FTE allotted to CD).

- One faculty member serves as director for Curriculum Development Programs within the FDP and is responsible for all internal administration and coordination of the longitudinal program (4% FTE) and special programs/workshops (3% FTE).

Facilities, Equipment, Materials:

- Space: Large conference room with one to two breakout rooms for workshops; small conference room for meetings of project teams with facilitators.

- Other: LCD projector, flip charts, Web site for posting curricular materials, text, share of Xerox machine for handouts. Equipment for taping and videoconferencing added to conference rooms in 2007, increasing opportunities for distant learning.

Funding: The Bureau of Health Professions, Health Resources and Services Administration, U.S. Public Health Service provided grant support in all but one year from 1987 to 2006. In 1993, we started charging tuition to partly cover expenses. In all years, the Johns Hopkins Bayview Medical Center has provided meeting space and secretarial support. Beginning in 2006, the program became financially independent. We adjusted tuition to cover faculty and food expenses and a 15% continuing education office charge. CD participants who are on faculty at Johns Hopkins receive tuition support for the program as part of their benefit package.

Support	The institution and department chair welcomed the program at its inception because it was supported by a competitively awarded external grant. Over the years, a large number of faculty and many educational leaders at Johns Hopkins have been trained in the program, including the associate dean for curriculum. As the program has become financially independent and has trained faculty and fellows from all divisions and departments, it has become a resource for the medical school curricular reform effort and for the Johns Hopkins Medical Institutions in general. It is well known to the vice dean for education and the faculty development office.
Administration	See above under Resources/*Personnel.*
Barriers	Initial barriers with respect to funding were overcome by external funding. Subsequently the program used existing mechanisms of tuition support to become financially independent of external support. Tuition is still a barrier for participants from other institutions. All participants must protect one-half day per week for the duration of the program, which has made participation difficult for some. The FDP has developed alternative shorter programs and a limited longitudinal program for individuals who cannot commit to the full longitudinal program. For the first 21 years, the program was held on the same Thursday mornings, which was a barrier for some interested faculty. Starting in 2008 the day of the week began alternating from year to year between Wednesday and Thursday mornings. A sufficient number of faculty have now been trained to facilitate individual projects during years when there are a relatively large number of projects enrolled. There has been no major competition for resources or participants by other faculty development programs.
Introduction	The program was introduced in 1987 with external funding to faculty and fellows in the funded division, who were interested and had their time protected for participation. Based on informal feedback and formal evaluation, changes were made each year in the program. Information about the program spread by word of

mouth and through the provision of separate workshops. Gradually faculty and fellows from other divisions, departments, and institutions participated, a trend that accelerated after transition from external grant support (which focused on primary care faculty development) to a tuition-supported program.

Step 6: Evaluation

Evaluation was stimulated by demands of the funding agency and the motivations of the involved faculty. Early planning for the evaluation permitted identification of desired outcomes and evaluation questions, construction of useful questionnaire instruments, and the inclusion of a comparison group for cohorts 2 through 9 of the program. External funding was helpful but resources limited, so that we had to rely primarily on self-report for assessment of skill attainment and subsequent behaviors. Some objective measures, such as implementation of curricular projects and publications, were able to be included with minimal cost. To reduce data collection effort and boost response rates, we administered and collected questionnaire data during the program, whenever possible. We provided a desirable clinical text, produced by our department and available to us at much reduced cost, to participants and controls as an incentive to boost response rates for the long-term follow-up study. GIM medical education fellows, supported by division grants, used evaluation of the program as mentored research projects that resulted in first authored publications (40, 41).

Users	Predominantly curriculum faculty, but also the funding agency, CME office, and prospective participants.
Uses	Ongoing program improvement, documentation of effectiveness for CME office, dissemination. Formative information for the curriculum coordinator and facilitators to guide improvement of the curriculum and their teaching; summative information for the curriculum coordinator, facilitators, external funding agency, and CME office on program effectiveness/worthiness of continued support; summative information for dissemination.
Resources	External grant support in all but one year from 1987 to 2006.
Evaluation Questions	1) Do participants in the program improve their self-assessed skills in CD compared to nonparticipants?
	2) Do participants produce and implement curricula as a result of participation? What types of curricula are produced? Is work related to their curricula published?
	3) How are the program, its facilitators, and various components of the program rated by participants? What are its strengths and weaknesses?
	4) Do participants continue to rate their skills more highly than nonparticipants years after completion of the program?

5) Are participants more active in CD than nonparticipants years after completion of the program?

6) What is the perceived impact of the program on its participants years after completion of the program?

Evaluation Design		
1)	E	O_1 - - - X - - - O_2
	C	O_1 - - - - - - - - O_2
2)		O_1 - - - X - - - O_2
3)		X - - - O_2
4)	E	O_1 - - - X - O_3
	C	O_1 - O_3
5	E	X - O_3
	C	- O_3
6)		X - O_3

Evaluation Methods and Instruments	1 and 4) Self-ratings of skills in CD, implementation, and evaluation by questionnaire.
	2) Questionnaire assessing curricular work at baseline, assessment of whether curricular projects were implemented through contact with participants and knowledge of facilitators. Classification of curricula produced by learner type and topic. Count of number of publications related to curricula produced.
	3) In a postprogram questionnaire, participants rate the program's quality, methods, and facilitation on a five-point scale. Open-ended questions ask the participants to assess the program's strengths and weaknesses and to comment on constraints that might inhibit their curricular work.
	5 and 6) Long-term follow-up questionnaire asked participants to rate their skills in CD, implementation, and evaluation; describe CD-related behaviors and activities in the past 5 years; rate the impact the faculty development program had on their career and professional lives and on their personal lives; and describe the impact in an open-ended question.
Ethical Concerns	A Johns Hopkins institutional review board determined that the immediate pre-post evaluation qualified for exemption from review under guidelines regarding education program evaluation and approved the long-term follow-up study. Responses were confidential, and findings were presented only in aggregate in a manner that maintained respondent confidentiality. Identifying information was removed from completed questionnaires and

stored separately in a locked cabinet. Access to this identifying information was limited to a designated administrative assistant.

Data Collection	Pre-post data collection is integrated into meeting time. The FDP administrative assistant follows up until questionnaires are completed by participants who were unable to complete the questionnaires during meeting time. The long-term follow-up study of FDP participants used a single questionnaire for teaching skills and CD participants, many of whom completed both programs. The principal investigator for this study followed up until satisfactory response rates (>75%) were obtained. Respondents for the long-term follow-up questionnaire received a free clinical text on completion and return of the questionnaire.
Data Analysis	The administrative assistant, under the supervision of the curriculum coordinator, collates and performs descriptive statistics on the immediate pre-post data for local formative and summative evaluation. Data entry and analysis were performed by study principal investigators for the dissemination studies, with assistance from a statistical consultant.
Reporting of Results	Collated evaluation results, with simple descriptive statistics, are compiled and distributed yearly to the curriculum coordinator and facilitators shortly after completion of the program, and in time for use in the planning of the following year's program. Analysis for and preparation of manuscripts for dissemination of multiyear evaluations took place over many months by a study team of fellows who were graduates of the program, the curriculum coordinators, and curriculum facilitators. They were submitted to peer-reviewed journals for publication (40, 41).

Curriculum Maintenance and Enhancement

Curriculum maintenance and enhancement are supported by ongoing faculty development, an experienced and committed faculty, affirmation through strong evaluations and program successes, periodic meetings, faculty interactions with educational leaders beyond the institutions, dissemination and scholarly work, and the development of ongoing funding for the program.

Understanding the Curriculum	The curriculum coordinator maintains a good understanding of the curriculum through presence at all total group meetings, periodic review of the progress of each curriculum project team with other facilitators, review of all evaluation results, informal discussions with participants and other facilitators, and once to twice yearly formal planning meetings.

Management of Change	Changes during the course of the year are made by the curriculum coordinator after electronic or in-person communication with that year's facilitators. Current and some past facilitators meet once yearly to review formal evaluation results and make plans for the following year.

Examples of changes based on yearly evaluations:

- Sessions added over the years include 1) writing for publication, Internet resources for curriculum development, finding and applying for funding in 2002; 2) searching educational databases and obtaining institutional review board (IRB) approval in 2004; 3) survey design in 2007; and 4) simulation center in 2008.

- As years passed, facilitators focused increasingly on the implementation step of curriculum development. For the first 16 cohorts, 84% of curricula developed were fully or partly implemented (40). In 2003, facilitators began screening the proposed projects of potential applicants to the program before accepting them, to ensure support within the participants' institutions and further increase the likelihood of successful implementation.

- In recent years there has been increasing emphasis on dissemination by program facilitators and participants.

Faculty Development	Development of an expert faculty has been crucial to curriculum maintenance and enhancement.

- All but one of the current facilitators in the program were trained in the program. Graduates of the program who have become facilitators cofacilitated with an experienced facilitator during their first year as faculty.

- Over the years, the faculty have gained much experience and expertise through teaching in the program, mentoring projects, and disseminating work (see below).

Sustaining the Curriculum Team	Several methods are used:

- CD facilitators receive salary support for their contributions to the program.

- Periodic meetings, as mentioned above, help maintain a sense of ownership and responsibility for the curriculum.

- Review of collated evaluation results, final papers, and abstract presentation by the teams mentored by the facilitators provide feedback of facilitator and team success.

- Occasionally a facilitator is included on a project team publication or grant.

- Ongoing funding has been secured by developing the program as a CME product with the help of our institutional CME office and charging tuition, which is enabled by our institution's benefit structure.

Networking, Innovation, and Scholarly Activity	CD facilitators have done the following:
	- presented workshops, courses, and abstracts on developing curricula and interacted with educational leaders at other institutions nationally and internationally;
	- presented workshops on disseminating curricular work and edited a medical education issue of a major journal that included curriculum-related publications with colleagues from other institutions;
	- authored several publications related to or stimulated by this curriculum (see below).

Dissemination

Dissemination has occurred in the forms of both CME activities and publications.

Target Audience	Educational program directors and other medical faculty who plan educational experiences, often without having received training or acquired experience in such endeavors, and often in the presence of limited resources and significant institutional constraints.
Reasons for Dissemination	- Improve the quality of medical education.
	- Help curriculum developers (ourselves and others) achieve recognition and academic advancement for curriculum-related work.
Content	- National survey on status of faculty development (20).
	- CD principles and a communication of a practical, theoretically sound approach to developing, implementing, evaluating, and continually improving educational experiences in medicine (22).
	- Description and Evaluations of the Longitudinal Program in Curriculum Development (40, 41).
Methods	- Workshops and courses on CD at other institutions in the United States and other countries.
	- Book (22).
	- Peer-reviewed journal articles (20, 40, 41).

Resources   ■ Faculty expertise developed through review of existing literature, interaction with colleagues from other institutions, years
of experience teaching in the Longitudinal Program in CD and
in workshops/courses, and publishing work on the subject.

■ Semiprotected academic time of some faculty and reimbursement for travel, supported by a Division of General Internal
Medicine fund and external grant support.

■ Funding for statistical consultant from external grant support
and a Division of General Internal Medicine fund.

■ External grant support until 2006 (see above).

REFERENCES

1. Baldwin DC Jr., Daugherty SR, Rowley BD. Unethical and unprofessional conduct observed by residents during their first year of training. *Acad Med.* 1998;73:1195–1200.
2. Beckman HB, Frankel RM. The effect of physician behavior on the collection of data. *Ann Intern Med.* 1984;101:692–96.
3. Feinstein RE, Blumenfield M, Orlowski B, Frishman WH, Ovanessian S. A national survey of cardiovascular physicians' beliefs and clinical care practices when diagnosing and treating depression in patients with cardiovascular disease. *Cardiol Rev.* 2006;14:164–69.
4. Hanlon JT, Schmader KE, Ruby CM, Weinberger M. Suboptimal prescribing in older inpatients and outpatients. *J Am Geriatr Soc.* 2001;49:200–9.
5. Moscucci M. Behavioral factors, bias, and practice guidelines in the decision to use percutane-ous coronary interventions for stable coronary artery disease. *Arch Intern Med.* 2007 Aug 13–27;167(15):1573–75.
6. Shah BR, Hux JE, Laupacis A, Zinman B, Zwarenstein M. Deficiencies in the quality of diabetes care: comparing specialist with generalist care misses the point. *J Gen Intern Med.* 2007 Feb;22(2):275–79.
7. Yao DC, Wright SM. The challenge of problem residents. *J Gen Intern Med.* 2001;16:486–92.
8. Institute of Medicine. *Crossing the Quality Chasm: A New Health System for the 21st Century.* Washington, D.C.: National Academy Press; 2001.
9. Report of the Ad Hoc Committee of Deans. *Educating Doctors to Provide High Quality Medical Care: A Vision for Medical Education in the United States.* Washington, D.C.: American Association of Medical Colleges; 2004.
10. Institute of Medicine. *Health Professions Education. A Bridge to Quality.* Washington, D.C.: National Academy Press; 2003.
11. Institute of Medicine. *Academic Health Centers: Leading Change in the 21st Century.* Washington, D.C.: National Academy Press; 2004.
12. Blue Ridge Academic Health Group. *Reforming Medical Education: Urgent Priority for Academic Health Centers in the New Century.* Atlanta: Robert W. Woodruff Health Sciences Center; 2003.
13. Accreditation Council on Graduate Medical Education. *Common Program Requirements,* February 2004. Available at www.acgme.org. Accessed March 12, 2009.
14. Liaison Committee on Medical Education. *Functions and Structure of a Medical School: Standards for Accreditation of Medical Education Programs Leading to an M.D. Degree.* Available at www.lcme.org. Accessed March 12, 2009.

15. American Academy of Continuing Medical Education. AACME Accreditation Standards and Policies. Available at www.aaocme.org. Accessed March 12, 2009.

16. Britton CV. American Academy of Pediatrics Committee on Pediatric Workforce. Ensuring culturally effective pediatric care: implications for education and health policy. *Pediatrics.* 2004;114(6):1677–85.

17. Accreditation Council for Graduate Medical Education. ACGME outcome project: enhancing residency education through outcomes assessment. Chicago: Accreditation Council for Graduate Medical Education; 2000. Available at www.acgme.org/Outcome/. Accessed March 12, 2009.

18. Epstein R, Hundert E. Defining and assessing professional competence. *JAMA.* 2002;287(2):226–35.

19. Wilkerson L, Irby DM. Strategies for improving teaching practices: a comprehensive approach to faculty development. *Acad Med.* 1998;73(4):387–96.

20. Clark JM, Houston TK, Kolodner K, Branch WT Jr, Levine RB, Kern DE. Teaching the teachers: national survey of faculty development in departments of medicine of U.S. teaching hospitals. *J Gen Intern Med.* 2004;19(3):205–14.

21. Sheets KJ, Anderson WA. The reporting of curriculum development activities in the health professions. *Teach Learn Ed.* 1991;3(4):221–26.

22. Kern DE, Thomas PA, Howard DM, Bass EB. *Curriculum Development for Medical Education: A Six-Step Approach.* Baltimore: Johns Hopkins University Press; 1998.

23. Kern DE. Achievements and challenges in medical education. *SGIM Forum.* 2003;26(8):1, 6–7.

24. Institute of Medicine. *Academic Health Centers: Leading Change in the 21st Century.* Washington, D.C.: National Academies Press; 2003.

25. Reed D, Kern DE, Levine RB, Wright SM. Costs and funding for published medical education research. *JAMA.* 2005;294:1052–57.

26. Reed DA, Cook DA, Beckman TJ, Levine RB, Kern DE, Wright SM. Association between funding and quality of published medical education research. *JAMA.* 2007;298:1002–9.

27. Taba H. *Curriculum Development: Theory and Practice.* New York: Harcourt, Brace, & World; 1962. Pp. 1–515.

28. Tyler RW. *Basic Principles of Curriculum and Instruction.* Chicago: University of Chicago Press; 1950. Pp. 1–83.

29. Yura H, Torres GJ, eds. *Faculty-Curriculum Development: Curriculum Design by Nursing Faculty.* New York: National League for Nursing; 1986. Publication No. 15–2164. Pp. 1–371.

30. Sheets KJ, Anderson WA, Alguire PC. Curriculum development and evaluation in medical education: annotated bibliography. *J Gen Intern Med.* 1992;7(5):538–43.

31. McGaghie WC, Miller GE, Sajid AW, Telder TV. *Competency Based Curriculum Development in Medical Education: An Introduction.* Geneva: World Health Organization; 1978. Pp. 1–99.

32. Golden AS. A model for curriculum development linking curriculum with health needs. In: Golden AS, Carlson DG, Hogan JL, eds. *The Art of Teaching Primary Care.* New York: Springer Publishing Co.; 1982. Pp. 9–25.

33. Anderson WA, Stritter FT, Mygdal WK, Arndt JE, Reid A. Outcomes of three part-time faculty development programs. *Fam Med.* 1997;29(3):204–8.

34. Armstrong EG, Doyle J, Bennett NL. Transformative professional development of physicians as educators: assessment of a model. *Acad Med.* 2003;78(7):702–8.

35. Steinert Y, Nasmith L, McLeod PJ Conochie L. A teaching scholars program to develop leaders in medical education. *Acad Med.* 2003;78(2):142–49.

36. Rosenbaum ME, Lenoch S, Ferguson KJ. Outcomes of a teaching scholars program to promote leadership in faculty development. *Teach Learn Med.* 2005;17(3):247–52.

37. Snyder S. A program to teach curriculum development to junior faculty. *Fam Med.* 2001;33(5):382–87.

38. Gruppen LD, Frohna AZ, Anderson RM, Lowe KD. Faculty development for educational leadership and scholarship. *Acad Med.* 2003;78(2):137–41.
39. Saha S, Christakis DA, Saint S, Whooley MA, Simon SR. A survival guide for generalist physicians in academic fellowships part 1: getting started. *J Gen Intern Med.* 1999;14(12):745–49.
40. Windish DM, Gozu A, Bass EB, Thomas PA, Sisson SD, Howard DM, Kern DE. A ten-month program in curriculum development for medical educators: 16 years of experience. *J Gen Intern Med.* 2007;22:655–61.
41. Gozu A, Windish DM, Knight AM, Thomas PA, Kolodner K, Bass EB, Sisson SD, Kern DE. Long-term follow-up of a ten-month program in curriculum development for medical educators: A cohort study. *Med Educ.* 2008;42:684–92.

APPENDIX B

Curricular, Faculty Development, and Funding Resources

Patricia A. Thomas, M.D., and David E. Kern, M.D., M.P.H.

Lists of specific and annotated general references appear at the end of each chapter. These lists provide the reader with access to predominantly published resources on curriculum development and evaluation. This appendix supplements the chapter references by providing a selected list of resources for the steps of curriculum development, such as general needs assessment, learning objectives, educational strategies, and evaluation, including already developed curricula. It also provides a selected list of resources for faculty development and funding. Not meant to be all-inclusive, the lists include resources that have been relatively stable over time and useful to the authors. All Web sites were accessed in March 2009.

CURRICULAR RESOURCES

When searching for additional resources related to medical education curricula, we recommend the following approach (1):

a. Review Web sites and publications of the major accrediting bodies for medical accreditation standards that might apply to the curriculum once implemented and for other resources.
b. Review resources and organizations devoted to particular topics or fields.
c. Review general educational resources within medicine.
d. Review general educational resources beyond medicine.

Many of these organizations sponsor meetings and peer-reviewed publications, a potential resource for the dissemination of the curriculum or its evaluation.

Oversight and Accreditation Organizations

- The *Association of American Medical Colleges (AAMC):* Available at www.aamc .org. The AAMC represents 147 U.S. and Canadian medical schools and hundreds of teaching hospitals and health systems, as well as professional societies. The Group on Educational Affairs (GEA) sponsors meetings and scholarship related to medical education. AAMC also sponsors a number of databases that provide national information, such as the *CurrMIT* curriculum management system and the annual *Graduation Questionnaire*, which surveys medical school graduates. The AAMC publishes *Academic Medicine* and other publications helpful as general needs assessment resources.
- *Accreditation Council for Continuing Medical Education (ACCME):* The ACCME is a voluntary accreditation body for CME-related activities and sets the standards for qualifying educational programs. Its site contains faculty development materials for those attempting to meet standards. Available at www.accme.org.
- *Accreditation Council for Graduate Medical Education (ACGME):* Available at www .acgme.org. The ACGME is charged with accreditation of clinical residency training programs and is made up of five sponsoring organizations, including the American Hospital Association, the American Medical Association (AMA), AAMC, American Board of Medical Specialties, and the Council of Medical Specialty Societies. The Web site lists specific program requirements for each specialty. ACGME sponsors the *Journal of Graduate Medical Education*. In addition, the Outcome Project page has useful information defining the six core competencies, listing example curricula, faculty development resources, and a toolbox of evaluation methods at www .acgme.org/Outcome/.
- *American Medical Association (AMA):* The largest professional organization of physicians in the United States, the AMA has particular interest in professionalism and ethics (publication *Virtual Mentor*) and is currently sponsoring a 27-school educational research project to improve medical education. Its Council on Medical Education formulates educational policy and makes recommendations to the AMA. Professional resources and information are available at www.ama-assn.org. There is an annual edition of the journal *JAMA* devoted to medical education.
- *General Medical Council (GMC):* The GMC registers and provides oversight for all practicing physicians in the United Kingdom. The GMC has published its standards for undergraduate medical education, *Tomorrow's Doctors,* which is available from its Web site, www.gmc-uk.org, under "Education," "Undergraduate education."
- *Liaison Committee on Medical Education (LCME):* This is a joint committee of the AMA and the AAMC (above) that has been recognized by the U.S. Department of Education as the official accreditation body for the M.D. degree. The LCME has developed curricular standards for the undergraduate program that are available in the document *Functions and Structure of a Medical School*, available at www.lcme .org under "Accreditation Standards."

Topic-related Resources and Organizations

Basic Science

- *International Association of Medical Science Educators (IAMSE):* IAMSE is concerned with basic science medical education. It sponsors an online peer-reviewed journal, the *Journal of the International Association of Medical Science Educators*, and an annual meeting and hosts faculty development resources. The site is an excellent source of content related to basic science education and a potential resource for dissemination. Available at www.iamse.org.

Clinical Sciences

- *Alliance for Clinical Education (ACE):* Available at www.allianceforclinicaleducation .org. This is an umbrella organization for seven specialty medical student clerkship organizations. Its site contains links to all of these organizations, as well as a faculty development resource, the *Guidebook for Clerkship Directors*, and panel presentations from AAMC meetings, such as "Portfolios in Clinical Medical Education." Curriculum developers working in a particular clerkship should review that specialty's site for developed core curricula that have been nationally peer-reviewed. Examples are the *Clerkship Directors in Internal Medicine Core Curriculum Guide* (available at www.im.org under "CDIM") and the *Educational Clearinghouse* for the American Society of Surgical Educators (available at www.surgicaleducation .com/).

Communication, Behavioral and Psychosocial Medicine

- *American Academy on Communication in Healthcare:* A society dedicated to advocating patient-centered health care communication (see Faculty Development resources below). AACH hosts an interactive online curriculum to teach communication skills and sponsors a newsletter, *Medical Encounter*. Available at www .aachonline.org.
- *Association for the Behavioral Sciences and Medical Education (ABSAME):* An interdisciplinary professional society dedicated to strengthening behavioral science teaching in medical schools, in residency programs, and in continuing medical education. ABSAME publishes *Annals of Behavioral Science and Medical Education* and provides access to some publications, reports, and a curricular guide in this content area. Available at www.absame.org.

Family Medicine

- *Society of Teachers in Family Medicine (STFM):* Curricula available in sports medicine, substance abuse, clinical nutrition, innovative primary care curricula for first- and second-year medical students, third-year family medicine clerkship, and other areas. Web site at www.stfm.org.

Geriatrics/Palliative/End-of-Life Care

- *End-of-Life/Palliative Education Resource Center (EPERC):* This organization serves as a clearinghouse for educational materials related to end-of-life and palliative care. Sample curricula in palliative care education are available on the site. A bibliography of pertinent articles and links to online and audio meetings are also posted. Available at www.eperc.mcw.edu.
- *Portal of Geriatric Online Education (POGOe):* This is an online clearinghouse for educators sponsored by the Association of Directors of Geriatric Academic Programs. It includes a list of minimum geriatric competencies for medical students, faculty development materials, and links to other geriatric educational resources. Available at www.pogoe.org/.

Informatics

- *American Medical Informatics Association (AMIA):* AMIA is concerned with advancement of informatics professionals. It sponsors a peer-reviewed publication, *Journal of the American Medical Informatics Association (JAMIA),* and annual meetings related to the use of informatics for health care and for educational purposes. The organization has developed some informatics standards for educational programs. Available at www.amia.org.

Internal Medicine

- *Alliance for Academic Internal Medicine (AAIM):* Consortium of five academically focused specialty organizations representing departments of internal medicine at medical schools and teaching hospitals in the United States and Canada: Association for the Professors of Medicine (APM), Association of Program Directors in Internal Medicine (APDIM), Clerkship Directors in Internal Medicine (CDIM), Association of Subspecialty Professors (ASP), and the Administrators in Internal Medicine (AIM). AAIM provides links to constituent organizations and access to educational materials under "educational tools," such as an Internal Medicine Subinternship Curriculum and the most recent edition of the Guidebook for Clerkship Directors. Available at www.im.org.
- *American College of Physicians (ACP):* The largest professional organization for internists maintains active educational resources for all levels of learners. By clicking on Education and Recertification, then Medical Educator Resources, one can access resources such as the FCIM (Federal Council in Internal Medicine) Curriculum Guide for internal medicine residency training. Available at www.acponline.org.
- *Society of General Internal Medicine:* This society offers annual meeting precourses, workshops, task force groups, and a monthly journal, the *Journal of General Internal Medicine,* on a variety of topics, including teaching curricula/programs directed toward medical students, residents, practicing physicians, and patients. There is an annual medical education issue. There are numerous topic-oriented interest groups that one can join. Curricular materials are available under Education Resources, including the third-year medicine clerkship curriculum guide. Available at www.sgim.org.

Neurology

- *Consortium of Neurology Clerkship Directors/American Academy of Neurology (CNCD):* Contains a Core Clerkship Curriculum Guide and access to other curricula under the "Clerkship Directors, Curricula" link. Available at www.aan.com/go/education/clerkship/consortium.

Pediatrics

- *Academic Pediatric Association (APA):* Formerly the Ambulatory Pediatric Association. Curricular materials are available in areas such as substance abuse, training residents to serve the underserved, guidelines for residency training, a general pediatric clerkship curriculum and resource manual, etc. (Not a member of ACE). APA publishes *Academic Pediatrics* (formerly *Ambulatory Pediatrics*). Available at www.ambpeds.org.
- *Council on Medical Student Education in Pediatrics (COMSEP):* COMSEP provides access to the APA/COMSEP General Pediatric Clerkship Curriculum, faculty development, and other teaching (including multimedia) resources. Available at www.comsep.org/index.htm.

Preventive Medicine

- *Association for Prevention Teaching and Research (APTR):* This Web site includes numerous curricular materials, reached by clicking "Resources", then "Curriculum". Available at www.aptrweb.org.

Public Health

- *American Public Health Association (APHA):* APHA publishes the *American Journal of Public Health* and an online newspaper, *The Nation's Health*, which may be a source of content for general needs assessment. Available at www.apha.org.
- The *Centers for Disease Control and Prevention (CDC):* The CDC has public health statistics (GNA) and has set standards for public health (Ideal Approach). The site also links to the *Office of Minority Health and Health Disparities* and the *Office of Women's Health,* which have statistical information as well as clinical guidelines. Available at www.cdc.gov/.

Surgery

- *Association for Surgical Education:* The site contains an educational clearinghouse in areas of the surgical clerkship, educational research, evaluation, and faculty development, including a Manual of Surgical Objectives and a case-based, self-directed study guide for medical students. Its Center for Excellence in Surgical Education, Research and Training (CESERT) sponsors a grants program. Available at www.surgicaleducation.com.

Women's Health

- *Association of Professors of Gynecology and Obstetrics (APGO):* A nonprofit, membership-based organization for women's health educators that focuses primarily on medical student education. Numerous resources, including the most recent edition of the APGO *Medical Student Educational Objectives*, are available at the Web site. Requires membership for access to resources. Available at www.apgo.org/home/.

Curriculum developers should contact *professional societies in their relevant specialty/subspecialty* that are not listed above because they may maintain curricular guidelines, curricular materials, or other resources helpful in developing specific curricula.

General Education Resources within Medicine

- *Best Evidence Medical Education (BEME):* A collaboration of individuals and institutions devoted to the dissemination of high-quality information through the production and publication of systematic reviews of medical education. The site also provides links to other resources. Available at www.bemecollaboration.org/.
- *MedEdPORTAL:* Initiated by the AAMC, MedEdPORTAL is designed to provide online access to peer-reviewed medical education curricular resources across the continuum of medical education. Content can be browsed by discipline or by keyword. Available at www.aamc.org/mededportal.
- *National Board of Medical Examiners (NBME):* The NBME administers the U.S. Medical Licensing Examinations (USMLE). Information on the annual Stemmler Medical Education Research Fund and publications related to medical education can be found under "Research" on its Web site. Previously funded Stemmler proposals with abstracts are available and serve as a useful resource for understanding the "state of the art." Available at www.nbme.org.
- *National Guideline Clearinghouse:* This project of the Agency for Health Care Research and Quality (AHRQ) provides a searchable clearinghouse of evidence-based practice guidelines that may serve as resources for "ideal approach." Available at www.guidelines.gov.
- *Medbiquitous:* The Medbiquitous consortium creates technology standards for health care education. It sponsors an annual meeting and also workshops to train faculty in use of SCORM (the Sharable Content Object Reference Model, a technical specification that governs how online training or "e-learning" is created and delivered to learners). Under Resources (www.medbiq.org/resources/) are located a number of online curricula, termed "learning objects," available for download. The home page is available at www.medbiq.org.

General Educational Resources beyond Medicine

- *American Education Research Association (AERA):* A national research society devoted to advancing knowledge about education, teaching, and learning. AERA sponsors an annual meeting for educational researchers. Available at www.aera.net.
- *The Carnegie Foundation for the Advancement of Teaching:* The foundation has sponsored a century of scholarship related to teaching and learning. Its interest in medical education dates to the 1910 Flexner Report. It is currently assessing the issues related to medical education under the "Preparation for the Professions Program." Available at www.carnegiefoundation.org.
- *Educational Resource Information Center (ERIC):* Sponsored by the U.S. Department of Education, ERIC provides online access to a bibliography of educational publica-

tions, with links to many. Can be particularly useful when researching new educational methods or evaluation methods, such as "reflective writing," not limited to medical education. Available at www.eric.ed.gov.

FACULTY DEVELOPMENT RESOURCES

Listed below are selected programs, courses, and written resources that address the development of clinician-educators in general and educators for specific content areas. As medical education has become increasingly professionalized, many educators are seeking advanced degrees in education, and example degree programs are also noted.

Faculty Development Programs/Courses

- *American Academy on Communication in Healthcare (AACH):* AACH offers national and regional faculty development courses for teachers of medical interviewing and psychosocial medicine. Available at www.aachonline.org.
- *Association of American Medical Colleges (AAMC):* The AAMC hosts a section of its Web site devoted to faculty development and leadership, including an online publication, *Faculty Vitae,* and publications such as *National Leadership Development Programs* and *Society-based Professional Development Programs.* Available at www.aamc.org/members/facultydev/start.htm.
- *Harvard Macy Institute:* Sponsors a number of programs for health professional educators presented by multidisciplinary national and international faculty. Information at www.harvardmacy.org.
- *Johns Hopkins University Faculty Development Program:* Offers longitudinal programs in both teaching skills and curriculum development in Baltimore for physicians in the Mid-Atlantic region. Program faculty are also available to consult, develop, and present on-site programs in teaching skills and curriculum development for client institutions in any location. Information at www.hopkinsbayview.org/fdp.
- *Medical Education Research Certificate (MERC) Program:* Sponsored by the AAMC and intended to provide individuals with skills to foster educational research. Participants must complete six workshops to receive certification. Workshops are presented at the annual AAMC meeting and regionally. Information at www.aamc .org/members/gea/merc.htm.
- *McMaster University Faculty in Health Sciences Program for Faculty Development:* Offers a series of faculty development programs in three pathways: basic educators, advanced skills, and leadership. Information at fhs.mcmaster.ca/facdev/.
- *Michigan State University, Office of Medical Education Research and Development:* Offers a longitudinal on-campus/at-home Primary Care Faculty Development Fellowship Program for Family Medicine, General Internal Medicine, and General Pediatrics faculty. There are tracks in curriculum development, educational leadership, and research. Each fellow completes a project. Information at http://omerad .msu.edu/fellowship/.
- *Stanford University Faculty Development Program:* Offers four-week programs in Stanford, California, in principles and skills of clinical teaching and in teaching professionalism in contemporary practice. Participants agree to return to their home

institutions and disseminate what they have learned. The program has recently released a free Internet-based facilitator-training course in end-of-life care. The site maintains bibliographic databases for each of its programs that can be downloaded. Available at http://sfdc.stanford.edu/.

- *University of California, San Francisco, Office of Medical Education:* Runs a series of Faculty Development workshops, which are posted on its Web site at www.med school.ucsf.edu/workshops/.
- *University of Southern California, Division of Medical Education:* Offers fellowships in Teaching and Learning and in Educational Leadership. Information at www.usc .edu/schools/medicine/departments/medical_education/.

In addition to the above, individuals may want to contact *professional societies* in their field and *health professional or educational schools* in their area, which may offer faculty development programs or courses.

Degree Programs

- *New York University School of Medicine and the NYU Steinhardt School of Education*: Master of Science in Medical Education (M.S.). Offered as a fellowship in the Division of General Medicine, NYU Medical Center. Information available at www.med.nyu.edu/medicine/dgim/education/fellowship/general.html.
- *University of Cincinnati College of Education and the Division of Community and General Pediatrics at Cincinnati Children's Hospital:* Masters in Medical Education (M.Ed.). A joint degree online program. Information available at www.cincinnatichil drens.org/ed/clinical/grad/masters/.
- *University of Houston/Texas Medical Center:* Master of Education in Teaching Program with Emphasis in the Health Sciences. (M.Ed.) Information available at http://discovery.coe.uh.edu/medical/admissions.htm.
- *University of Illinois, Department of Medical Education:* Master of Health Professions Education (MHPE). Offered in both online and on-campus formats. Information available at www.uic.edu/com/mcme/mhpeweb/.
- *University of Iowa, Office of Consultation and Research in Medical Education:* Masters in Medical Education (MME), a 30 credit hour degree. Information available at www.healthcare.uiowa.edu/ocrme/masters/mastersprogram.htm.
- *University of Michigan School of Education and the Medical School of the University of Michigan:* Masters Concentration in Medical and Professional Education (M.A.), a 30 credit hour degree program. Information available at www.soe.umich.edu/ highereducation/medicaleducation/.
- *University of New England College of Osteopathic Medicine and Maine Medical Center:* Master of Science (M.S.) in Medical Education Leadership, a 33 credit hour curriculum. Also offers certificates in program development and leadership development. Information available at www.une.edu/com/mmel/.
- *University of Pittsburgh, Institute for Clinical Research Education:* Master of Science (M.S.) in Medical Education, a 30 credit program. Also offers a 15 credit certificate program in medical education. Information available at www.icre.pitt.edu/degrees/ degrees.html.
- *University of Southern California, Keck School of Medicine in collaboration with the schools of dentistry and pharmacy:* Master of Academic Medicine. Information at www.usc.edu/schools/medicine/departments/medical_education/.

Written Resources for Faculty Development

- *Center for Ambulatory Teaching Excellence (CATE):* Housed in the Department of Family and Community Medicine at the Medical College of Wisconsin, CATE hosts a number of written faculty development materials related to the Educators Portfolio, Mentoring Guidebook for Academic Physicians, precepting skills and teaching skills. Available at www.mcw.edu/display/router.asp?docid=1083.
- The Clinician-Educator: Resurgence of a Tradition. *J Gen Intern Med.* 1997;12(Suppl 2):S1–110. This supplement contains guidelines for promotion of clinician-educators, as well as articles on an evidence-based approach to keeping up with the medical literature, continuing medical education resources, incorporating research advances into practice, clinical practice guidelines, practical tips on teaching in the outpatient setting, inpatient teaching, strategies for learning and teaching communication and the medical interview, teaching procedural skills, faculty development, institutional change, recruiting and retaining clinician-educators, career satisfaction, teaching in managed care settings, and the economics of teaching in ambulatory settings.
- Simpson D, Fincher RM, Hafler JP, Irby DM, Richards BF, Rosenfeld GC, Viggiano TR. Advancing educators and education by defining the components and evidence associated with educational scholarship. *Med Educ.* 2007;41:1002–9.

FUNDING RESOURCES

Funds for most medical education programs are provided through the sponsoring institution from tuition, clinical, or other revenues, or government support of the educational mission of the institution. When asked to take on curriculum development, maintenance, or evaluation activities, it is advisable to think through the resources that will be required for implementation (Chapter 6) and maintenance (Chapter 8) and negotiate with one's institution for the support that will be required to do the job well. Notwithstanding, institutional funding is often limited. It is often desirable to obtain additional funding to protect faculty time, to hire support staff, and to enhance the quality of the educational intervention and evaluation. Unfortunately, the funding that is provided by external sources for direct support of the development, maintenance, and evaluation of specific educational programs is small, compared to sources that provide grant support for clinical and basic research. Some government and private entities that do provide direct support for medical education, usually in targeted areas, are listed below. Information is current at the time of writing, but Web sites should be checked carefully as funding priorities change over time. Additional funding not only can increase the quality the educational intervention but also enhances the quality of related evaluation/research (2) and adds to the academic portfolio of the curriculum developer.

General Information

- *Community of Sciences (COS) Funding Alert:* A weekly e-mail notification service with a customized list of funding opportunities based on specified criteria provided by COS members. Available at www.cos.com.

U.S. Government Resources

- *Agency for Healthcare Research and Quality (AHRQ):* Focus is on research to improve the quality, safety, efficiency, and effectiveness of health care for all Americans. AHRQ supports research not only on the organization, financing, and delivery of health care services and the effectiveness and appropriateness of clinical practice but also on the promotion of improvements in clinical practice. AHRQ uses mechanisms of grants, cooperative agreements, and contracts to carry out research projects, demonstrations, evaluations, and dissemination activities. Sometimes research on the promotion of improvements in clinical practice and dissemination activities can be framed in curriculum development terms. Having had research training and having a funded mentor for the application process are very helpful. Available at www.ahrq.gov; click on "Funding Opportunities".

- *Fund for the Improvement of Postsecondary Education (FIPSE):* Nonmedical focus on college- and graduate-level curriculum and faculty development, assessment, graduate and teacher training, student-centered, and technology-mediated strategies. FIPSE looks for innovative ideas that address significant issues and problems in postsecondary education, action-oriented and risk-taking projects (rather than basic educational research) with the potential of developing into national models, the likelihood of continuing to operate after funding ends, and the leverage of funding. There is no reason why medical curricula that fit these criteria cannot be funded. Applications must be organizational rather than individual. Available at www .ed.gov/about/offices/list/ope/fipse/index.html.

- *Grants.gov:* Guide to U.S. government grants. This site allows individuals/organizations to find grant opportunities electronically from all federal grant-making agencies. Grants.gov is the single access point for more than 1,000 grant programs offered by 26 federal grant-making agencies. The U.S. Department of Health and Human Services is the managing partner for Grants.gov. You can also register to receive all e-mail notifications of new grant postings from FedGrants.gov. Available at www.grants.gov/.

- *GrantsNet:* This Web-based application tool was created by the DHHS Office of Grants Management and Policy (OGMP) for finding and exchanging information about more than 300 HHS and other federal grant programs. Available at www.hhs .gov/grantsnet/.

- *Health Resources and Services Administration (HRSA), Bureau of Health Professions (BHPr):* In the past, the Bureau of Health Professions at HRSA has funded residency training and faculty development programs under Title VII, section 747 of the Public Health Service Act, in the areas of primary care medicine and dentistry, geriatrics, nursing, public health/preventive medicine, and health administration. Grants have been substantial. For some grant programs, only applicants that satisfied a funding preference were funded. The funding preferences were defined differently for each type of grant, but all were related to the placement of graduates in practices/settings that serve defined, underserved patient populations. Current status of these programs is uncertain. Available at http://bhpr.hrsa.gov.

- *National Institutes of Health (NIH):* Most funding is directed toward clinical, basic science, or disease-oriented research, and awarded through disease-oriented institutes. Sometimes educational research and development can be targeted toward specific disease processes and fall within the purview of one of the institutes. The

NIH's increased interest in translating research into practice may create opportunities for educators to incorporate educational initiatives into grant proposals. Career development K awards can provide substantial support to individuals for periods of 3–5 years to develop as research scientists. R25 (Education Projects), K07 (Academic/Teacher Award), and K30 (Clinical Research Curriculum Awards) awards provide opportunity for curriculum development. NIH grants provide generous funding but are very competitive. Having had research training and having a funded mentor are very helpful. One can subscribe to a weekly electronic notice of new postings by joining an NIH Guide LISTSERV. Available at www.nih.gov; click on Grants.

- *National Science Foundation:* The NSF funds research and education in science and engineering, through grants, contracts, and cooperative agreements. The foundation accounts for about 20% of federal support to academic institutions for basic research. It might be a source for basic science curricula. The ADVANCE program focuses on increasing the participation and advancement of women in academic science and engineering careers and could support systematic faculty development efforts in basic science departments. Available at www.nsf.gov/index.jsp.
- *Veterans Administration:* Faculty at VA hospitals in the United States should explore VA career development awards, as well as funding opportunities for individual projects.

Applying for government grants in the United States is, in general, a very competitive process. Having a mentor who has served on a review board or been funded by the type of grant being applied for is strongly recommended. It is advisable for readers from other countries to acquaint themselves with the government funding resources within their countries.

Private Foundations

- *Commonwealth Fund:* The fund supports independent research on health and social issues and makes grants to improve health care practice and policy. It is dedicated to helping people become more informed about their health care and improving care for vulnerable populations such as children, elderly people, low-income families, minorities, and the uninsured. The fund predominantly supports health services research, but some needs assessment, educational intervention studies, and conferences might be supported. Available at www.commonwealth fund.org/index.htm.
- *Arthur Vining Davis Foundations:* The foundation has identified Health Care (Caring Attitudes) as one of their numerous foci. They are particularly interested in supporting programs leading to organizational and transformational change in medical education, addressing the "hidden curriculum," and designed to integrate caring attitudes throughout the curriculum. Grants made in this program area normally range from $100,000 to $200,000. Available at www.avdf.org/.
- *Fogarty International Center:* International Research Ethics Education and Curriculum Development Awards (BIOETH) support domestic and international educational and research institutions to develop or expand current graduate curricula and training opportunities in international bioethics related to performing research on acute and chronic diseases in low- and middle-income nations. Available at www.fic.nih.gov/programs/training_grants/bioethics/index.htm.

- *The Foundation Center:*, A guide to private foundations. Available at www.fdn center.org.
- *Arnold P. Gold Foundation for Humanism in Medicine:* The foundation funds curriculum development projects related to humanism, ethics and compassion, and research focused on an aspect of humanism in medicine, at up to $25,000, with an opportunity for renewal for a second year. They also provide partial funding for 1–3 years for assistant and associate professors to protect time for teaching and research related to the humanistic practice of medicine. Available at www.human ism-in-medicine.org.
- *John A. Hartford Foundation:* The Harford Foundation funds numerous programs related to geriatric education and health services, usually in conjunction with other organizations. Support for unsolicited individual projects is limited and by invitation only after submission of a 1–2 page letter of inquiry. Available at www.jhartfound .org.
- *William Randolph Hearst Foundations:* The foundations fund programs in the areas of education, health, social service, and culture/the arts. Preference is given to institutions of higher education, particularly in the fields of teaching and health care, both undergraduate and graduate. They support efforts that ensure students access to a quality education. The foundations are also committed to supporting programs that seek to improve and assure access to quality health care for underserved populations in both urban and rural areas. Available at www.hearstfdn.org/.
- *W. K. Kellogg Foundation:* Funding priorities change over time. In the past, medical education has constituted a small proportion of grants. They also have funding initiatives to promote health among vulnerable individuals and communities. Available at www.wkkf.org.
- *Josiah Macy, Jr. Foundation:* The foundation has focused its resources specifically on improving the education of health professionals, particularly physicians' mission "to develop, monitor, and evaluate projects which demonstrate new approaches to addressing problems in health professions education." The foundation has defined four areas of particular emphasis in grant making. They are 1) projects to improve medical and health professional education in the context of the changing health care system, 2) projects that will increase diversity among health care professionals, 3) projects that demonstrate or encourage ways to increase teamwork between and among health care professionals, and 4) educational strategies to increase care for underserved populations. Available at www.josiahmacyfoundation.org/.
- *NBME (National Board of Medical Examiners)/Edward J. Stemmler, M.D. Medical Education Research Fund:* The NBME accepts proposals from LCME- or AOA-accredited medical schools. The goal of the Stemmler Fund is to provide support for research or development of innovative assessment/evaluation approaches. Expected outcomes include advances in the theory, knowledge, or practice of assessment at any point along the continuum of medical education, from undergraduate and graduate education and training through practice. Pilot and more comprehensive projects are both of interest. Collaborative investigations within or among institutions are eligible, particularly as they strengthen the likelihood of the project's contribution and success. Awards are for about $150,000 for a project period of up to 2 years. Available at www.nbme.org.
- *Pew Charitable Trusts:* They have programs in public policy, informing the public and supporting civic life. In the past they have funded a Partnership for Quality

Education program (subsequently funded by RWJ Foundation), which funded eight academic health centers and managed care organizations to work together to better prepare physicians to practice high-quality, cost-effective care, and the ACP Community-Based Teaching Project. Medical education, however, is a small part of their focus. Available at www.pewtrusts.org.

- *Donald W. Reynolds Foundation:* Program on Aging & Quality of Life: grants aimed at improving the training of physicians in geriatrics. Available at www.dwreynolds.org/.
- *RGK Foundation:* Small grants (~$5,000 to $50,000). The foundation's programmatic areas of interest have broadened over the years to include Education, Community, and Health/Medicine. The range of projects funded has been broad. Available at www.rgkfoundation.org/.
- *Robert Wood Johnson Foundation:* RWJF seeks to improve the health and health care of all Americans. Current program areas include the following: Building Human Capital, Childhood Obesity, Coverage, Pioneer (bold, innovative solutions at the cutting edge of health and health care), Public Health, Quality/Equality, Vulnerable Populations. Available at www.rwjf.org/.

Other Funding Resources

- *Fees/Tuition:* For curricula serving multiple institutions, a user or subscriber fee can be charged (3, 4). Charging tuition may be an option for faculty development programs (faculty often have tuition benefits).
- *Institutional Grant Programs:* Educational institutions often have small grant programs available internally. One should learn about grants offered by one's own institution.
- *Professional Organizations:* For specialty-oriented curricula, contact the relevant specialty organization. Here are two examples:
  - The American College of Rheumatology Research and Education Foundation, www.rheumatology.org/ref/awards/index.asp, offers a Clinician Scholar Educator Award.
  - The Association for Surgical Education (ASE) Foundation of the Association for Surgical Education (ASE), www.surgicaleducation.com/, has Center for Excellence in Surgical Education, Research and Training (CESERT) grants available in the range of $25,000 to $50,000 annually. Multiyear proposals are also considered (three year maximum), but total grant size may not exceed $100,000. Priorities are listed on the Web site.

REFERENCES

1. Thomas PA, Kern DE. Internet resources for curriculum development in medical education: an annotated bibliography. *J Gen Intern Med.* 2004;19:598–604.
2. Reed DA, Cook DA, Beckman TJ, Levine RB, Kern DE, Wright SM. Association between funding and quality of published medical education research. *JAMA.* 2007;298:1002–9.
3. Sisson SD, Rastegar DA, Rice TN, Hughes MT. Multicenter implementation of a shared graduate medical education resource. *Arch Intern Med.* 2007;167:2476–80.
4. American Academy on Communication in Healthcare produces doc.com, an interactive curriculum in communication skills. Available at www.aachonline.org/.

Index

Note: When numerous pages are indexed, the most relevant pages are *italicized*.